JUICE PROCESSING

Quality, Safety and Value-Added Opportunities

T0225529

Contemporary Food Engineering

Series Editor

Professor Da-Wen Sun, Director

Food Refrigeration & Computerized Food Technology
National University of Ireland, Dublin
(University College Dublin)
Dublin, Ireland
http://www.ucd.ie/sun/

Juice Processing: Quality, Safety and Value-Added Opportunities, *edited by Víctor Falguera; Albert Ibarz* (2014)

Engineering Aspects of Food Biotechnology, *edited by José A. Teixeira and António A. Vicente* (2013)

Engineering Aspects of Cereal and Cereal-Based Products, *edited by Raquel de Pinho Ferreira Guiné and Paula Maria dos Reis Correia* (2013)

Fermentation Processes Engineering in the Food Industry, *edited by Carlos Ricardo Soccol, Ashok Pandey, and Christian Larroche* (2013)

Modified Atmosphere and Active Packaging Technologies, *edited by Ioannis Arvanitoyannis* (2012)

Advances in Fruit Processing Technologies, *edited by Sueli Rodrigues and Fabiano Andre Narciso Fernandes* (2012)

Biopolymer Engineering in Food Processing, *edited by Vânia Regina Nicoletti Telis* (2012)

Operations in Food Refrigeration, *edited by Rodolfo H. Mascheroni* (2012)

Thermal Food Processing: New Technologies and Quality Issues, Second Edition, *edited by Da-Wen Sun* (2012)

Physical Properties of Foods: Novel Measurement Techniques and Applications, *edited by Ignacio Arana* (2012)

Handbook of Frozen Food Processing and Packaging, Second Edition, *edited by Da-Wen Sun* (2011)

Advances in Food Extrusion Technology, *edited by Medeni Maskan and Aylin Altan* (2011)

Enhancing Extraction Processes in the Food Industry, *edited by Nikolai Lebovka, Eugene Vorobiev, and Farid Chemat* (2011)

Emerging Technologies for Food Quality and Food Safety Evaluation, *edited by Yong-Jin Cho and Sukwon Kang* (2011)

Food Process Engineering Operations, *edited by George D. Saravacos and Zacharias B. Maroulis* (2011)

Biosensors in Food Processing, Safety, and Quality Control, *edited by Mehmet Mutlu* (2011)

Physicochemical Aspects of Food Engineering and Processing, *edited by Sakamon Devahastin* (2010)

Infrared Heating for Food and Agricultural Processing, *edited by Zhongli Pan and Griffiths Gregory Atungulu* (2010)

Mathematical Modeling of Food Processing, *edited by Mohammed M. Farid* (2009)

Engineering Aspects of Milk and Dairy Products, *edited by Jane Sélia dos Reis Coimbra and José A. Teixeira* (2009)

Innovation in Food Engineering: New Techniques and Products, *edited by Maria Laura Passos and Claudio P. Ribeiro* (2009)

Processing Effects on Safety and Quality of Foods, *edited by Enrique Ortega-Rivas* (2009)

Engineering Aspects of Thermal Food Processing, *edited by Ricardo Simpson* (2009)

Ultraviolet Light in Food Technology: Principles and Applications, *Tatiana N. Koutchma, Larry J. Forney, and Carmen I. Moraru* (2009)

Advances in Deep-Fat Frying of Foods, *edited by Serpil Sahin and Servet Gülüm Sumnu* (2009)

Extracting Bioactive Compounds for Food Products: Theory and Applications, *edited by M. Angela A. Meireles* (2009)

Advances in Food Dehydration, *edited by Cristina Ratti* (2009)

Optimization in Food Engineering, *edited by Ferruh Erdoğdu* (2009)

Optical Monitoring of Fresh and Processed Agricultural Crops, *edited by Manuela Zude* (2009)

Food Engineering Aspects of Baking Sweet Goods, *edited by Servet Gülüm Sumnu and Serpil Sahin* (2008)

Computational Fluid Dynamics in Food Processing, *edited by Da-Wen Sun* (2007)

JUICE PROCESSING

Quality, Safety and Value-Added Opportunities

EDITED BY

Víctor Falguera
Albert Ibarz

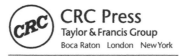

CRC Press
Taylor & Francis Group
Boca Raton London New York

CRC Press is an imprint of the
Taylor & Francis Group, an **informa** business

CRC Press
Taylor & Francis Group
6000 Broken Sound Parkway NW, Suite 300
Boca Raton, FL 33487-2742

First issued in paperback 2016

Version Date: 20130923

ISBN 13: 978-1-138-03374-0 (pbk)
ISBN 13: 978-1-4665-7733-6 (hbk)

Library of Congress Cataloging-in-Publication Data

Juice processing : quality, safety, and value-added opportunities / edited by Victor
    Falguera and Albert Ibarz.
      pages cm -- (Contemporary food engineering ; 30)
    Includes bibliographical references and index.
    ISBN 978-1-4665-7733-6
    1. Fruit juices. I. Falguera, Victor, editor of compilation. II. Ibarz, Albert, editor of
compilation.

TP562.J85 2014
663'.63--dc23   2013037842

Visit the Taylor & Francis Web site at
http://www.taylorandfrancis.com

and the CRC Press Web site at
http://www.crcpress.com

Contents

Series Preface...ix
Series Editor...xi
Preface.. xiii
Editors... xv
Contributors xvii

Chapter 1 Squeezing Fruits in the Second Decade of the Twenty-First
Century: The Current Situation of the Juice Industry......................... 1

Víctor Falguera and Albert Ibarz

Chapter 2 Product Innovation: Current Trends in Fruit Juice Production
to Meet Market Demands.. 13

Miguel Ángel Cubero Márquez

Chapter 3 New Trends in Fruit Juices: Superfruits..27

Francisco López

Chapter 4 Recovery and Use of By-Products from Fruit Juice Production 41

*Nuria Martí, José Lorente, Manuel Valero, Albert Ibarz, and
Domingo Saura*

Chapter 5 Assessing Juice Quality: Measuring Quality and Authenticity 75

Núria Rafel, Xavier Costa, and Carlos Berdún

Chapter 6 Assessing Juice Quality: Advances in the Determination
of Rheological Properties of Fruit Juices and Derivatives................. 83

Pedro E. D. Augusto and Alfredo A. Vitali

Chapter 7 Assessing Juice Quality: Analysis of Organoleptic Properties
of Fruit Juices 137

Gemma Echeverría and María Luisa López

Chapter 8 Utilization of Enzymes in Fruit Juice Production............................ 151

Jordi Pagán

Chapter 9   Advances in Fruit Juice Conventional Thermal Processing 171

José Lorente, Nuria Martí, and Domingo Saura

Chapter 10   Emerging Technologies in Fruit Juice Processing 197

*María Victoria Traffano-Schiffo, Nuria Balaguer,
Marta Castro-Giráldez, and Pedro J. Fito-Suñer*

Chapter 11   Emerging Nonthermal Technologies in Fruit Juice Processing 217

*Olga Martín-Belloso, Ángel Robert Marsellés-Fontanet,
Robert Soliva-Fortuny, and Pedro Elez-Martínez*

Chapter 12   Pressure Treatments in Juice Processing: Homogenization
Pressures Applied to Mandarin and Blueberry Juices 237

*Juan Manuel Castagnini, Ester Betoret, Noelia Betoret,
and Pedro Fito-Maupoey*

Chapter 13   Membrane Processes in Juice Production 265

María Isabel Iborra, María Isabel Alcaina, and Silvia Álvarez

Chapter 14   Juice Packaging 301

*Maribel Cornejo-Mazón, Darío Iker Téllez-Medina, Liliana
Alamilla-Beltrán, and Gustavo Fidel Gutiérrez-López*

Chapter 15   Spoiling Microorganisms in Fruit Juices 311

Antonio J. Ramos and Sonia Marín

Chapter 16   Safety in Fruit Juice Processing: Chemical and Microbiological
Hazards 329

Sonia Marín and Antonio J. Ramos

Chapter 17   Public and Private Standards and Regulations Concerning
Fruit Juices 349

*Antonio Martínez, Dolores Rodrigo, Josep Arbós, and
Yvonne Colomer*

Index 373

Series Preface

CONTEMPORARY FOOD ENGINEERING

Food engineering is the multidisciplinary field of applied physical sciences combined with the knowledge of product properties. Food engineers provide the technological knowledge transfer essential to the cost-effective production and commercialization of food products and services. In particular, food engineers develop and design processes and equipment to convert raw agricultural materials and ingredients into safe, convenient, and nutritious consumer food products. However, food engineering topics are continuously undergoing changes to meet diverse consumer demands, and the subject is being rapidly developed to reflect market needs.

In the development of food engineering, one of the many challenges is to employ modern tools and knowledge, such as computational materials science and nanotechnology, to develop new products and processes. Simultaneously, improving food quality, safety, and security continues to be a critical issue in food engineering studies. New packaging materials and techniques are being developed to provide more protection to foods, and novel preservation technologies are emerging to enhance food security and defense. Additionally, process control and automation regularly appear among the top priorities identified in food engineering. Advanced monitoring and control systems are developed to facilitate automation and flexible food manufacturing. Furthermore, energy saving and minimization of environmental problems continue to be important food engineering issues, and significant progress is being made in waste management, efficient utilization of energy, and reduction of effluents and emissions in food production.

The Contemporary Food Engineering Series, consisting of edited books, attempts to address some of the recent developments in food engineering. The series covers advances in classical unit operations in engineering applied to food manufacturing as well as such topics as progress in the transport and storage of liquid and solid foods; heating, chilling, and freezing of foods; mass transfer in foods; chemical and biochemical aspects of food engineering and the use of kinetic analysis; dehydration, thermal processing, nonthermal processing, extrusion, liquid food concentration, membrane processes, and applications of membranes in food processing; shelf-life and electronic indicators in inventory management; sustainable technologies in food processing; and packaging, cleaning, and sanitation. These books are aimed at professional food scientists, academics researching food engineering problems, and graduate-level students.

The editors of these books are leading engineers and scientists from different parts of the world. All the editors were asked to present their books to address the market's needs and pinpoint cutting-edge technologies in food engineering.

All contributions are written by internationally renowned experts who have both academic and professional credentials. All authors have attempted to provide critical, comprehensive, and readily accessible information on the art and science of a relevant topic in each chapter, with reference lists for further information. Therefore, each book can serve as an essential reference source to students and researchers in universities and research institutions.

Da-Wen Sun
Series Editor

Series Editor

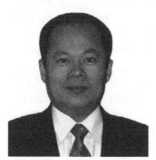

Born in Southern China, Professor Da-Wen Sun is a world authority in food engineering research and education; he is a member of the Royal Irish Academy (RIA), which is the highest academic honor in Ireland; he is also a member of Academia Europaea (The Academy of Europe) and a fellow of the International Academy of Food Science and Technology. His main research activities include cooling, drying, and refrigeration processes and systems, quality and safety of food products, bioprocess simulation and optimization, and computer vision technology. Especially, his many scholarly works have become standard reference materials for researchers in the areas of computer vision, computational fluid dynamics modeling, vacuum cooling, and so on. Results of his work have been published in over 600 papers including about 300 peer-reviewed journal papers (Web of Science h-index = 45; Google Scholar h-index = 52). He has also edited 13 authoritative books. According to Thomson Scientific's *Essential Science Indicators*[SM], based on data derived over a period of 10 years from the ISI Web of Science, there are about 2500 scientists who are among the top 1% of the most cited scientists in the category of agriculture sciences. For many years, Professor Sun has consistently been ranked among the top 100 scientists in the world (he was at 31st position in 2010).

He received a first class BSc Honors and MSc in mechanical engineering, and a PhD in chemical engineering in China before working in various universities in Europe. He became the first Chinese national to be permanently employed in an Irish university when he was appointed college lecturer at the National University of Ireland, Dublin (University College Dublin [UCD]), in 1995, and was then continuously promoted in the shortest possible time to senior lecturer, associate professor, and full professor. Dr. Sun is now a professor of Food and Biosystems Engineering and the director of the Food Refrigeration and Computerised Food Technology Research Group at the UCD.

As a leading educator in food engineering, Professor Sun has significantly contributed to the field of food engineering. He has trained many PhD students, who have made their own contributions to the industry and academia. He has also delivered lectures on advances in food engineering on a regular basis in academic institutions internationally and delivered keynote speeches at international conferences. As a recognized authority in food engineering, he has been conferred adjunct/visiting/consulting professorships from 10 top universities in China, including Zhejiang University, Shanghai Jiaotong University, Harbin Institute of Technology, China Agricultural University, South China University of Technology, and Jiangnan University. In recognition of his significant contribution to food engineering worldwide and for his outstanding leadership in the field, the International Commission of Agricultural and Biosystems Engineering (CIGR) awarded him the "CIGR Merit

Award" in 2000, and again in 2006, the Institution of Mechanical Engineers based in the United Kingdom named him "Food Engineer of the Year 2004." In 2008, he was awarded the "CIGR Recognition Award" in honor of his distinguished achievements as the top 1% of agricultural engineering scientists in the world. In 2007, he was presented with the only "AFST(I) Fellow Award" in that year by the Association of Food Scientists and Technologists (India), and in 2010, he was presented with the "CIGR Fellow Award"; the title of Fellow is the highest honor in CIGR and is conferred to individuals who have made sustained, outstanding contributions worldwide. In March 2013, he was presented with the "You Bring Charm to the World" Award by Hong Kong-based Phoenix Satellite Television. In July 2013, he received the "Frozen Food Foundation Freezing Research Award" from the International Association for Food Protection (IAFP) for his significant contributions to enhancing the field of food freezing technologies. This is the first time that this prestigious award was presented to a scientist outside the United States.

He is a fellow of the Institution of Agricultural Engineers and a fellow of Engineers Ireland (the Institution of Engineers of Ireland). He has also received numerous awards for teaching and research excellence, including the President's Research Fellowship, and has twice received the President's Research Award of the UCD. He is the editor-in-chief of *Food and Bioprocess Technology—An International Journal* (2012 Impact Factor=4.115), former editor of *Journal of Food Engineering* (Elsevier), and editorial board member for a number of international journals, including the *Journal of Food Process Engineering, Journal of Food Measurement and Characterization,* and *Polish Journal of Food and Nutritional Sciences.* He is also a chartered engineer.

On May 28, 2010, he was awarded membership in the RIA, which is the highest honor that can be attained by scholars and scientists working in Ireland; at the 51st CIGR General Assembly held during the CIGR World Congress in Quebec City, Canada, on June 13–17, 2010, he was elected incoming president of CIGR and became CIGR president in 2013–2014—the term of his CIGR presidency is six years, two years each for serving as incoming president, president, and past president. On September 20, 2011, he was elected to Academia Europaea (The Academy of Europe), which is functioning as the European Academy of Humanities, Letters and Sciences, and is one of the most prestigious academies in the world; election to the Academia Europaea represents the highest academic distinction.

Preface

Fruit juices and derivatives are food products that have wide consumer acceptance. They are consumed as soft, refreshing drinks, although their sugar and vitamin content is very appealing to many consumers from a nutritional point of view. Juice quality largely depends on the fruit from which it is made, although the manufacturing process is also very important. There are several different commercial products based on fruit juices, although the most common ones are clarified juices and those containing suspended pulp. Nowadays, consumers seek quality juices that contain the proper vitamins and nutritional components. These contents strongly depend on the process that the fruit has undergone through the different stages of industrial manufacturing. Therefore, in recent years new technologies have been developed that allow processing that maintains high amounts of these components in the final product, without neglecting safety. In this book, different innovative aspects of fruit juice processing are addressed, as well as other issues related to the use of the by-products generated by these industries. To fulfill this purpose, the book contains chapters that cover both new approaches to traditional issues and innovative approaches.

Thus, the first chapter highlights the importance of this sector within the food industry and describes the general process of fruit juice manufacturing. Within this process, the use of different types of enzymes that allow suitable processing, both in the optimization of clarification and in the early stages of extracting juice from the fruit itself, deserves special attention. Moreover, in recent times juice companies have been forced to develop new products in order to meet consumers' new demands for food with fresh-like properties that provide health benefits. Among these trends, juices from organically grown fruits and juices from fruits with large concentrations of bioactive compounds (*superfruits*) are nowadays at the forefront of market interest, as well as juice-derived beverages that enhance their nutraceutical features. At the same time, analysis methods to identify and assess the availability of these bioactive compounds (and to detect frauds) have undergone important evolution in recent years, as well as methods to evaluate organoleptic parameters.

Juice industries generate a large amount of waste, mainly from the exhausted fruit pulp, and it is therefore important to find an application for these by-products. Several interesting processes have been developed to extract different components that contain and take advantage of their functional properties. The use of these products represents a new way to obtain innovative foodstuffs that can also meet the aforementioned new demands of consumers.

Traditionally, juice concentrates have been obtained by means of multistage evaporation operations. In addition, those fluid fruit products that do not undergo a concentration process must be subjected to a pasteurization process to ensure the safety of the final product. Due to the high temperatures used in these processes, thermolabile components such as vitamins and other nutrients are negatively affected. However, recent advances in the design and engineering of evaporators and thermal processing equipment have greatly improved the quality of the final products. Such advances are mainly due to better knowledge of the properties of juices; rheology stands out in this field. In addition, regarding alternative techniques that can improve the final quality of fruit juices, there are chapters covering the application of both thermal and nonthermal emerging technologies, their fundamentals, and their main effects on the most important features of fruit juices.

All juice processing technologies are devoted to preventing spoilage and ensuring product safety while striving for the highest quality. Therefore, issues concerning spoiling microorganisms and biological and chemical hazards must also be addressed. In the last decade, these issues have led to several food scandals and scares, which in turn have led to important changes in food policy and regulation. In addition, both public and private standards have had to be reworked in order to integrate the new properties of today's food-related issues: new trends in food consumption, new processing technologies, rising global trade in food and agricultural products, the merging of food and pharmacy, and new disease vectors. Several new principles such as risk analysis, traceability, and an integrated food chain have had to be included, and the fruit juice industry must keep continuously up-to-date with all these new standards and regulations.

Editors

Víctor Falguera graduated in agricultural engineering at the University of Lleida, receiving an extraordinary award from the Spanish Ministry of Science and Education. After completing a research master's in food production systems, he carried out two PhDs simultaneously: one of them in agrifood science and technology at the University of Lleida and the other one in engineering and advanced technologies at the University of Barcelona (he completed both *cum laude*).

Dr. Falguera worked for several years at the Food Technology Department of the University of Lleida in topics related to fruit juice processing such as nonthermal technologies, fruit-derived enzymes, and the analysis of fluid food physical and chemical properties. Afterwards, he participated in a multidisciplinary group at the Institute for Food and Agriculture Research and Technology of the Government of Catalonia (IRTA), contributing his knowledge on fruit physiology and biochemistry. His main contributions to food and agricultural research have been devoted to the development of mathematical models and the application of advanced multivariate data analysis, as well as optimization of experimental procedures for assessing enzymatic activities. His expertise includes several projects developed in collaboration with researchers from Spain, France, Brazil, Mexico, Colombia, and the United States. Dr. Falguera is one of the founding members of the platform Agricultural Knowledge & Innovation Services (AKIS International), in which he manages the research division and the services related to food research, food engineering, and the food industry.

Albert Ibarz graduated and received a PhD in chemical engineering at the University of Barcelona. He is a technical engineer in the agricultural and food industries for the Polytechnic University of Catalonia. Dr. Ibarz is a professor of food technology at the University of Lleida. He has been visiting professor at the Universidad Nacional del Sur (Bahía Blanca, Argentina) (1989) and Universidad de las Américas (Puebla, Mexico) (1999–2001), adjunct faculty professor at Washington State University (Pullman, WA) (1995), honorary professor at the Universidad Nacional del Santa (Chimbote, Peru) (2004), and doctor honoris causa at the Universidad Nacional de Trujillo (Trujillo, Peru) (2013).

He has carried out administration positions as director at the Food Technology Department at the Polytechnic University of Catalonia (1987–1991), vice-director at the Superior Technical School of Agrarian Engineering of Lleida (1984–1985), and vice-chancellor for faculty affairs at the University of Lleida (1999–2003).

He has published more than two hundred scientific articles, mostly on rheology, chemistry, biochemistry and photochemistry kinetics, and UV treatments. He has presented more than one hundred and fifty communications to national and international congresses.

He is coauthor of the following books: *Unit Operations in Food Engineering*, Technomic, Lancaster, PA (1999) and Mundiprensa, Madrid (2005); *Experimental*

Methods in Food Engineering, Acribia, Zaragoza (2000); and *Unit Operations in Food Engineering*, CRC Press, Boca Raton, FL (2003). He is also author and coauthor of eight book chapters, including "Newtonian and Non-Newtonian Flow" in Volume 2 of *Food Engineering—Encyclopedia of Life Support Systems* (UNESCO). He has translated 11 books on diverse areas of knowledge in food engineering. He was coordinator and editor of the *Reports de Recerca of Catalunya* (1996–2002) and *Enginyeria Agronòmica, Forest i Alimentària* (Institut d'Estudis Catalans). He has been part of scientific committees of diverse national and international congresses and the president of the organizing committee of the Spanish Congress of Food Engineering II (Lleida, 2002).

Contributors

María Isabel Alcaina-Miranda
Chemical and Nuclear Engineering
    Department
Polytechnic University of Valencia
Valencia, Spain

Liliana Alamilla-Beltrán
Department of Food Science and
    Technology
National School of Biological Sciences
Mexico City, Mexico

Silvia Álvarez
Chemical and Nuclear Engineering
    Department
Polytechnic University of Valencia
Valencia, Spain

Josep Arbós
Zucasa
Huesca, Spain

Pedro E. D. Augusto
Department of Agri-food Industry,
    Food and Nutrition
University of São Paulo
Piracicaba, Brazil

Nuria Balaguer
Institute of Food Engineering for
    Development
Polytechnic University of Valencia
Valencia, Spain

Carlos Berdún
Nufri, S.A.T.
Mollerussa, Spain

Ester Betoret
Institute of Food Engineering for
    Development
Polytechnic University of Valencia
Valencia, Spain

Noelia Betoret
Institute of Food Engineering for
    Development
Polytechnic University of Valencia
Valencia, Spain

Juan Manuel Castagnini
Institute of Food Engineering for
    Development
Polytechnic University of Valencia
Valencia, Spain

Marta Castro-Giráldez
Institute of Food Engineering for
    Development
Polytechnic University of Valencia
Valencia, Spain

Yvonne Colomer
Triptolemos Foundation
Barcelona, Spain

Maribel Cornejo-Mazón
Department of Biophysics
National School of Biological
    Sciences
Mexico City, Mexico

Xavier Costa
Nufri, S.A.T.
Mollerussa, Spain

Miguel Ángel Cubero Márquez
Food Science and Technology Department
University of Lleida

and

Indulleida, S.A.
Alguaire, Spain

Gemma Echeverría
Institute of Food and Agricultural
  Research and Technology
Lleida, Spain

Pedro Elez-Martínez
Department of Food Technology
Lleida, Spain

Víctor Falguera
Agricultural Knowledge & Innovation
  Services
Albatàrrec, Spain

Pedro Fito-Maupoey
Institute of Food Engineering for
  Development
Polytechnic University of Valencia
Valencia, Spain

Pedro J. Fito-Suñer
Institute of Food Engineering for
  Development
Polytechnic University of Valencia
Valencia, Spain

Gustavo Fidel Gutiérrez-López
Department of Food Science and
  Technology
National School of Biological Sciences
Mexico City, Mexico

Albert Ibarz
Department of Food Technology
University of Lleida
Lleida, Spain

María Isabel Iborra
Chemical and Nuclear Engineering
  Department
Polytechnic University of Valencia
Valencia, Spain

Francisco López
Department of Chemical Engineering
University Rovira i Virgili
Tarragona, Spain

María Luisa López
Department of Food Technology
University of Lleida
Lleida, Spain

José Lorente
Molecular and Cellular Biology
  Institute
University Miguel Hernández of Elche
Elche, Spain

Sonia Marín
Department of Food Technology
University of Lleida
Lleida, Spain

Ángel Robert Marsellés-Fontanet
Department of Food Technology
University of Lleida
Lleida, Spain

Nuria Martí
Molecular and Cellular Biology
  Institute
University Miguel Hernández
  of Elche
Elche, Spain

Olga Martín-Belloso
Department of Food Technology
University of Lleida
Lleida, Spain

Antonio Martínez
National Research Council
Institute of Agrochemistry and Food
    Technology
Valencia, Spain

Jordi Pagán
Department of Food Technology
University of Lleida
Lleida, Spain

Núria Rafel
Nufri, S.A.T.
Mollerussa, Spain

Antonio J. Ramos
Department of Food Technology
University of Lleida
Lleida, Spain

Dolores Rodrigo
National Research Council
Institute of Agrochemistry and Food
    Technology
Valencia, Spain

Domingo Saura
Molecular and Cellular Biology Institute
University Miguel Hernández of Elche
Elche, Spain

Robert Soliva-Fortuny
Department of Food Technology
University of Lleida
Lleida, Spain

Darío Iker Téllez-Medina
Department of Food Science and
    Technology
National School of Biological
    Sciences
Mexico City, Mexico

María Victoria Traffano-Schiffo
Institute of Food Engineering for
    Development
Polytechnic University of Valencia
Valencia, Spain

Manuel Valero
Molecular and Cellular Biology Institute
University Miguel Hernández of Elche
Elche, Spain

Alfredo A. Vitali
Brazilian Institute of Food
    Technology
Campinas, Brazil

1 Squeezing Fruits in the Second Decade of the Twenty-First Century
The Current Situation of the Juice Industry

Víctor Falguera and Albert Ibarz

CONTENTS

1.1 Introduction 1
1.2 Brief Introduction to the History of the Juice Industry 3
1.3 Most Wanted: Current Trends in Consumption of Fruit Juices.....................4
1.4 Juices and Fruit Derivatives...7
1.5 Standard Juice Processing 8
References 12

1.1 INTRODUCTION

In recent decades, the global food industry that was created to satisfy the growing demand for food from the middle of the twentieth century has experienced a progressive shift toward a more complex system, in which *quality* rather than *quantity* has become the leading concept. But in fact, the quality concept is being continuously reformulated, making this adaptation increasingly more difficult. Therefore, food industry managers, producers, retailers, and also scientists and technologists must keep up-to-date by knowing which issues are at the forefront of quality. Nowadays, such issues may be classified into six main groups: nutritive value, organoleptic properties, market trends, effects on health, impact on society, and impact on the environment. Obviously, producers must ensure that their products meet all these requirements at a reasonable price.

For a long time, the industry focused only on the first three issues. However, with the advances in information technology, consumers' emphasis has shifted to nontraditional attributes of food, as they grow more concerned about the impact of their decisions on their own health, on the environment, and on social equity (Falguera et al., 2012). Indeed, quality aspects have become increasingly linked to an added-value basket of indirect and invisible food quality criteria, including movements such

1

as green marketing, animal welfare, and fair trade. In general, all these phenomena are described by social scientists as *reflexive consumption* (Giddens, 1991): people think of themselves as active, discerning consumers, whose choices contribute to their sense of identity and have an effect on the world beyond the individual level.

As an important part of the food industry, juice manufacturing has had to meet these new trends in consumers' demands that have led to technical, social, economic, and environmental changes. For example, using the best raw material produced without (or with the minimum amount of) pesticides and inorganic fertilizers, developing new processing technologies to maintain the original nutritive and organoleptic value of the fruit, and searching for new fruits that provide new tastes or new health benefits. As a result of these changes in consumers' attitudes (and the subsequent changes in producers' attitudes), both public regulations and private standards have also been forced to adapt to the new situation. From the industrial standpoint, the changes in the industry's own definition of *juice* and those of its related products must always be kept in mind, as well as what is and is not allowed in a certain market area. The Codex Alimentarius (FAO/WHO, 2005) defines *fruit juice* as "the unfermented but fermentable liquid obtained from the edible part of sound, appropriately mature and fresh fruit or of fruit maintained in sound condition by suitable means." In addition, the codex also states that juice must be prepared by suitable processes that "maintain the essential physical, chemical, organoleptical and nutritional properties of the juices of the fruit from which it comes." Although this basic definition may not pose any problem, juice manufacturers must be aware of the ever-changing national and international regulations, especially those concerning the allowed ingredients that may be added and the labeling specifications. As an example, in the European Union (EU), Directive 2012/12/EU of the European Parliament and of the Council introduced some more restrictive measures intended to elevate the good practices described in the codex to the status of law.

Beyond what is covered by the different regulations and the quality requirements imposed by private standards (both of which will be discussed in Chapter 17), the production and consumption of fruit juices have experienced a remarkable increase throughout history, mainly due to practical reasons. First, all fruits have a limited shelf life that determines the time at which they can be consumed and the distance that they can travel across the world. Moreover, even the best fruit for storage or transportation contains some pieces that are not suitable to be sold as fresh whole fruit due to their size, color, or shape. And transforming these pieces into juice is a simple way to solve these problems, obtaining products with enhanced conservation properties and safety attributes. Meanwhile, for consumers, the advantages of juices have made them one of the most popular beverages. They provide the same nutritive and health benefits as fresh fruit, their consumption is easier than that of an entire piece of fruit, and they may be more suitable for certain population groups such as children and the elderly. Furthermore, juice blends or juice-derived products can offer a broad, brand-new range of flavors and tastes. In this way, in addition to developing new processing technologies that can ensure the safety and fresh-like attributes of juices, and providing for today's quality requirements, a significant part of the job of juice-related professionals consists of finding new ways or products that encourage the consumption of juices and juice-based products.

1.2 BRIEF INTRODUCTION TO THE HISTORY OF THE JUICE INDUSTRY

The beginnings of juice production date back to antiquity. In fact, juices can be considered as old as (or even older than) agriculture itself, because transporting fruits at an adequate maturity stage for consumption might have easily resulted in the creation of juice. Later, tool-making skills and trial-and-error assays improved the manufacture and storage of juices (Bates et al., 2001). However, the shelf life of these products strongly limited their consumption until preservation methods such as natural chilling and fermentation were discovered. Some key findings, such as the acidification of grape juice produces vinegar, also provided new conservation methods for other fruits and vegetables, some of which could be stored and squeezed later. Nonetheless, even with such discoveries, there was limited time for the consumption of fruit juices.

According to some researchers, the first "modern" juice seems to have been lemonade, which was invented in the Middle East and imported to Italy during the sixteenth century (Wolf et al., 2007). In the eighteenth century, James Lind discovered that citrus fruits were useful to prevent scurvy, and more than 100 years later, carrying citrus juices on ocean voyages became a legal requirement for British vessels with the approval of the Merchant Shipping Act of 1867. But on an industrial scale, it is commonly accepted that the story of juices started in 1869, when Thomas Welch began bottling unfermented Concord grape juice at Vineland (New Jersey), applying the principles of heat sterilization (Brown et al., 1993). The procedure used by Welch included hot pressing crushed grapes, pulp, and suspended matter, which was allowed to settle in cold cellars, then poured into consumer-size bottles and pasteurized at 82.2°C–87.7°C. Although this method allowed the preservation of the grape juice for months, its widespread use did not occur until the late 1920s, after the Great Depression. Out of economic necessity, most families prepared their own canned fruits and vegetables at home, but these did not last for more than a few weeks. Meanwhile, the industry had provided a suitable solution and, as a consequence, it experienced remarkable growth. A decade later, the appearance of flash pasteurization (containers were filled completely, without any headspace, with hot product) improved the quality of the commercially available juices by means of a relatively cheap and simple procedure, thereby fostering consumer interest in these products during the late 1930s and early 1940s.

As with many other industrial sectors, World War II represented a major boost for juice production and distribution. As part of the U.S. program to ship food products to its allies, efforts focused on manufacturing an orange juice as close as possible to the quality of fresh orange juice and available year-round. It is often said that the original intention was to produce powdered orange juice, but reconstituting the powder did not work well (Wolf et al., 2007). The end result of this research was frozen concentrated orange juice (FCOJ). The Florida Citrus Commission and the U.S. Department of Agriculture (USDA) developed a system by which the concentration of single-strength orange juice was increased fivefold to eightfold by vacuum evaporation. The loss of the juice's aroma and taste was solved by diluting this concentrate with freshly extracted juice, up to a threefold or fourfold concentration. Then, the resulting product was frozen. This juice was stable during storage, and when it was reconstituted, its flavor was close to that of fresh juice (Morris, 2010). FCOJ was introduced in the domestic marketplace in 1945–1946 (Brown et al., 1993). Due to its price, stability, and ease of preparation in its ready-to-drink form (rather than squeezing oranges at home), this product soon became a major commodity in markets around the world. During the 1950s and 1960s, the growth in demand for FCOJ (also influenced by exports as part of the Marshall Plan) led to a dramatic increase in the number of citrus fruit producers and processors.

In the early 1970s, aseptic processing was introduced and commercialized on a large scale, which was an essential breakthrough that allowed the juice market to expand worldwide, thereby ensuring the safety of juices and reducing their production and marketing expenses. In addition, aseptic storage and packaging allowed new modes of transport, with a reduced risk of contamination and cost per unit. During that decade, another important issue also changed the direction of the juice industry. The aforementioned advantages of aseptic processing that made packaging and distribution easier and cheaper, along with consumer demand for quality and convenience, led to increased sales of chilled ready-to-serve (RTS) juice, despite it being 30% more expensive than FCOJ (Morris, 2010). However, this price gap narrowed when glass packaging was progressively replaced by paper envelopes. The chilled RTS market share growth was especially significant for orange and grapefruit juices. It is worth mentioning that, although chilled RTS juices may include either reconstituted concentrate or juice that has never been concentrated, in the 1970s most of the sales belonged to the former.

In the 1980s, not-from-concentrate (NFC) juices grabbed consumers' attention, although they were significantly more expensive than the RTS reconstituted juices. The ability of NFC juices to better conserve the flavor of fresh fruit because they had never been subjected to evaporation made them increasingly popular. Regarding the global market, in those years, severe weather freezes in the major orange and grapefruit supply areas of the United States had two main consequences: the emergence of Brazil as a world-leading producer and exporter of oranges and orange juice, and the increase in prices and the subsequent search for new beverage products that contained less than 100% juice. As an example, between 1980 and 1994, the juice beverages and juice blends share of the U.S. market increased from 24% to over 40%, while single-fruit juices sales decreased (Morris, 2010).

From then on, one of the major challenges of the current fruit industry has been (and still is) the search for new, exotic juices, blends, or juice-based products that provide new flavors and new healthy or functional benefits, according to the current expectations of consumers and the issues that are nowadays included in the definition of *quality*. A thorough approach to the understanding of market demands and the research and development of new products will be discussed in Chapter 2.

1.3   MOST WANTED: CURRENT TRENDS IN CONSUMPTION OF FRUIT JUICES

In 2011, global fruit juice and nectar sales recorded a slight decrease. Basically, this was caused by two main factors: a sharp fall in demand in North America due to high prices, and a steep drop in demand in Russia, East Europe's key consumption market (AIJN, 2012). However, in other countries the opposite trend was registered: in

Turkey, the consumption of juices and nectars increased by 8.7%. In addition to the overall data on quantities purchased, the definitive trend toward *premium* products continues in most areas (especially in Europe), since consumers' perception of the health benefits of juice is increasing. However, due to severe limitations on consumers' food and drink budgets, the highest increase has been seen in those producers that are able to sell affordable *premium* products, such as chilled or NFC juices. This fact leads to the conclusion that innovation will play a key role in the ability of juice and juice-derived producers to maintain or increase their market share in the coming years.

In 2011, 38,948 million liters of juice were consumed in the world, with West Europe (9,831 million liters) and North America (9,755 million liters) being the greatest consuming markets (AIJN, 2012). However, consumption per capita was higher in North America (28.3–23.7 L/person/year). Within West Europe, the most important market was Germany, in terms of both total volume (2733 million liters) and consumption per capita (34.0 L/person/year). The battle to achieve all-budget consumers led to several brands offering continuous promotions in order to reduce the difference in price with private-label juices.

In the European market, orange juices and nectars continue to lead the way with 38.5% of the EU share (Figure 1.1), representing more than 50% of the consumption of juices and nectars in Ireland (71.0%), the United Kingdom (62.3%), Finland (56.8%), Luxembourg (55.3%), Czech Republic (54.5%), and Slovakia (50.2%). Meanwhile, flavor mixes (beverages where no single flavor is perceived to be dominant) are consolidated in second place, being the preferred type of juice in Greece (55.0%), the Netherlands (43.5%), and Italy (19.4%). For decades, innovation in the juice industry focused on offering new blends of the most commonly consumed juices mainly for commercial (new product lines with different organoleptic features) and technological (to take advantage of some juices' properties, such as antioxidants) reasons. Subsequently, in accordance with the demand of the European and North American consumers, exotic fruits were introduced and blended with other juices in order to achieve a smoother flavor.

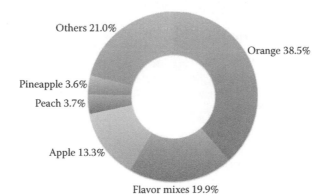

FIGURE 1.1   EU fruit juice and nectar share by flavor in 2011. (Adapted from AIJN, *2012 Liquid Fruit Market Report*, European Fruit Juice Association, Brussels, 2012.)

Apple takes third place in the flavor ranking, mainly due to its importance in Austria (33.1%) and Germany (22.3%). It is also the second most preferred flavor in Slovenia (31.1%), Denmark (29.4%), Switzerland (25.4%), Latvia (22.5%), Norway (22.2%), and Finland (20.9%). In the Turkish market, which had the largest increase in 2011, the most singular flavor distribution is found: the market is led by peach juices and nectars (share 32.4%), followed by cherry (19.7%), flavor mixes (16.3%), apricot (13.1%), and in fifth place, orange (11.1%).

Knowing the demand of each region and country is essential for a sector that moves billions of dollars every year. Juices have become a commodity with a global infrastructure specifically devoted to trade with these products, with huge cargo ships continuously crossing the oceans and large facilities acting as hubs distributed worldwide, ready to either prepare and package any product or resell it in a matter of minutes. However, part of this juice is reexported, which makes it difficult for consumers to know where the juice that they consume really comes from. In Europe, Belgium and the Netherlands are the major gateways, receiving, for instance, around 90% of EU imports of concentrated orange juice (AIJN, 2012). Most of this orange juice comes from Brazil, which is thought to supply more than 80% of the EU's orange juice in any year; 64% of the Brazilian orange juice exports (in value) goes to the EU (Figure 1.2). Despite the fact that Brazil is still the major foreign provider of orange juice for the United States, the American market only represents 13% of Brazilian exports.

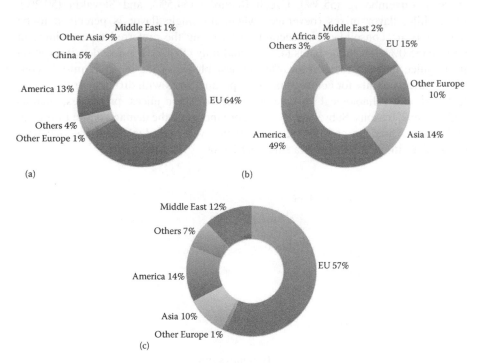

FIGURE 1.2 Value of Brazilian orange (a), Chinese apple (b), and Thai pineapple (c) juice exports in 2011. (Adapted from AIJN, *2012 Liquid Fruit Market Report*, European Fruit Juice Association, Brussels, 2012.)

As far as the apple juice market is concerned, China is the leading producer and exporter. Some 49% (in value) of China's exports goes to America, while 15% is sold to the EU, and 14% to other Asian countries. The EU imported 228,000 tons of apple juice in 2011, 50% of which came from China. However, in recent years the European industry has increased its sourcing within Europe itself, mainly due to the increase in the price of apple juice from China and the higher acidity of the apple juice produced in countries such as Poland (which is a highly appreciated property in this market). Pineapple juice, which has high consumption rates in some European countries such as Spain (share 20.1%), is mainly imported by the EU from Costa Rica (42% of the 232,000 tons imported in 2011) and Thailand (36%). For Thailand, which tops the exports of this juice, commerce with the EU represents 57% of its trade (in value).

1.4 JUICES AND FRUIT DERIVATIVES

The processes for obtaining juice from fruit consist of different unit operations that depend mainly on the type of juice that is desired and on the fruit itself. Therefore, initially, it is worth highlighting the different kinds of juice that can be obtained in the fruit processing industry. Globally, there are three basic kinds of juice: clarified and depectinized juices, cloudy juices, and purees. Many of the unit operations that are applied in the preparation of these juices are common to all of them, but there are specific operations that are used for each type of juice.

Depending on the type of fruit from which the juice is extracted, certain stages of development will differ depending on whether the fruit is stone fruit, pome fruit or berries. Furthermore, it is also important to note that the processing steps depend on whether the fruits are soft or hard, or whether the fruit or only the fruit pulp is completely edible. It is usually considered that the *juice* is the fluid obtained from the fruit by means of a crushing and pressing process. The liquid thus obtained may be a clear, cloudy, or mushy juice. To obtain clarified juices, the pulp and pectin must be removed, so that the final product contains mostly water with soluble solids. In the case of *cloudy* juices, the pulp is removed, but the pectin remains in suspension, giving the mixture a cloudy appearance. Fruit purees contain pulp and have high consistency values that make them flow slowly. These differences in the rheological properties among the three kinds of juice lead to different equipment design needs for each type of juice, an issue that will be further addressed in Chapter 6.

Juices obtained from fruits are not always marketed directly. In some cases, some components may be added to facilitate their commercialization. They may be diluted with water, mixed with sugar (or sweetener) syrups, or both in order to obtain a final product that is more consistent with consumer demand. Although (as previously commented) market trends are changing, nowadays, concentrated juices are still manufactured in most processing industries with the purpose of enhancing their shelf life and facilitating their storage and transportation. Many commercial juices found in supermarkets are obtained from concentrates, to which water has been added in order to obtain a product with a soluble solids content approximately equal to the initial juice (commonly called *single strength*). Other fruit derivatives are marketed as nectars, which are obtained from clarified or pulpy juice with added water and sugar. The minimum percentage of juice and/or puree in a nectar is speci-fied by the Codex Alimentarius and ranges between 25% and 50%, depending on the type of fruit used. A juice or puree that is rediluted below 10% and has other added ingredients is called a *juice drink*, *juice cocktail*, or *juice punch*.

1.5 STANDARD JUICE PROCESSING

As stated, the steps that make up the process for obtaining fruit juices differ depend-ing on the type of final product to be obtained. Figure 1.3 shows a standard process flow diagram for clarified juices and concentrates. The fruit to be processed is ini-tially subjected to a *washing* step with clean and chlorinated water in order to remove dirt from its surface. This step eliminates many of the pesticide/fungicide traces from field treatments and treatments carried out before cold storage to prevent fungal attack. This stage must ensure that the fruit is cleaned, and that no dirty fruit enters the next processing step. To facilitate the removal of dirt and contaminants adhered

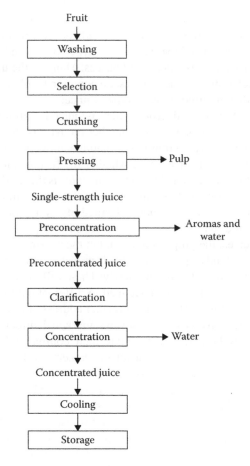

FIGURE 1.3 Standard flow diagram for a process to obtain clarified and concentrated juices.

to the fruit's surface, brushes and air jets can be used, which can also reduce the amount of washing water, with the subsequent economic and environmental benefits.

Then, the clean fruit undergoes a *selection* step, allowing foreign bodies and bad pieces of fruit to be removed. The fruits that are to be processed must meet the requirements of food safety and quality to ensure that the final juice satisfies consumer expectation. Also in this stage, bioburden content and the levels of mycotoxins and pesticides should be checked. Selection may be performed manually or automatically, using suitable sensors that determine the color, shape, and size of the fruit, thereby eliminating the defective fruits.

Once the selection has been made, the fruit is subjected to a *grinding* step. However, it is important to consider the type of fruit that is being processed, since treatment differs significantly between fruits. For example, pome fruit (such as apples and pears) can be processed without pretreatment, but in stone fruits (such as peaches and plums) it is necessary to apply a step for removing the stone before grinding. Figure 1.4 shows a standard processing line for stone fruit. For other types of fruit, such as oranges, tangerines, grapefruits, and bananas, the skin must be removed previously or by means of a special juice extractor.

When the fruit has been crushed, it undergoes a *pressing* step where the juice is extracted from the fruit. This extraction step is performed using the appropriate equipment for each case, which separates the pulp from the fruit's own juice, basically using suitably sized sieves to retain particulates and let the juice flow. Depending on the type of fruit and its ripeness, in some cases maceration enzymes that facilitate the extraction of the juice can be used, thereby increasing the yield of juice extraction. The use of enzymes in the different processing steps will be discussed in Chapter 8. Generally, the maceration step is carried out in batches, in heated tanks that maintain the crushed fruit at a temperature that must correspond to the optimum temperature of the enzymes used (typically around 50°C).

After pressing, a juice with a soluble solids content that corresponds to the maturity state of the fruit from which it comes (usually around 12°Brix for most pome and stone fruits) is obtained. Since this juice is less stable than the entire fruit, it may easily undergo chemical, enzymatic, and microbial processes that could impair its quality and make it unsuitable for drinking in a short period of time. In order to destroy microorganisms and inactivate the enzymes that are present, the juice undergoes a pasteurization step, which is usually carried out by means of heat processes. This operation is performed in an evaporator that, while stabilizing the juice, leads to a product with a suitable concentration for the clarification stage (usually 15°Brix). Therefore, this step is the *preconcentration* step, where part of the water is removed from the juice. At the same time, most of the aromatic molecules of the fruit are also removed. This stream of water and aroma can be recovered by means of a distillation step and reincorporated into the juice in the redilution and packaging steps.

The juice obtained in the preconcentration stage is usually turbid, since it contains particulate matter formed by fiber and pectin. To obtain a clarified juice, it is necessary to remove the turbidity, which can be achieved in a *clarification* stage in different ways. One way is to destabilize the colloidal system that keeps the fiber in suspension by means of pectinolytic enzymes. Such enzymes attack pectin chains, favoring the formation of aggregates that are large enough to settle at the bottom of

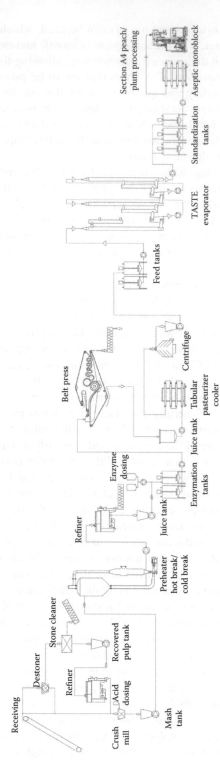

FIGURE 1.4 Peach/plum processing line. Thermally accelerated short time evaporator (TASTE). (Courtesy of John Bean Technologies Corp.)

the tank. The upper juice fraction is pumped through a candle filter in order to obtain a particle-free filtered juice, while the lower part (with juice containing sediment) is brought to a vacuum filter that removes the sediment, and the resultant filtrate is also brought to the candle filter to obtain a clarified juice stream. This operation usually lasts for 8–10 h, which may lead to quality problems due to nonenzymatic browning and the possible growth of microorganisms. To avoid these problems, the clarification can be performed in a single step using ultrafiltration membranes. In this way, semipermeable membranes are used to produce a permeate stream that contains water- and juice-soluble components, mainly sugars and organic acids. The retentate stream containing the insoluble part of the juice is removed. Because pectins remain in this latter stream, a polarization layer with a high pectin content is progressively formed on the ultrafiltration membrane. If the concentration of pectins is high enough, it can lead to gel formation, creating a new resistance against the juice flow through the membrane wall. When this flow is below a given value, cleaning the membrane is essential. To avoid stopping production, industries usually have two ultrafiltration modules installed in parallel, so that while one is working, the other one is being cleaned. Pectinolytic enzymes can be used to retard this cleaning operation, so that the concentration of insoluble pectin decreases and the polarization layer takes longer to form.

The clarified juice has a soluble solids content of around 15°Brix, and therefore it is still susceptible to attack by microorganisms if it is not stored under aseptic conditions. Processing industries often obtain juices with a soluble solids content of about 70°Brix, which are more easily stored and transported. Water removal from clarified juice is usually carried out in a multiple-stage *evaporation* process, usually with four to six evaporators. The evaporation chamber of the last effect often works under vacuum at a temperature of about 60°C, which prevents the most concentrated juice from being subjected to an excessive temperature (which, in turn, could cause nonenzymatic browning). Nevertheless, in the concentration by evaporation the juice continuously changes its soluble solids content and temperature as it passes from one evaporator to another, and this heat treatment can cause both a reduction in quality and the loss of juice nutrients. Therefore, alternative concentration technologies may also be used, such as cryoconcentration or reverse osmosis. With this type of technology, the juice does not reach temperatures that can damage its properties, but it has the disadvantage that the maximum concentration that can be reached is about 30°Brix. However, these *cold* technologies might be used as a preconcentration step, combined with conventional concentration by heat processes in other batches to obtain an intermediate-strength product after blending.

In most factories, the concentrated juice leaving the evaporator is at a temperature of about 60°C, so it must be lowered in a *cooling* step prior to storage since this temperature is high enough to cause chemical deterioration reactions. The final concentrated juice has a sufficiently low water activity to avoid the growth of microorganisms and, at the same time, reduces the necessary storage volume. However, a high concentration of soluble solids favors nonenzymatic browning reactions, and to minimize this effect the concentrated juice must be stored under refrigeration, usually at about 5°C. The concentrated juice has high density and viscosity values, and at low temperatures special equipment is needed to ease the juice flow through these heat exchangers.

If the desired final product is a puree, the processing steps are different from those used for clarified juice. The early stages of the washing and crushing processes are similar to those described above. However, purees contain the whole fruit pulp, so once crushed the obtained mass is brought to a sieve (*finisher*), which gives a suitable particle size. Afterward, the mash is subjected to a pasteurization step to eliminate microorganisms and to inactivate enzymes. As the soluble solids content of the puree is that of the fruit itself, it is necessary to pack and store it under aseptic conditions. To avoid deterioration by chemical reactions, the storage temperature is usually about 5°C, and in some cases it is even frozen.

Sometimes, a final product with the entire pulp and a higher soluble solids content than that of the fruit is desired. With this aim, the mash exiting the finisher is subjected to a water removal step, generally by evaporation. It is worth mentioning that concentrated purees have a significantly lower soluble solids content than clarified and concentrated juices, mainly due to technical reasons: purees contain fiber and pectin, and if their concentration was very high, the high viscosity values would make it impossible for them to circulate through the evaporators. Since the soluble solids content of these concentrated purees is not high enough to avoid deterioration, they must also be packed and stored under aseptic conditions.

REFERENCES

AIJN (2012). *2012 Liquid Fruit Market Report*. Brussels: European Fruit Juice Association.

Bates, R.P., Morris, J.R. and Crandall, P.G. (2001). Principles and practices of small- and medium-scale fruit juice processing. *FAO Agricultural Services Bulletin* 146: 3–9.

Brown, M., Kilmer, R.L. and Bedigian, K. (1993). Overview and trends in the fruit juice processing industry. In: Nagy, S., Chen, S.C. and Shaw, P.E. (eds), *Fruit Juice Processing Technology*. Auburndale, FL: Agscience, pp. 1–22.

Falguera, V., Aliguer, N. and Falguera, M. (2012). An integrated approach to current trends in food consumption. Moving toward functional and organic products? *Food Control* 26: 274–281.

FAO/WHO (2005). *Codex General Standards for Fruit Juices and Nectars (Codex STAN 247-2005)*.

Giddens, A. (1991). *Modernity and Self-Identity: Self and Society in the Late Modern Age*. Cambridge: Polity Press.

Morris, R.A. (2010). The U.S. orange and grapefruit juice markets: History, development, growth, and change. EDIS document FE834. Gainesville, FL: Food and Resource Economics Department, University of Florida.

Wolf, A., Bray, G.A. and Popkin, B.M. (2007). A short history of beverages and how our body treats them. *Obesity Reviews* 9: 151–164.

2 Product Innovation
Current Trends in Fruit Juice Production to Meet Market Demands

Miguel Ángel Cubero Márquez

When we go to any supermarket and take a look at the products they sell, it is clearly evident that the fruit juice industry has come a long way from orange and apple juices, which are two of the key items on any supermarket shelf. We can clearly see that all brands, even the ones known as trade brands, market many different items and kinds of products.

Even with the simplest item we can see lots of variation and diversity. Take orange juice as an example. In a supermarket, we can find oranges (which we can use to make our own homemade orange juice), orange juice, orange juice with pulp, orange nectar, orange nectar with added pulp, orange drinks, and so on (Figure 2.1). What, long ago, was a simple item has grown and changed from its original concept. So, we can see that the product has evolved and adapted, and for that process, product innovation is needed. Even private and trader labels are now bringing innovative concepts to the market.

Two meanings for "innovation" may be found in a dictionary:

- Something newly introduced, such as a new method or device
- The act of innovating, understanding *innovating* as "to invent" or "to begin to apply" (methods, ideas, and so on)

It is clear, then, that the possibilities for product innovation are huge, but we also have to understand why the industry needs to innovate. We can think about new products as the lifeblood and drivers of growth for the industry, and that industries that are innovative are those that are growing and are a standard for the market.

In the last few decades and years, many new products have reached the market, as can easily be seen in any supermarket in any country. The motivations for those innovations have been diverse but clear. Innovation can be generated by the introduction of a new ingredient, the shortage of a raw material, the desire to obtain a larger market share, and so on. As an example, from the data that Mintel gathered and presented during the Food Ingredients Fair, we can see from Figure 2.2 that new introductions, just for the fruit juices category, were in the hundreds in 2009 and

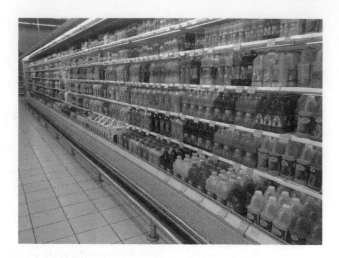

FIGURE 2.1   Shelves of fruit juices and drinks at a supermarket.

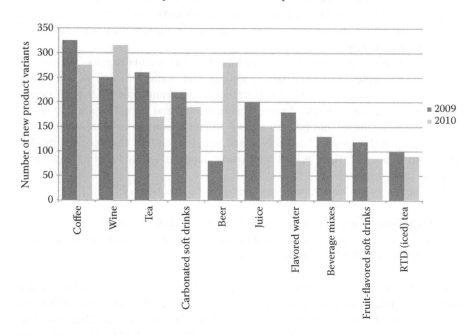

FIGURE 2.2   Data for new introductions in the U.S. market for 2009 and 2010.

2010. If fruit-based drinks and soft drinks are also considered, the number of new items doubles.

So, it can be concluded that the root cause of innovation in the food and drink sector is, mainly the desire to make good food. To fulfill that desire, firstly, food has to be delicious, giving us the desire to consume it and, primarily, to do so a number of times; if the food is not good, a consumer is not going to buy it again. Secondly, food must be healthy, as this is a trend in the market because consuming large quantities of unhealthy food has caused a lot of problems in the recent past. Thirdly, food has to be sustainable, as raw material sources are becoming increasingly scarce and the population is growing year after year, so, ultimately, we need to be able to replenish the sources of our food to be able to eat it over the next few years. Actually, fruit and vegetables fit perfectly into these three objectives, as they normally have a nice, sweet taste; nobody argues that they are not healthy; and they are obtained from harvesting trees or bushes, which can normally continue to produce over several years.

An easy way to introduce innovative products into the fruit and vegetable juices sector is to use fruits that have not previously been processed in the industry, such as some of the exotic juices that have been introduced in Europe over the last few years, or to develop processes to obtain different products from those that are already on the market. A clear example of the first kind of innovation is the goji berry, as an exotic product, which can normally be found as part of a blend, or the pomegranate, which has hit the market due to its unique characteristics. An example of the second case is the apple: in addition to the original clarified juice that was processed during the twentieth century, we can now find several different products on the shelves, such as cloudy juice, apple puree, or, on the French market, apple compote.

The use of blends to introduce price and formula stability is not new to the market (Bhardwaj and Pandey 2011) and it is a good way of creating innovative flavors or products for the market. Normally, this kind of innovation is driven by the need to ensure a low-cost product, as the use of a blend can lead to an adjustment of the quantities of the various fruits or vegetables composing the drink, depending on the intended final cost.

A good opportunity to find new and innovative products is international fairs, such as Food Ingredients, which has several versions all over the world (Europe, Latin America, India, China, etc.), or more specific fairs such as Anuga, SIAL, Vitafoods, or Alimentaria.

When thinking of achieving a healthy innovation, fruits and vegetables are normally a good option with which to begin. A good example of such a healthy innovation is smoothies, which were a big success a few years ago. The first company to introduce the concept of smoothies was Innocent Drinks, which was bought some years ago by Coca-Cola, after being hugely successful in the market. From their public data, we can see how successful innovation can be for a company, as its revenue increased to more than £100 million in less than a decade (Figure 2.3).

But, why are smoothies a good example of product innovation? Actually, smoothies are a product that is not clearly defined in law, and the best definition we can think of for them is "a functional product which is made only with natural ingredients." As we know, a functional product is one that, along with its nutritional facts, also gives some little extra to the customer for several reasons. Normally, it offers a promise concerning health or an additional ingredient that can bring a new dimension to the food product. A clear example of this kind of product is Danone's Actimel, for instance. We will return later to the concept of functional foods, as it is an important issue for innovation at the present.

So, smoothies were a quite interesting concept for innovation, making a blend that was aimed at a specific market; additionally, Innocent Drinks added an interesting marketing idea, making the products not only nutritious, but also fun. As an example,

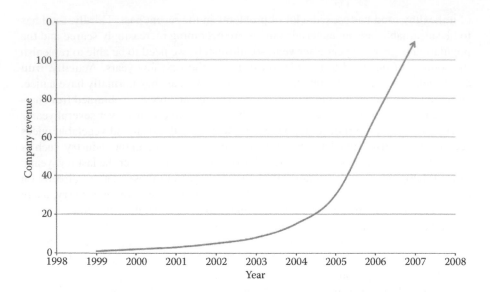

FIGURE 2.3   Increase in revenue of Innocent Drinks from its foundation in 1999 until 2007. (Adapted from Innocent. 2008. The first ever Innocent annual report, Innocent, London, 2008. http://www.innocentdrinks.co.uk/AGM/annual_report/.)

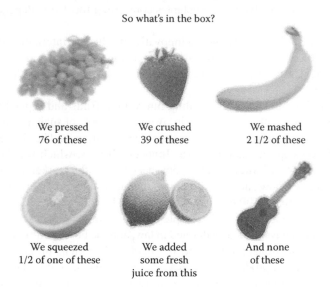

FIGURE 2.4   Label from an Innocent Drinks smoothie.

they have a concept called smoothie of the month, which can only be bought during a specific month and may not be repeated. Thus, the question that should arise is: Why are smoothies so successful in the market? Plainly, because they are tasty, people think of them as natural and healthy, and they are packaged with a good story (Figure 2.4), which also includes sustainability. How did they achieve that last part?

If we analyze one of their labels, we can see how they present their products to the final customers: easy, natural, and good. Even the list of ingredients is intended to be fun and easy to read.

Thus, with smoothies as an example, we can understand why companies want to be innovative: when they are innovative they achieve a better share of the market and, normally, better profits. Innocent Drinks is a clear example of that, as we have seen. But other companies are also good examples of it. If companies are innovative, invariably they are copied, as other companies want a piece of their success. Innocent Drinks invented the smoothie concept back in 1999, but nowadays a lot of companies have created their own range of smoothies, even changing the original idea, as we can see by the fact that the original concept always required minimally treated products, but within some of the copies we can sometimes find highly treated ingredients and even not so natural ones.

Therefore, it can also be said that when a company produces a very innovative product, other companies will copy it. When the company sees others copying its concepts and ideas, it should come to the clear conclusion that it has innovated successfully. Normally the copies need some time to get close to the original, and in the meantime the investment made on the development has been returned and used to create more innovative products, to stay ahead of our competitors. That is the clear idea and emphasis on the market.

During our discussion of smoothies, another important issue arises: that of natural products. One of the most clear and current trends in the market is "back to basics." Consumers are tired of products such as fruit drinks or nectars with a long list of ingredients that they are concerned are not natural. Therefore, formulas now have fewer ingredients and include more natural ones instead of the dreaded E numbers. E numbers are codes assigned by the European Union health and safety authorities, which have received relevant scientific information about a specific ingredient and, therefore, have approved its use and created rules for it. So, we can easily see that the E numbers were created for protecting consumers from unsafe ingredients. It is easy to find a list of E numbers on the internet, for example, at the UK Food Guide site (2013).

Unfortunately, people see E numbers as artificial additives that are unsafe, although they were created just for the opposite reason. In addition, E numbers are only European, and other agencies have created other ways of identifying and using additives, such as the U.S. Food and Drug Administration (FDA), which created the generally recognized as safe (GRAS) concept. This means that if an additive is stated as GRAS it can be used in the United States, and that with all the information gathered on it, no negative effects have been found. Not all E numbers are approved additives in countries outside Europe, and even some additives unauthorized by the European Union are legally used in such countries. So, part of the problem that makes consumers uneasy about additives is the lack of worldwide harmonization of food ingredients and their use, which has been planned but is still pending. Furthermore, we can easily find on the labels and packages declarations that some particular kinds of ingredients have not been used, such as preservatives, artificial colors, and so on. In some cases, we can call this the "free from" trend for those products, as they prefer to declare what they do not have, rather than what they really offer to the consumer, as the former is more important from a marketing point of view.

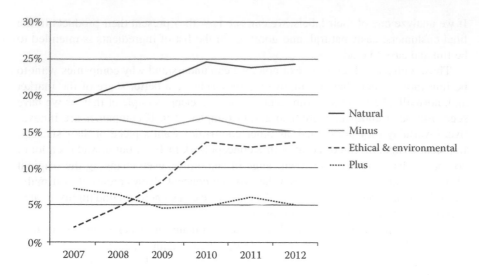

FIGURE 2.5   Global new product introductions by claim category as percentage of total. (From Mintel. 2012. HiE: What's new in natural. Presented at Health Ingredients Fair, Frankfurt.)

Because of those trends, several years ago a tendency to use food as an ingredient was created. Food is understood as an ingredient when, instead of using a legal additive, a product that is in fact a food by itself is added to a food matrix. For example, instead of adding ascorbic acid (which is E number 300), acerola juice or acerola juice concentrate is added, which is a food with a high natural content of ascorbic acid. This has been an increasing trend over the last few years, as shown in Figure 2.5.

This kind of product has led to the concept of "clean label," which can be defined as the avoidance of any kind of additive in a food formula. We must be aware that included in the ingredients normally used for a beverage or a fruit juice (among others) we can normally find aromatic ingredients, colorants, preservatives, and so on. So, a really clean label product is an "all natural" product, for example, a freshly squeezed orange juice, which declares itself to be 100% juice on the label. But when we look at a nectar or a fruit-based drink, we may find a long list of ingredients.

Due to their high amounts of appealing components, many fruit juices can be used as an ingredient in other foods. A clear example of this is the use of fruit and vegetable concentrates as food colorings, which some companies have already placed on the market. In Tables 2.1 and 2.2, we present examples of red coloring shades. Actually, many fruits and vegetables are a good source of food colorings, and companies such as GNT, Naturex, Chr. Hansen, among others, are offering them as a natural and clean label alternative for different food matrices, such as beverages, bakery products, and so on.

Therefore, we have arrived at a great source of innovation in the fruit juice industry: the development of ingredients based on fruits, vegetables, and their juices. A lot of the chemical components present in vegetables can be used in different food matrices with different goals. The use of fruit concentrates as colorants has been seen before, but they are now also used as aromatics, texturizing agents, and

TABLE 2.1

Chr. Hansen Red Colors: E Numbers

Pigment	Source	Status
Carmine	Cochineal	Natural color E120
Lycopene	Tomatoes	Natural color E160d
Betanin	Red beets	Natural color E162
Anthocyanins	Fruits and vegetables	Natural color E163
Carmoisine	Synthesis	Azoic color E122
Ponceau 4R	Synthesis	Azoic color E124
Allura red	Synthesis	Azoic color E129

Source: Chr. Hansen (n.d.) http://www.chr-hansen.com/ (accessed December 2012).

TABLE 2.2

Chr. Hansen Natural Alternatives to Red Color E Numbers

Source	Product	Shade
Grape	Grape anthocyanins and grape juice concentrates	Intense purple
Chokeberry	Chokeberry extracts and chokeberry concentrates	Orange
Elderberry	Elderberry anthocyanins and elderberry juice concentrates	Reddish-orange
Black carrot	Black carrot anthocyanins and black carrot juice concentrates	Reddish-brown
Sweet potato	Sweet potato anthocyanins	Red
Purple carrot	Anthocyanins and concentrates	Violet
Red cabbage	Red cabbage anthocyanins	Intense violet

Source: Chr. Hansen (n.d.) http://www.chr-hansen.com/ (accessed December 2012).

functional ingredients (Sun-Waterhouse 2011). This is an interesting option, as we can generate not only food, but also ingredients for complex food matrices. Another option is the development of ingredients from food industry by-products, which is a line of work that scientists and industries are following nowadays with good results (Urrecho and Romo 2009).

There is also another clear line of work driven by the *natural* trend, which is created by novel technologies. Such technologies can be used to process fruit and vegetable products with less heat, obtaining a product with more nutritional benefits. Among these technologies, there are several different ones that are starting to be used (Urrecho and Alonso 2011), such as pulsed electric fields (PEF) (Soliva-Fortuny et al. 2009), which can be used both as a pasteurization process and to cause electroporation in order to increase the recovery of some chemical compounds located in the interior of the cell (Turk et al. 2010); ultrasound-assisted processing, which has the same uses (Chemat et al. 2011); high-pressure processing for preservation (Olsen et al. 2010); ionic resin technologies for the recovery of selected components (Kammerer et al. 2011); ohmic heating for preservation; and freeze concentration, which can recover concentrates with more flavor and taste than heat concentration. There is a huge range of possibilities for the application of novel technologies to the fruit and vegetable processing industry, and although not many can be seen in the market, examples of them can begin to be seen, as shown in Table 2.3. It is also a research trend the industry is following, as advances in these subjects can lead to a whole new range of product categories.

When considering the valorization of by-products, a lot of opportunities arise, as there is normally a high amount of unused biomass from the transformation processes within the fruit industry. We can use as an example the case of the company Indulleida, where this line of work has been developed for years. The company always takes the position that its real benefit comes from the profits from this valorization of by-products.

Another choice for improvement is to increase the shelf life or the transport costs of the obtained ingredients. As an example, a development that has been carried out by the industry is to be able to dry purees to apply them to different food products, normally focusing on baby-food products or those for seniors. The product is easily reconstituted with water to a puree, or mixed with more dried products to obtain or improve soups, sauces, and so on. We can see from this example that going beyond the standard industry process can lead to new markets, normally of higher value and with fewer competitors, due to the need for development and knowledge; so taking some risks based on experience leads to greater success and benefits due to the know-how that already exists.

From fruits and vegetables, we can obtain valuable products, such as fruit fiber, fruit flakes, citrus cells, from the named fruit (FTNF) aromas, essential oils, phenolic fractions, and so on. Fruit fiber (as an example, citrus fiber is shown in Figure 2.6) is another good example of a fruit-derived ingredient. It comes from a cleaning process that produces pulp and peels without sugars or other unwanted components. These fibers are rich in dietetic fiber, as they are composed mainly of pectin, pectates, hemicelluloses, celluloses, and lignins. The origin of the fruit clearly indicates its composition. This product can be used also to help to texturize several food matrices such as meat or bakery products, with a clean label concept, as they can be declared only as fruit fiber with no need for E numbers. Companies such as Indulleida (mentioned above), Fiberstar, Hausman, and some others have developed products that follow this idea.

Refined juice sacs that are obtained when removing excess from the fruit, or from fruits of a large size, can also be used as a food ingredient (Figure 2.7). Some companies are introducing them to fruit-based drinks or nectars to give them a pulpy feeling, or even a "just-made" sensation. To obtain a quality ingredient from this source, development has been carried out to remove the unwanted particles that are present within it, such as peel particles, albedo particles, or even insects and worms, which can be found in the inner part of the fruit, untouched by normal processing.

TABLE 2.3
Examples of Fruit Products Obtained by Novel Technologies

Product Type	Product	Country	Pathogens Control	Shelf-Life Increase	Preservative-Free	Organic	Functional	Shelf-Stable
Juices and Smoothies	Citrus juices	France	✓	✓	✓	–	–	–
	Apple, plum, strawberry, pear juices	Italy	✓	✓	✓	–	–	–
	Juices and smoothies	Northern Ireland	✓	✓	✓	–	–	–
	Orange juice and smoothies	Spain	✓	✓	✓	–	–	–
	Organic apple juices	Portugal	✓	✓	✓	✓	–	–
	Smoothies and organic orange juice	Australia	✓	✓	✓	✓	–	–
	Broccoli and apple, carrot juices	Czech Republic	✓	✓	✓	–	✓	–
	Pomegranate juice	Australia	✓	✓	✓	–	✓	–
	Juices and superfood smoothies	United States	✓	✓	✓	✓	✓	–
Purees, Coulis, and Sauces	Avocado pulp and guacamole	Mexico	✓	✓	✓	–	–	–
	Guacamole (regular and organic)	United States	✓	✓	✓	✓	–	–
	Mexican-style tomato sauces	United States	✓	✓	✓	–	–	–
	Tofu and dressings	United States	✓	✓	✓	✓	–	–
	Hummus and salsas	United States	✓	✓	✓	✓	–	–
	Fruit puree and coulis	Australia	✓	✓	✓	–	–	–
	Apple and strawberry jams	Italy	✓	✓	✓	–	–	–
	Blended apple fruit purees	Canada	✓	✓	✓	✓	–	✓

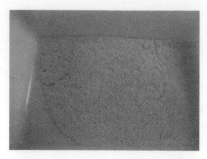

FIGURE 2.6   Citrus fruit fiber.

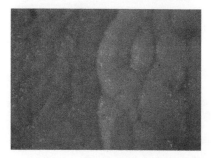

FIGURE 2.7   Citrus cells.

Companies such as Orangina-Schweppes, JBT, and Granini are using this new range of ingredients to bring innovative products to the market.

Instead of throwing away all the biomass remnants as a residue, they can be used as an animal feed (Figure 2.8). Using them directly is an option, but as the industry grows larger, the need arises to stabilize such products to be able to transport them over long distances. So, dried pellets can be made from them, but even what seems to be an easy process to put into place needs study and development to be successful, as peels are still high in sugars and unwanted components, which are not easy to dry.

As has been observed, the highest content of phenols present in fruits and vegetables is normally in the peel, as it is suspected that they perform their function in that specific area (Brouillard 1983). As fruit and vegetable processing is designed to separate the peel from the pulp, it seems clear that this raw material can be a good option, as it is a cheap and concentrated source for the recovery of potentially interesting bioactive compounds. Figure 2.9 shows phenolic extracts recovered from the by-products of juice processing.

Following this discussion, it should be clear that a product line that in the consumer's mind is easy and simple may have a large amount of innovation within it, sometimes with much help from marketing and sometimes without, but with the aim of benefitting the final customers. The main point about functional ingredients is that two things have to be proved: the content of the new ingredient and its usefulness. This is the key, where we must bring together science and industry to reach our goals.

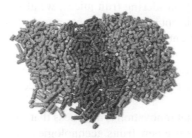

FIGURE 2.8 Animal feed obtained from unused biomass.

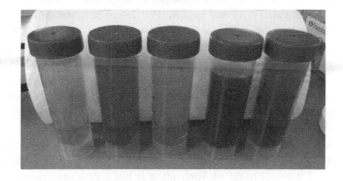

FIGURE 2.9 Phenolic fractions recovered from unused by-products.

The functional ingredients trend hit the market several years ago, but due to the European health claims regulations, the innovation that was driven by this concept was stopped in order to adapt to it, although in the United States and Japan the regulations are completely different and easier for the industries to adapt to and apply (Lalor and Wall 2012). It was clear that the consumer was in need of protection, as there existed strange health claims or those with little scientific backing. It was for that reason that the European Union, through the European Food Safety Agency (EFSA) and national agencies (such as the Spanish Food Safety and Nutrition Agency [AESAN]) decided to establish and evaluate the truth and facts behind the health claims, assuming that, in the end, they would greatly benefit the final consumer. EU Regulation no. 1924/2006 came into force in 2007, and finally, in 2012, a list of 222 approved health claims was issued. We must also understand that these claims are not written in stone, and that agencies have an active role in evaluating new proposals for claims as new scientific evidence is created and gathered. One significant point about fruit and vegetable juices within the health claims regulations is that it is understood that they are suitable matrices to add functional ingredients, as they are generally judged to be healthy, in contrast to matrices such as high-fat sausages, for example. We can recognize that the process has been long and slow, as the amount of information for every claim is clearly large. Also, the EFSA was overwhelmed with the number of claims as thousands of files were presented to them during 2007.

In this section, while considering fruit juices, we also have to consider so-called superfruits. This is a concept which represents a fruit that is very rich in chemical compounds that are present in it naturally, not artificially added, which may have several healthy effects on our bodies. A lot of scientific work has been done on those fruits and is still in progress, in order to discover their real components and capacities. The superfruits that concentrate most of the juice industry's attention will be described in Chapter 3.

We must remember that innovation is a process that can be applied every day, and that it does not really require new fruits, technologies, or research. Also, innovation in management is required and desired, as new standards and needs arise every year, because consumers nowadays are more concerned and reactive about what they eat than in the past, and we must follow their needs to be able to supply to the market safe products that are also tasty and healthy. For that reason, the industry is evolving from the International Organization for Standardization (ISO) 9001:2008 standard to more complex and safe ones, such as the British Retail Consortium (BRC) standard, the International Food Safety (IFS) standard, and ISO 22000:2005, which are all linked and related to food safety issues. All of us can remember some food safety scandals that have happened all over the world, even in the countries most advanced in food safety, such as Germany and the United States. So, innovation also has to take into account those events.

We can clearly see that the fruit and vegetable juice industry has a good opportunity to fulfill its customers' requests by using innovation, and to be different from its competitors if it wants to do so. Innovation is not only a one-man task or a task to be undertaken weekly; it is a philosophy that must be applied at all levels of an organization and followed by all workers. Industry leaders can show their companies the path to be taken, but the need for a close relationship between academic research and industry is easily observed, as what is developed by the former finally reaches the supermarket shelves after some years.

REFERENCES

Bhardwaj, R.L. and Pandey, S. (2011). Juice blends: A way of utilization of under-utilized fruits, vegetables and spices: A review. *Critical Reviews in Food Science and Nutrition* 51(6): 563–570.

Brouillard, R. (1983). The *in vivo* expression of anthocyanin colour in plants. *Phytochemistry* 22: 1311–1323.

Chemat, F.F., Huma, Z., and Khan, M.K. (2011). Applications of ultrasound in food technology: Processing, preservation and extraction. *Ultrasonics Sonochemistry* 18(4): 813–835.

Chr. Hansen (n.d.) http://www.chr-hansen.com/ (accessed December 2012).

Innocent (2008). The first ever Innocent annual report. London: Innocent. http://www.innocentdrinks.co.uk/AGM/annual_report/ (accessed December 2012).

Kammerer, J., Carle, R., and Kammerer, D.R. (2011). Adsorption and ion exchange: Basic principles and their application in food processing. *Journal of Agricultural and Food Chemistry* 59(1): 22–42.

Lalor, F. and Wall, P.G. (2012). Health claims regulations: Comparison between USA, Japan and European Union. *British Food Journal* 113(2): 298–313.

Mintel (2012). HiE: What's new in natural. Presented at Health Ingredients Fair, Frankfurt.

Olsen, N.V., Grunert, K.G., and Sonne, A.M. (2010). Consumer acceptance of high-pressure processing and pulsed-electric field: A review. *Trends in Food Science and Technology* 21(9): 464–472.

Soliva-Fortuny, R., Balasa, A., Knorr, D., and Martín-Belloso, O. (2009). Effects of pulsed electric fields on bioactive compounds in foods: A review. *Trends in Food Science and Technology* 20(11–12): 544–556.

Sun-Waterhouse, D. (2011). The development of fruit-based functional foods targeting the health and wellness market: A review. *International Journal of Food Science and Technology* 46(5): 899–920.

Turk, M.F., Baron, A., and Vorobiev, E. (2010). Effect of pulsed electric fields treatment and mash size on extraction and composition of apple juices. *Journal of Agricultural and Food Chemistry* 58(17): 9611–9616.

UK Food Guide (2013). E number index. http://www.ukfoodguide.net/enumeric.htm (accessed July 2013).

Urrecho, A. and Alonso, M. (2011). *El Libro Del Zumo*. Madrid: Asozumos.

Urrecho, A. and Romo, A. (2009). *Aprovechamiento de Residuos de Frutas*. Madrid: Asozumos.

3 New Trends in Fruit Juices
Superfruits

Francisco López

CONTENTS

3.1 Introduction 28
3.2 Superfruits 29
    3.2.1 Açaí...29
    3.2.2 Acerola...29
    3.2.3 Avocado 29
    3.2.4 Blackberry 29
    3.2.5 Blackcurrant...29
    3.2.6 Blueberry 30
    3.2.7 Cherry...30
    3.2.8 Cranberry..30
    3.2.9 Date...30
    3.2.10 Fig 31
    3.2.11 Goji 31
    3.2.12 Grape 31
    3.2.13 Guava 31
    3.2.14 Guarana 31
    3.2.15 Kiwifruit 32
    3.2.16 Mango 32
    3.2.17 Mangosteen...32
    3.2.18 Noni 33
    3.2.19 Orange 33
    3.2.20 Papaya..33
    3.2.21 Pomegranate 33
    3.2.22 Raspberry...34
    3.2.23 Seabuckthorn 34
    3.2.24 Strawberry 34
3.3 Superjuices...34
3.4 The Market for Superjuices 36
References...37

3.1   INTRODUCTION

The consumption of fruit is positive in a healthy diet, especially due to nutrients and compounds they contain that have healthy properties. In recent years, due to the characterization of their properties, a series of fruits have been established that are especially rich in nutrients and bioactive compounds: *superfruits*. These fruits are desirable to the consumer, especially exotic fruits. Although there is no clear scientific definition, in general a superfruit complies with the following constraints (Gross, 2010):

- Nutrient diversity and density
- Phytochemical diversity and density
- Basic research intensity
- Clinical research progress
- Popularity based on sensory appeal and market demand

However, Crawford and Mellentin (2008) say that superfruits are the product of a strategy: they do not just grow on trees, but are the result of a convergence of science and marketing in order to create a new value-added product in the nutrition market. They define six elements for superfruit success: (1) sensory appeal, (2) novelty, (3) convenience, (4) control of supply, (5) health benefit, and (6) marketing.

These exotic and healthy fruits have attracted the interest of nutritionists, scientists, and physicians, and research on them has increased in recent years, especially regarding their antioxidant capacity (AOC) and positive effects on the risks of certain diseases. The health benefits of superfruits are mainly due to their content of antioxidants, especially vitamins C and E, as well as polyphenol compounds. These antioxidants destroy free radicals, which are unstable molecules of oxygen formed during the normal processes of the body. Free radicals, if not controlled, can damage healthy cells and cause health problems such as Alzheimer's disease, cancer, heart disease, and inflammation (Tomás-Barberán and Andrés-Lacueva, 2012).

Some fruits that are now being called superfruits in reality are not, as no claims about their antioxidant health benefits have actually been established by science or allowed by regulatory authorities (Mackay, 2007; Gross, 2010). Superfruits can be defined as fruits whose regular intake as whole foods provides healthy nutrients. Processed, blended, and diluted juices are not included because most of the juices that stimulated the concept of superfruits are highly processed so that there is little left in them except color and taste (Gross, 2010; Grace et al., 2012).

Interest in superfruits and their derivatives has increased since companies, especially those producing juices, have accentuated their properties, making them attractive for consumers. Their AOC and effects on various diseases have been highlighted. All this has led the scientific community to increase research on the characterization of these superfruits, both traditional ones and exotic ones, mainly from tropical climates.

There are many lists of superfruits, especially on the Internet, which has much information on them. There is a consensus on a number of fruits, which appear in all lists, but some new fruits have only recently been included in this category.

3.2 SUPERFRUITS

This section contains a review of the main fruits considered superfruits.

3.2.1 Açaí

Açaí (*Euterpe oleracea* Mart., cabbage palm berry) is a palm tree fruit found throughout the Amazon estuary flood plains. The fruit, a small berry, is a round, black-purple drupe with a circumference of about 25 mm, similar in appearance to but smaller than a grape and with less pulp. The berries are produced in branched panicles of 500–900 fruits. Açaí is rich in vitamins A, C, B1, and B2, calcium, iron, magnesium, and antioxidants. The high antioxidant concentration of açaí helps combat premature aging, with 10 times more antioxidants than red grapes and 10–30 times more anthocyanins than red wine (Rufino et al., 2010, 2011).

3.2.2 Acerola

Acerola (*Malpighia emarginata* DC., Barbados cherry) is a fruit from a small tree cultivated in tropical and subtropical regions (Central America and the southwestern United States). The fruit is a bright red drupe 10–30 mm in diameter. Drupes are in pairs or groups of three, and each contains three triangular seeds. The drupes are juicy. Acerola is well known as an excellent food source of vitamin C, and it also contains phytochemicals such as carotenoids and polyphenols (Mezadri et al., 2008). Its vitamin C content is more than 30 times higher than that of oranges.

3.2.3 Avocado

Avocadoes (*Persea americana* Mill., palta, aguacate) are egg-shaped, green-brown on the outside, and green-yellow on the inside. This fruit is native to Mexico and throughout history has been cultivated in Central and South America (Galindo Tovar et al., 2008). It contains healthy monounsaturated fat, which has been linked to a reduced risk of cancer, heart disease, and diabetes (D'Ambrosio et al., 2011; Yasir et al., 2010).

3.2.4 Blackberry

The blackberry (*Rubus fruticosus* L. agg.) is an edible fruit produced by many species in the *Rubus* genus in the Rosaceae family. The (usually) black fruit is not a true berry; botanically it is termed an aggregate fruit, composed of small drupelets. It is a widespread and well-known group of over 375 species. Blackberries are notable for their high nutritional content of dietary fiber, vitamin C, vitamin K, folic acid (a B vitamin), and the essential mineral manganese. Blackberries also have a high abundance of healthy antioxidants and salicylic acid (Kaume et al., 2012).

3.2.5 Blackcurrant

Blackcurrant (*Ribes nigrum* L.) is a temperate fruit crop native to central and northern Europe and northern Asia, and is widely cultivated both commercially and domestically for its abundant berries. The ripe fruit is around 10 mm in diameter, very dark purple in color, almost black, with a glossy skin and a persistent calyx at the apex, and contains several seeds dense in nutrients. The fruit has extraordinarily high vitamin C content, good levels of potassium, phosphorus, iron, and vitamin B5, and a broad range of other essential nutrients (Hummer and Barney, 2002).

3.2.6 BLUEBERRY

The blueberry (*Vaccinium angustifolium* L., *V. corymbosum* L.) fruit is a berry of 5–16 mm in diameter with a flared crown at the end. The skin is smooth and soft and ranges from light blue to dark blue when ripe. Blueberries have a sweet taste when mature, with variable acidity. They are native to North America but also grown in Australia, New Zealand, and South American countries. They are rich in flavonoids, manganese, vitamins B, C, E, and K, calcium, iron, magnesium, and zinc. The health benefits for the vascular system and brain are mediated in part by their flavonoid content (Dastmalchi et al., 2011). This fruit is also related to anti aging and improved vision (Liu et al., 2011). Blueberries are also a source of fiber, which helps to maintain a healthy digestive system (Basu et al., 2010; Willis et al., 2011).

3.2.7 CHERRY

Cherry (*Prunus avium* L., *P. cesarus* L.) fruits are roughly round with a depression at the apex (top) of the fruit. The skin is smooth and shiny and usually ranges from pale to very dark red, although yellow and white cultivars exist. The cherry is the fruit with a fleshy drupe (stone fruit). Sweet and sour cherries are the two common types of cherries. Cherries contain anthocyanins, the red pigment in berries (Damar and Eks, 2012).

3.2.8 CRANBERRY

Cranberries (*Vaccinium macrocarpon* Ait.) are berries of 6–18 mm in size; their skin is smooth and shiny, and color varies from bright to dark red when ripe. They grow on a perennial dwarf shrub that grows in cold areas of the Northern Hemisphere.

Cranberries are rich in vitamins C, A, and K, calcium, magnesium, manganese, phosphorus, potassium, and antioxidants. Cranberries offer a wealth of health benefits because they contain proanthocyanidins (PACs; or condensed tannins), which can be used to prevent or treat urinary tract infections (Grace et al., 2012; Feghali et al., 2012).

3.2.9 DATE

Dates (*Phoenix dactylifera* L.) are the fruit of the date palm. They are dark reddish brown, oval, and about 20–30 mm long. Date skin is wrinkled and coated with a sticky, waxy film. Date fruits are rich in natural antioxidants that might be more widely used by both the general population and the food industry as a source of bioactive human health promoter phytochemicals (Amira et al., 2012).

3.2.10 FIG

Fig (*Ficus carica* L.) fruits are bell-shaped, with a wide, flat bottom narrowing to a pointed top. The fruit size is around 30–50 mm. When the fruit ripens, the top may bend, forming a "neck." Figs can be brown, purple, green, yellow, or black, and vary in size. The skin is slightly wrinkled and leathery. Figs are among the richest plant sources of calcium and fiber. Figs have a laxative effect and contain many antioxidants and they are a good source of flavonoids and polyphenols (Vallejo et al., 2012).

3.2.11 GOJI

Goji (*Lycium barbarum* L., wolfberry) is a red berry that is usually found dried. The fruit is closely related to the nightshade family and is native to southeastern Europe and Asia. It is cultivated in China, Mongolia, and the Himalayas in Tibet. Goji contains vitamin A (from β-carotene) that acts as an antioxidant, and this fruit is also rich in vitamins C and B, calcium, magnesium, potassium, iron, zinc, selenium, and polyphenols (anthocyanins, ellagic acid). This fruit is well known in traditional Chinese medicine and currently is widely used as a popular functional food. Research interest in goji has recently increased due to its immunomodulation and antitumor activity (Miller and Shukitt-Hale, 2012).

3.2.12 GRAPE

Grapes (*Vitis vinifera* L.) are berries rich in vitamins B, C, and K, calcium, potassium, iron, magnesium, manganese, phosphorus, sodium, and zinc. *V. vinifera* L. contains many phenolic compounds and anthocyanins that impart their color to the berries (generally in the skin). Grapes and red wines are rich sources of phenolic compounds such as anthocyanins, catechins, PACs, flavonols, stilbenes, and other phenolics, all of which are potent antioxidants that show cardioprotective properties (Tenore et al., 2012).

3.2.13 GUAVA

Guava fruit (*Psidium guajava* L.) are usually 40–120 mm long, and round or oval, depending on the species. The outer skin may be rough, often with a bitter taste, or soft and sweet. The skin varies between species; it can be any thickness, and is usually green before maturity, evolving to a yellow or brown color. Guavas are native to Mexico, Central America, and northern South America. Guavas are rich in dietary fiber, vitamins A and C, folic acid, and the dietary minerals, potassium, copper, and manganese. This fruit also contains bioactive compounds, such as phenolic acids and flavonoids, and has been used to treat inflammation, hepatotoxicity, and hypertension, among others (Contreras-Calderon et al., 2011; Menezes et al., 2012).

3.2.14 GUARANA

Guarana (*Paullinia cupana* Mart.) fruit is obtained from a climbing plant of the maple family that grows in the Amazon basin. The guarana fruit's color ranges from brown to red and it contains black seeds that are partly covered by white arils. The fruit is rich in caffeine and protein, and it is used in sweetened, energy, and carbonated soft drinks (Smith and Atroch, 2010). The functional properties of guarana, which are similar to those of green tea, are related to metabolic disorders (Bittencourt et al., 2013). In addition, guarana has a cardioprotective effect due to its inhibition of plate-let aggregation (Portella et al., 2013).

3.2.15 KIWIFRUIT

Kiwifruit (*Actinidia deliciosa* Planch., *A. chinensis* Planch.) can be produced in tem-perate climates with adequate summer heat. Kiwifruits are egg-shaped with bright green (or golden) flesh and tiny black seeds. The fruit is covered in a fuzzy, dark green coat, which helps to preserve freshness and adds to its appeal. Kiwifruit juice contains many nutrients, including high amounts of vitamin C and vitamin E (Sun-Waterhouse et al., 2009). It also contains dietary minerals such as potassium. A single kiwifruit is said to supply more than the normal daily adult requirement of vitamin C (more than oranges). Vitamin E is also an antioxidant that has several functions, including helping protect cells in the body from damaging compounds (Park et al., 2013).

3.2.16 MANGO

Mangoes (*Mangifera indica* L.) are a fruit obtained from the tree with the same name, originally from India, and are cultivated in tropical and subtropical regions. Mango fruits are oval and egg-shaped with smooth, soft skin. The skin is usually a combination of green, red, and yellow. The interior flesh is bright orange and soft with a large, flat pit in the middle. Mangoes are rich in vitamins A (mostly in the form of β-carotene), B, and C, calcium, iron, potassium, magnesium, phosphorus, zinc, and antioxidants. Vitamin C is an antioxidant that has been shown to improve the immune system, fight cancer, and decrease the risk of heart disease (Noratto et al., 2010). Vitamin A is essential for normal vision, gene expression, reproduction, embryonic development, growth, and immune function (Abu et al., 2005). This fruit is used traditionally to produce juices.

3.2.17 MANGOSTEEN

Mangosteen (*Garcinia mangostana* L.) is a fruit with a sweet–sour white flesh, obtained from a tropical evergreen tree originating in Indonesia, which can be cultivated in countries with a hot, humid climate such as Thailand, Malaysia, Singapore, Vietnam, and Indonesia. Unrelated to the mango, mangosteen has a thick purple skin covering an edible white pulp and a size of 30–50 mm. Its rind contains xanthones, which can neutralize free radicals (Kondo et al., 2009). Mangosteen is the latest superfruit, featuring in a range of functional juices and dietary supplements, which claim to have a high concentration of xanthone (Muñoz-Acuña et al., 2012).

3.2.18 NONI

Noni (*Morinda citrifolia* L., cheese fruit, ach, mengkudu) is an oval-shaped and prickly fruit. The tree is related to the coffee family and is native to Southeast Asia. Noni is rich in vitamins C, B, and A, iron, proteins, potassium, sodium, and calcium. Due to the high level of antioxidants, the juice can help reduce high blood pressure and relieve arthritic pain, but due to its high potassium level, caution is advised in people with reduced kidney function (Ulloa et al., 2012; Brown, 2012).

3.2.19 ORANGE

Oranges (*Citrus sinensis* L.) are oval- to sphere-shaped fruits with leathery, porous skin. Their color ranges from orange to red-orange. Inside, the fruit is divided into segments, which have thin tough skins that hold together many little sections with juice inside. There are usually 10 segments in an orange, but sometimes there are more. It is believed that the orange is native to tropical and subtropical areas of Asia, including China, India, and the Malay Archipelago. Aside from their refreshing flavor and distinct taste, oranges are one of the most nutrient-dense fruits. They contain phytonutrients, which are nourishing components that occur naturally in certain plants, as well as essential nutrients such as vitamin C and folate (Liu et al., 2012). Vitamin C is an antioxidant that has many functions such as the promotion of healthy skin and gums and the ability to increase iron absorption. Folate is important in fetal development and in making healthy red blood cells.

3.2.20 PAPAYA

The papaya is the fruit of the plant *Carica papaya*. It is native to the tropics of America, southern Mexico, and Central America. Papayas are bell-shaped, with one end much smaller than the other. Their skin is smooth and leathery, and changes from green to yellow-orange as the fruit ripens. The interior flesh is golden yellow and surrounds a large cluster of seeds. The papaya is a big fruit, between 150 and 450 mm in length and 100–300 mm in diameter. Papaya fruit is a rich source of nutrients such as provitamin A carotenoids, vitamins C and B, lycopene, dietary minerals, and dietary fiber (Gayosso-García Sancho, 2011).

3.2.21 POMEGRANATE

Pomegranate (*Punica granatum* L.) is a fruit that is obtained from a small tree native to Iran and is currently cultivated in different countries, especially in the Mediterranean area. The fruit has between 200 and 1400 seeds that can vary from white to dark red. Pomegranate has become a very popular superfruit in recent years due to its high AOC (anthocyanins, polyphenols, tannins, and vitamin C) and its rich, tart flavor (Fischer et al., 2011). Pomegranate is known to improve blood lipid profiles by enhancing high-density lipoprotein (HDL) levels while reducing harmful low-density lipoproteins (LDL), helping to prevent plaque buildup in the arteries and reduce blood pressure (Rosenblat et al., 2010). Traditionally, pomegranate has been valued as an agent for improving inflammation-related skin conditions and for accelerating skin repair after sun damage. Pomegranate is also rich in calcium, iron, magnesium, phosphorous, potassium, and zinc.

3.2.22 RASPBERRY

The raspberry (*Rubusidaeus* L.) is a compound fruit composed of many small fruits. The skin of the fruit is smooth and fragile and is red, dark purple, or yellow in color. The core of the fruit is hollow, distinguishing raspberries from blackberries. Raspberries are an important commercial fruit crop, widely grown in all temperate regions of the world. Raspberries are a rich source of vitamin C, manganese, and dietary fiber (Verbeyst et al., 2012).

3.2.23 SEABUCKTHORN

Seabuckthorn (*Hippophae rhamnoides* L., sandthorn, seaberry) is a yellow-orange berry that grows on a thorny vine. The berries are 6–9 mm in diameter, soft, and juicy, with a high content of vitamin C; some varieties have a high content of vitamin A, vitamin E, and essential oils. Native to Europe and Asia, seabuckthorn berries are a valuable source of bioactives such as tocopherols, carotenoids, and flavonoids (Kagliwal et al., 2012). It is said to boost the immune system as it is rich in vitamin C. This fruit is usually available in juice or tea form (Mishra et al., 2008).

3.2.24 STRAWBERRY

Strawberry (*Fragaria × ananassa* Duch.) fruits are aggregates made up of several small fruits, each with one seed called an achene. The flesh of the strawberry is actually an enlarged receptacle made of nonreproductive material. The fruit is widely appreciated for its characteristic aroma, bright red color, juicy texture, and sweetness. Strawberries are an excellent source of vitamin C and flavonoids (Verbeyst et al., 2012).

3.3 SUPERJUICES

In the scientific literature, there are numerous studies that show that regular consumption of fruits and vegetables helps reduce the risk of several chronic diseases such as coronary heart disease and probably certain kinds of cancer (World Cancer Research Fund, 2007; Nikolic et al., 2008; Kris-Etherton et al., 2002). The hypothesis is that antioxidant ingredients such as polyphenols and water-soluble vitamins are the crucial factors that improve human health (Liu, 2003). This scientific evidence is translated worldwide into public health initiatives such as "five a day" and school fruit programs that aim to increase daily consumption of fruits and vegetables. Encouraged by these policy-driven actions, the food industry is strongly engaged in launching novel fruit (and vegetable)-based products onto the market. Blended juices, juice concentrates, and smoothies rich in polyphenols and water-soluble vitamins such as ascorbic acid are marketed as health-supporting foods specifically preventing radical-driven chronic diseases (Ellinger et al., 2012; Faraoni et al., 2012).

One of the problems encountered in these new products is the determination and quantification of this bioactive capacity (Huang et al., 2005; Prior et al., 2005). Polyphenolics contribute to the antioxidant properties of foods, juices, and beverages, and are essential to the human diet (Müller et al., 2010). The total phenols in foods and beverages are currently measured with the Folin–Ciocalteu method, through its reducing capacity. Medina (2011) developed a novel method to quantify polyphenols or phenolic compounds through direct interactions of polyphenols with Fast Blue BB in an alkaline medium and the absorbance was measured at 420 nm. The novel method demonstrated that gallic acid equivalent values were higher with the Fast Blue BB method than with the Folin–Ciocalteu method. Müller et al. (2010) recommends using at least two methods to measure the AOC in any given sample.

The second problem is maintaining the human health benefits from consumption of fruit derivatives because when they are processed by techniques such as pressing, canning, concentrating, or drying, a number of these natural components may be compromised or inactivated due to physical separation, thermal degradation, or oxidation (Grace et al., 2012; Hollands et al., 2008; Gross, 2010). For this reason, introducing additional bioactive compounds into products from other sources is one strategy to maintain and increase health beneficial properties in juices and other products. Törrönen et al. (2012) fortified blackcurrant juice with crowberry powder, observing that this juice doubled the polyphenol content and improved postprandial glycemic control in healthy subjects compared with a basic blackcurrant juice.

Nevertheless, in the development of functional foods and ingredients containing polyphenols, the relevance of the food matrix and the solubility of the polyphenols are important aspects (Roopchand et al., 2012). Technological treatments to mask undesirable sensory aspects often associated with some polyphenols (bitterness, astringency, etc.) or to ensure the stability of the active metabolites in the food during storage, processing, and transit through the gastrointestinal tract must be developed (Tomás-Barberán and Andrés-Lacueva, 2012).

Current trends and developments around the world regarding new foods and functional products aim to demonstrate their significant bioactivity. This applies especially to work on fruit, and in particular tropical or exotic fruits that are more attractive to consumers, although their health properties have not been scientifically tested. For instance, papaya has recently been featured in a number of packaged foods, beverages, dietary supplements, and beauty products, especially an enzyme that is extracted from it, called papain (Bengoechea, 2010). Papain is claimed to have several health benefits, especially in the field of digestive health, but the effectiveness of papain has not yet been scientifically proven. This poses a potential problem for papaya as it is expressly marketed as a health aid in many countries. Nevertheless, this fruit is used to give a more exotic taste to a new range of juices with flavor blends.

To increase the intake of phytochemicals, the food industry offers smoothies as an alternative or addition to the consumption of fresh fruits and vegetables. Smoothies belong to fruit juices and this term has been used for 70 years, primarily in the United States and United Kingdom, and recently also in Germany. Their production is based on the usage of the total fruits, which are processed to pulp or puree, partially with pieces (Müller et al., 2010). In most fruit products the majority of the AOC is generated by polyphenolic compounds, except acerola puree and orange juice. Very good correlations between total phenolic content and AOC were found in the single-fruit products; however, not in fruit and vegetable smoothies. Müller et al. (2010) found that most of the smoothies analyzed in their work were able to supply nearly the recommended dietary intake (RDI) of vitamin C for adults (100 mg/day) with one package.

Blending traditional fruit juice with exotic fruits can be another way to obtain new products with superfruit labels. Gironés-Vilaplana et al. (2012) designed new blends based on lemon juice mixed with different edible berries of exotic and local origin such as maqui, açaí, and blackthorn. The beverage based on lemon juice and maqui berry was the most interesting blend in terms of AOC. All juices presented an inhibitor effect of cholinesterases. The results suggested that lemon juice enriched with berries could be of potential interest in the design of new drinks with a nutrition-related function in combating chronic diseases. Vázquez-Araújo et al. (2010) studied the quality parameters of a commercial pomegranate juice mixed with other fruit juices such as blueberry, blackberry, or raspberry. The main characteristics in these juices were a high maturity index, low acidity, and the presence of aromatic compounds typical in blueberries. Some juice formulations had higher acceptance among consumers; total phenolic content was significantly higher in the pomegranate/blackberry sample and could be a positive determinant for consumers interested in purchasing healthful products.

3.4   THE MARKET FOR SUPERJUICES

The market for products with high antioxidant content is difficult to quantify, since these compounds are found in all kinds of foods, beverages, and health products. Euromonitor International (http://www.euromonitor.com) has selected a number of pertinent categories whose dynamism is primarily founded on the fact that they are rich sources of antioxidants. These are green tea, dark chocolate, superfruit juice, and dietary supplements. Combined global sales of these categories totaled $32 billion in 2009, exceeding the global value of organic packaged food and beverages ($26 billion). Japan, the United States, and China are the biggest markets for antioxidant-fortified food and drinks (Hudson, 2010a). Healthy superfruit juice sales amounted to $2.6 billion in 2009. The largest market continues to be the United States, where cranberry juice is extremely popular, accounting for 80% of global sales. In Western Europe, superfruit juice posted an 8% compound annual growth rate (CAGR) for the review period. Sales of superfruit juice grew even faster in Eastern Europe, posting an 11% current value CAGR for 2004–2009.

In 2007 alone, more than 6000 new products were introduced using the above-named superfruits as ingredients (Ark, 2010). The most frequent use is in beverages, a category that accounts for no less than 35% of the new products introduced. In second and third place are snacks (12%) and bakery products (11%).

According to Alzheimer's Disease International, dementia affects one in 20 people over the age of 65. Euromonitor International countries and consumers data show that over-65s amounted to around 541 million consumers globally in 2010, and by

2014 this will have risen to almost 600 million—a potentially enormous target group for easy-to-consume juice products (Hudson, 2010b).

In the future, antioxidant-rich products, with or without health claims, will continue to infiltrate and spread within new categories, such as flavored waters, concentrates, on-the-go single-serve drinks in bottles and cartons, bakery products, snack foods, and ice cream. Convenience and impulse products will stand to benefit a great deal.

REFERENCES

Abu, J., Batuwangala, M., Herbert, K., and Symonds, P. (2005). Retinoic acid and retinoid receptors: Potential chemopreventive and therapeutic role in cervical cancer. *Lancet Oncol.* 6: 712–720.

Amira, E., Behija, S.E., Beligh, M., Lamia, L., Manel, I., Mohamed, H., and Lotfi, A. (2012). Effects of the ripening stage on phenolic profile, phytochemical composition and antioxidant activity of date palm fruit. *J. Agric. Food Chem.* 60: 10896–10902.

Ark, R. (2010). Fashion foods: Superfruits open up new vistas. *Nutraceutical Bus. Technol.* 6(6): 48–49.

Basu, A., Rhone, M., and Lyons, T.J. (2010). Berries: Emerging impact on cardiovascular health. *Nutr. Rev.* 68(3): 168–177.

Bengoechea, I. (2010). Papaya: The superfruit suspect. *Asia Pac. Food Ind.* 22: 40–42.

Bittencourt, L.S., Machado, D.C., Machado, M.M., Dos Santos, G.F.F., Algarve, T.D., Marinowic, D.R., Ribeiro, E.E., et al. (2013). The protective effects of guaraná extract (*Paullinia cupana*) on fibroblast NIH-3T3 cells exposed to sodium nitroprusside. *Food Chem. Toxicol.* 53: 119–125.

Brown, A.C. (2012). Anticancer activity of *Morinda citrifolia* (Noni) fruit: A review. *Phytother. Res.* 26: 1427–1440.

Contreras-Calderon, J., Calderon-Jaimes, L., Guerra-Hernandez, E., and Garcia-Villanova, B. (2011). Antioxidant capacity, phenolic content and vitamin C in pulp, peel and seed from 24 exotic fruits from Colombia. *Food Res. Int.* 44: 2047–2053.

Crawford, K. and Mellentin, J. (2008). *Successful Superfruit Strategy: How to Build a Superfruit Business*. London: New Nutrition Business.

Damar, I. and Eks, A. (2012). Antioxidant capacity and anthocyanin profile of sour cherry (*Prunus cerasus* L.) juice. *Food Chem.* 135: 2910–2914.

D'Ambrosio, S.M., Han, C., Pan, L., Kinghorn, A.D., and Ding, H. (2011). Aliphatic acetogenin constituents of avocado fruits inhibit human oral cancer cell proliferation by targeting the EGFR/RAS/RAF/MEK/ERK1/2 pathway. *Biochem. Biophys. Res. Commun.* 409: 465–469.

Dastmalchi, K., Flores, G., Petrova, V., Pedraza-Peñalosa, P., and Kennelly, E.J. (2011). Edible neotropical blueberries: Antioxidant and compositional fingerprint analysis. *J. Agric. Food Chem.* 59: 3020–3026.

Ellinger, S., Gordon, A., Kurten, M., Jungfer, E., Zimmermann, B.F., Zur, B., Ellinger, J., Marx, F., and Stehle, P. (2012). Bolus consumption of a specifically designed fruit juice rich in anthocyanins and ascorbic acid did not influence markers of antioxidative defense in healthy humans. *J. Agric. Food Chem.* 60: 11292–11300.

Faraoni, A.S., Ramos, A.M., Guedes, D.B., Oliveira, A.N., Ferreira de Lima, T.H.S., and de Sousa, P.H.M. (2012). Desenvolvimento de um suco misto de manga, goiaba e acerola utilizando delineamento de misturas. *Ciência Rural* 42: 911–917.

Feghali, K., Feldman, M., La, V.D., Santos, J., and Grenier, D. (2012). Cranberry proanthocyanidins: Natural weapons against periodontal diseases. *J. Agric. Food Chem.* 60: 5728–5735.

Fischer, U.A., Carle, R., and Kammerer, D.R. (2011). Identification and quantification of phenolic compounds from pomegranate (*Punica granatum* L.) peel, mesocarp, aril and differently produced juices by HPLC-DAD-ESI/MSn. *Food Chem.* 127: 807–821.

Galindo-Tovar, M.E., Ogata-Aguilar, N., and Arzate-Fernández, A.M. (2008). Some aspects of avocado (*Persea americana* Mill.) diversity and domestication in Mesoamerica. *Genet. Resour. Crop. Evol.* 55: 441–450.

Gayosso-García Sancho, L.E., Yahia, E.M., and González-Aguilar, G.A. (2011). Identification and quantification of phenols, carotenoids, and vitamin C from papaya (*Carica papaya* L., cv. Maradol) fruit determined by HPLC-DAD-MS/MS-ESI. *Food Res. Int.* 44: 1284–1291.

Gironés-Vilaplana, A., Valentao, P., Moreno, D.M., Ferreres, F., García-Viguera, C., and Andrade, P.B. (2012). New beverages of lemon juice enriched with the exotic berries maqui, açaí, and blackthorn: Bioactive components and *in vitro* biological properties. *J. Agric. Food Chem.* 60: 6571–6580.

Grace, M.H., Massey, A.R., Mbeunkui, F., Yousef, G.G., and Lila, M.A. (2012). Comparison of health-relevant flavonoids in commonly consumed cranberry products. *J. Food Sci.* 77: H176–H183.

Gross, P. (2010). *Superfruits*. New York: McGraw-Hill.

Hollands, W., Brett, G.M., Radreau, P., Saha, S., Teucher, B., Bennett, R.N., and Kroon, P.A. (2008). Processing blackcurrant dramatically reduces the content and does not enhance the urinary yield of anthocyanins in human subjects. *Food Chem.* 108: 869–878.

Huang, D., Ou, B., and Prior, R.L. (2005). The chemistry behind antioxidant capacity assays. *J. Agric. Food Chem.* 53: 1841–1856.

Hudson, E. (2010a). The antioxidant industry: Where is it all going? *Nutraceutical Bus. Technol.* 6(6): 30–32.

Hudson, E. (2010b). Healthy options still relevant in a depressed economic climate. *Drinks Int.* May: 34–36.

Hummer, K.E. and Barney, D.L. (2002). Crop reports: Currants. *Hort. Technol.* 12: 377–387.

Kagliwal, L.D., Pol, A.S., Patil, S.C., Singhal, R.S., and Patravale, V.B. (2012). Antioxidant-rich extract from dehydrated seabuckthorn berries by supercritical carbon dioxide extraction. *Food Bioproc. Technol.* 5: 2768–2776.

Kaume, L., Howard, L.R., and Devareddy, L. (2012). The blackberry fruit: A review on its composition and chemistry, metabolism and bioavailability, and health benefits. *J. Agric. Food Chem.* 60: 5716–5727.

Kondo, M., Zhang, L., Ji, H., Kou, Y., and Ouj, B. (2009). Bioavailability and antioxidant effects of a xanthone-rich mangosteen (*Garcinia mangostana*) product in humans. *J. Agric. Food Chem.* 57: 8788–8792.

Kris-Etherton, P.N., Hecker, K.D., Bonanome, A., Coval, S.M., Binkoski, A.E., Hilpert, K.F., Griel, A.E., and Etherton, T.D. (2002). Bioactive compounds in foods: Their role in the prevention of cardiovascular disease and cancer. *Am. J. Med.* 113: 71S–88S.

Liu, R.H. (2003). Health benefits of fruit and vegetables are from additive and synergistic combinations of phytochemicals. *Am. J. Clin. Nutr.* 78: 517S–520S.

Liu, Y.Q., Heying, E., and Tanumihardjo, S.A. (2012). History, global distribution, and nutritional importance of citrus fruits. *Compr. Rev. Food Sci. Food Safety* 11: 530–545.

Liu, Y.X., Song, X., Han, Y., Zhou, F., Zhang, D., Ji, B.P., Hu, J.M., et al. (2011). Identification of anthocyanin components of wild Chinese blueberries and amelioration of light-induced retinal damage in pigmented rabbit using whole berries. *J. Agric. Food Chem.* 59: 356–363.

Mackay, D. (2007). Superfruits: Heroes of health. *Nutraceutical Bus. Technol.* Jan/Feb: 28–31.

Medina, M.B. (2011). Determination of the total phenolics in juices and superfruits by a novel chemical method. *J. Funct. Foods* 3: 79–87.

Menezes, C.C., Carneiro, J.D.S., Borges, S.V., da Silva, V.S.N., Brigagao, M.R.P.L., and Azevedo, L. (2012). Development of low-calorie guava preserves with prebiotics and evaluation of their effects on carcinogenesis biomarkers in rats. *Food Chem. Toxicol.* 50: 3719–3724.

Mezadri, T., Villaño, D., Fernández-Pachón, M.S., García-Parrilla, M.C., and Troncoso, A.M. (2008). Antioxidant compounds and antioxidant activity in acerola (*Malpighia emarginata* DC.) fruits and derivatives. *J. Food Compos. Anal.* 21: 282–290.

Miller, M.G. and Shukitt-Hale, B. (2012). Berry fruit enhances beneficial signaling in the brain. *J. Agric. Food Chem.* 60: 5709–5715.

Mishra, K.P., Chanda, S., Karan, D., Ganju, L., and Sawhney, R.C. (2008). Effect of seabuckthorn (*Hippophae rhamnoides*) flavone on immune system: An *in-vitro* approach. *Phytother. Res.* 22: 1490–1495.

Müller, L., Gnoyke, S., Popken, A.M., and Böhm, V. (2010). Research note: Antioxidant capacity and related parameters of different fruit formulations. *LWT—Food Sci. Technol.* 43: 992–999.

Muñoz-Acuña, U., Dastmalchi, K., Basile, M.J., and Kennelly, E.J. (2012). Edible quantitative high-performance liquid chromatography photo-diode array (HPLC-PDA) analysis of benzophenones and biflavonoids in eight *Garcinia* species. *J. Agric. Food Chem.* 59: 3020–3026.

Nikolic, M., Nikic, D., and Petrovic, B. (2008). Fruit and vegetable intake and the risk for developing coronary heart disease. *Cent. Eur. J. Public Health* 16: 17–20.

Noratto, G.D., Bertoldi, M.C., Krenek, K., Talcott, S.T., Stringheta, P.C., and Mertens-Talcott, S.U. (2010). Anticarcinogenic effects of polyphenolics from mango (*Mangifera indica*) varieties. *J. Agric. Food Chem.* 58: 4104–4112.

Park, Y.S., Im, M.H., Ham, K.S., Kang, S.G., Park, Y.K., Namiesnik, J., Leontowicz, H., Leontowicz, M., Katrich, E., and Gorinstein, S. (2013). Nutritional and pharmaceutical properties of bioactive compounds in organic and conventional growing kiwifruit plant. *Foods Hum. Nutr.* 68: 57–64.

Portella, R.D., Barcelos, R.P., da Rosa, E.J.F., Ribeiro, F.F., da Cruz, I.B.M., Suleiman, L., and Soares, F.A.A. (2013). Guaraná (*Paullinia cupana* Kunth) effects on LDL oxidation in elderly people: An *in vitro* and *in vivo* study. *Lipids Health Dis.* 12: 1–9.

Prior, R.L., Wu, X., and Schaisch, K. (2005). Standardized methods for the determination of antioxidant capacity and phenolics in foods and dietary supplements. *J. Agric. Food Chem.* 53: 4290–4302.

Roopchand, D.E., Kuhn, P., Poulev, A., Oren, A., Lila, M.A., Fridlender, B., and Raskin, I. (2012). Biochemical analysis and in vivo hypoglycemic activity of a grape polyphenol–soybean flour complex. *J. Agric. Food Chem.* 60: 8860–8865.

Rosenblat, M., Volkova, N., Attias, J., Mahamid, R., and Aviram, M. (2010). Consumption of polyphenolic-rich beverages (mostly pomegranate and black currant juices) by healthy subjects for a short term increased serum antioxidant status, and the serum's ability to attenuate macrophage cholesterol accumulation. *Food Funct.* 1(1): 99–109.

Rufino, M.S.M., Alves, R.E., Brito, E.S., Pérez-Jiménez, J., Saura-Calixto, F., and Mancini-Filho, J. (2010). Bioactive compounds and antioxidant capacities of 18 non-traditional tropical fruits from Brazil. *Food Chem.* 121: 996–1002.

Rufino, M.S.M., Pérez-Jiménez, J., Arranz, S., Alves, R.E., Brito, E.S., Oliveira, M.S.P., and Saura-Calixto, F. (2011). Açaí (*Euterpe oleraceae*) 'BRS Pará': A tropical fruit source of antioxidant dietary fiber and high antioxidant capacity oil. *Food Res. Int.* 44: 2100–2106.

Smith, N. and Atroch, A.L. (2010). Guarana's journey from regional tonic to aphrodisiac and global energy drink. *Evid. Based Complement. Alternat. Med.* 7: 279–282.

Sun-Waterhouse, D., Chen, J., Chuah, C., Wibisono, R., Melton, L.D., Laing, W., Ferguson, L.R., and Skinner, M.A. (2009). Kiwifruit-based polyphenols and related antioxidants for functional foods: Kiwifruit extract-enhanced gluten-free bread. *Int. J. Food Sci. Nutr.* 60: 251–264.

Tenore, G.C., Manfra, M., Stiuso, P., Coppola, L., Russo, M.T., Gomez-Monterrey, I.M., and Campiglia, P. (2012). Antioxidant profile and *in vitro* cardiac radical-scavenging versus pro-oxidant effects of commercial red grape juices (*Vitis vinifera* L. cv. Aglianico N.). *J. Agric. Food Chem.* 60: 9680–9687.

Tomás-Barberán, F.A. and Andrés-Lacueva, C. (2012). Polyphenols and health: Current state and progress. *J. Agric. Food Chem.* 60: 8773–8775.

Törrönen, R., McDougall, G.J., Dobson, G., Stewart, D., Hellström, J., Mattila, P., Pihlava, J.M., Koskela, A., and Karjalainen, R. (2012). Fortification of blackcurrant juice with crowberry: Impact on polyphenol composition, urinary phenolic metabolites, and postprandial glycemic response in healthy subjects. *J. Funct. Foods* 4: 746–756.

Ulloa, J.A., Ulloa, P.R., Ramírez-Ramírez, J.C., and Ulloa-Rangel, B.E. (2012). El noni: Propiedades, usos y aplicaciones potenciales. *Revista Fuente* 10(3): 44–49.

Vallejo, F., Marín, J.G., and Tomás-Barberán, F.A. (2012). Phenolic compound content of fresh and dried figs (*Ficus carica* L.). *Food Chem.* 130: 485–492.

Vázquez-Araújo, L., Chambers IV, E., Adhikari, K., and Carbonell-Barrachina, A.A. (2010). Sensory and physicochemical characterization of juices made with pomegranate and blueberries, blackberries, or raspberries. *J. Food Sci.* 75: S398–S404.

Verbeyst, L., Hendrickx, M., and Van Loey, A. (2012). Characterisation and screening of the process stability of bioactive compounds in red fruit paste and red fruit juice. *Eur. Food Res. Technol.* 234: 593–605.

Willis, H.J., Thomas, W., Willis, D.J., and Slavin, J.L. (2011). Feasibility of measuring gastric emptying time, with a wireless motility device, after subjects consume fiber-matched liquid and solid breakfasts. *Appetite* 57: 38–44.

World Cancer Research Fund/American Institute for Cancer Research (2007). *Food, Nutrition, Physical Activity, and the Prevention of Cancer: A Global Perspective*. Washington, DC: AICR.

Yasir, M., Das, S., and Kharya, M.D. (2010). The phytochemical and pharmacological profile of *Persea americana* Mill. *Pharmacogn. Rev.* 4(7): 77–84.

4 Recovery and Use of By-Products from Fruit Juice Production

*Nuria Martí, José Lorente, Manuel Valero,
Albert Ibarz, and Domingo Saura*

CONTENTS

4.1 Introduction 41
4.2 Citrus Industry 43
    4.2.1 Pectin 43
        4.2.1.1 Industrial Production of Pectin 44
    4.2.2 Fruit Fiber from the Citrus Industry 47
        4.2.2.1 Industrial Production of Fiber from Oranges and Lemons.... 48
        4.2.2.2 Industrial Fiber from Tangerines 52
    4.2.3 Industrial Citrus Pulp Production 52
    4.2.4 Citrus Essential Oil Recovery: New Approach 57
        4.2.4.1 Comparison of Extraction Systems with
                One and Two Centrifuges 57
    4.2.5 Other By-Products from the Citrus Industry 60
        4.2.5.1 Limonene 60
        4.2.5.2 Bioethanol from Citrus By-Products 62
4.3 By-Products from the Grape Juice Industry and Wineries 63
    4.3.1 Grape Skin 63
    4.3.2 Grape Seed 65
    4.3.3 Lees 66
    4.3.4 Stalks 66
References 67

4.1 INTRODUCTION

In the Health section of the *New York Times* (Rabin, 2012), the case of a patient with a slowing heart rate and falling blood pressure was described. Blood tests showed she had an amount of medication in her system five times the safe level, but it was not due to a drug overdose; she had overdosed on grapefruit juice.

This is an example of the fact that certain substances in fruits and juices can have powerful physiological effects. In fact, that interaction was first described by

Bailey et al. (1991), a Canadian researcher, two decades ago. Recently, he released an updated list of more than 85 drugs and medications affected by grapefruit (Bailey, 2010; Bailey et al., 2012).

Since then, several cases have followed, describing interactions of drugs with different substances (Bailey et al., 1994; Mazi-Kotwal and Seshadri, 2013) found not only in citrus fruits, but also in fruits and vegetables in general (Bailey and Dresser, 2004; Bailey, 2010), showing certain biochemical mechanisms of interaction at membrane transporter involved in intestinal tissue (Li et al., 2010; Li et al., 2012; Li and Paxton, 2013).

For years, these substances have been the basis of the pharmaceutical industry, but now we are discovering to what degree their levels in our diet are also an influence. In addition, our focus on the physiological importance of this type of substance, called nutraceuticals, is increasing as progress is made in scientific research (Mazza, 1998; Bidlack et al., 2000; Gibson and Williams, 2003; Johnson and Williamson, 2003; Watson, 2003; Wildman, 2007; Gilbert and Şenyuva, 2008).

In this sense, the findings of Barker (1999; Godfrey and Barker, 2000, Alastalo et al., 2013), which relate various aspects of child nutrition, including that of infants, and fetal nutrition, and their impact on later health as adults, lead to relevant conclusions from nutritional and human health points of view. Apparently, the diet of the pregnant mother, and diet in infancy and early childhood, not only in terms of calories but also the proportion of food eaten as fruits and vegetables (Pesonen et al., 2010; Perälä et al., 2012; Barker, 2012; Eriksson et al., 2013), determine the future adult's ability to maintain homeostatic balance and affect future cardiovascular health (Roseboom et al., 1999; Raghupathy et al., 2010; Barker et al., 2010a, 2012; Eriksson et al., 2011; Perälä et al., 2011), incidence of diabetes (Barker, 1999; Kajantie et al., 2010), obesity (Ravelli et al., 1999) and metabolic syndrome (Sachdev et al., 2009), bone stability (Javaid et al., 2011), and the occurrence of lung cancer (Eriksson et al., 2010; Barker et al., 2010b) and Hodgkin's lymphoma (Barker et al., 2013; Barker et al., 2013).

In this chapter we consider the presence of these substances in the waste of the fruit juice industry and the opportunity to obtain and purify these substances as new products, thus adding value to what has traditionally been considered as troublesome.

One of the challenges of the modern food industry is to exploit the waste generated by food production, thus reducing environmental impact and increasing profit margins in fruit juice companies, which need more than ever to leverage all possible resources that technology allows. Another challenge is to provide a stable and reliable source of nutraceuticals that increase the health and welfare of the general population. Use of the by-products off the juice industry is one of the best methods to overcome these two challenges simultaneously.

On the other hand, increasing the nutritional quality of processed food is fundamental to the challenge of global warming, which will reduce crops, resulting in a shortage of available food. Food processing and preservation technology can help to mitigate this problem.

The development of technologies that can extract these compounds from by-products and purify them, thus achieving a nonpolluting global purification process, lower energy costs and greater profitability, represents a fundamental human technological development. In this chapter we will detail our experience in this area as technicians and scientists in the food industry over the years, mainly in the citrus and grape juice industries.

4.2 CITRUS INDUSTRY

Thousands of published works document the importance of citrus fruits from nutritional and economic points of view. Traditional methods of manufacture in the citrus juice industry continue today, with interdigital cups technology being the most widely used process. However, the most common by-products of this industry (Figure 4.1), essential oils (EOs) and cattle feed, although the most important, are complemented by a broader range of products that are becoming more important (Baker, 1999, 2004). Very active specific technology for the extraction and purification of commercially interesting substances from the industry's waste are also beginning to be developed. A discussion of these technologies for each product follows.

4.2.1 PECTIN

Polysaccharides have provided an almost limitless source of products for a wide range of applications. Most natural carbohydrates are polysaccharides or oligosaccharides. They contain a great variety of molecular structures—and reveal a wide variety of chemical and biochemical properties. They are easily modified by chemical or biochemical processes, and these processes are used commercially to improve their properties and enhance their usefulness.

Many studies have looked at the structural characteristics of pectin and further studies continue today. Some of the best studies are Kertesz (1951), O'Neill et al. (1990), May (1992) and Viser and Voragen (1996).

Commercial pectin varies in many of its characteristics: its gel strength is typically 150 SAG, its gel temperature is widely variable but typically between 35°C and 45°C, and its gel time may vary from slow to rapid set with middling graduations. The pH of a solution of 1% pectin in deionized water may vary between 2.9 and 3.4

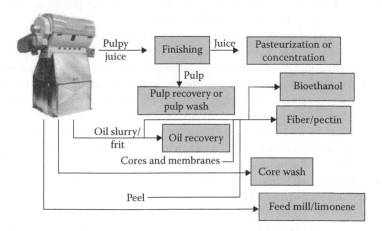

FIGURE 4.1 Products from citrus juice extractor.

for high-methoxyl pectin and 4.0–5.0 for low-methoxyl pectin. These properties are typically specified in commercial pectin (Transformación de Aditivos, 1998). Other characteristics include grade of esterification—high (69%–75% DE) and low (29%– 34%), with medium-grade DE pectin also available; and grade of amidation—only specified for low-methoxyl pectin obtained by NH_3 treatment and typically 16%– 20% soluble at 4% in deionized water at 60°C, with adequate agitation, particle size, calcium reactivity, dry loss, insoluble acid ash, color, and smell.

Europe is one of the main consumers of pectin (600 t/year), but consumption is climbing rapidly in Asian nations (300 t/year). Supplies are covered by major producers such as Copenhagen Pectin, Danisco Pectin México, Sanofi Bio-Industries, and Cargill.

Unlike other polysaccharide industries, no crops are specifically developed for obtaining pectin. Similarly to gelatin (a protein), pectin is basically produced from subproducts and these depend on previous operations in the juice industry (May, 1994).

4.2.1.1 Industrial Production of Pectin

In the 1920s and 1930s, various companies began to profit from the residues of the fruit juice and cider industries. In the beginning, these companies produced an extract of concentrated pectin that they subsequently stored in barrels with chemical preservatives. This practice continues today, although transport costs are a strongly limiting factor (May, 1990). Those producers using citrus peels quickly discovered that their pectin concentrate could not be used in most applications because of its very disagreeable smell. For this reason, they produced solid pectin manufactured by precipitation with alcohol or salts. The current situation in the industry is a result of this evolution toward the production of powdered pectin. In recent years, American producers of pectin from apples have suffered higher costs than producers of pectin from citrus fruit. The result has been that producers of pectin from citrus fruit dominate the market (The Copenhagen Pectin Factory, 1998). In addition, recent economic factors, such as an increase in environmental restrictions and costs, have led to an abandonment of production by the major American producers and severe reductions in output by European producers (May, 1990).

The current global structure of the business and production reflects a combination of these factors. European companies, which started producing pectin from apples, have subsequently switched to importing dried citrus peel from around the world and have thus eliminated many of the environmental costs of water consumption and effluent treatment (D'Amico, 2005). This situation has occurred against a background of strong growth in demand for pectin, and this has resulted in the opening of many factories associated with the major American and European producers. These factories either take advantage of the phenomena of delocalization to operate in citrus-producing regions with less environmental pressure, or encourage the development of extraction processes from residues produced by processing other vegetable products (El-Nawawi et al., 1995a,b; Norsker et al., 2000; Berardini et al., 2005; Rouilly et al., 2006; Alemzadeh, 2010; Liang et al., 2012).

Currently, a fundamental factor in the design of pectin factories is the process of washing and the treatment of the citrus peel prior to drying, as well as the drying process itself (Johnston, 2002). These processes, together with the processes of coagulation and purification, constitute the critical points in the production process from the environmental point of view—and this project is aimed at contributing to the resolution of this problem.

Citrus peel is a good example of an agricultural subproduct that is very common and insufficiently valued. For example, the Spanish citrus juice industry produces an average of 400,000 t of residue—mostly peel. This volume of material is highly polluting and is frequently sold as a low-value subproduct; and these residues pose an added problem when locating a factory of this type. For these reasons, it is worthwhile to reduce the environmental risks by using industrial processes that create fewer residues and, above all, more useable subproducts. The citrus processing industry has a considerable environmental impact: nearly 28% of the fruit weight is discarded as peel—without adding other parts of the fruit such as the core, heart, and peel shavings or frit (Marti, 2004). There are currently several products that can be profitably extracted from these residues: chippings, pellets, and bioalcohol, with several specific applications (Kimball, 1999). Nevertheless, transformation technologies must be selected while taking into consideration the use of existing equipment and other complementary technologies that are harmless to the environment. Lemon and lime are the best citrus fruits for producing pectin (Rouse and Crandall, 1976, 1979; Crandall et al., 1978a,b; Ros et al., 1995; Piñera et al., 1996).

The traditional production process is shown in Figure 4.2. The references describe several techniques that specify the production stages according to the various technologies used such as centrifuges and centrifugal decanters as exclusive separation

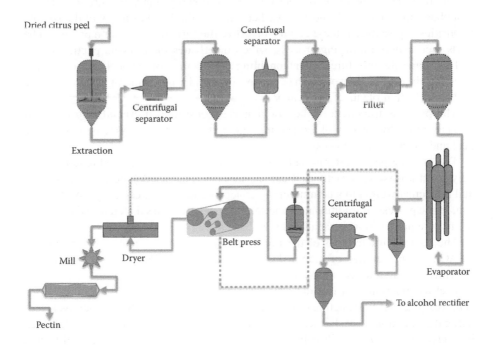

FIGURE 4.2   Flow chart for the industrial production of citrus pectin.

procedures (Wesfalia Separator, 1996) and various alternative continuous treatments (Kertesz, 1951; May, 1990, 1992; Chakravarty, 1997). Processes can be grouped together in stages that are common to all the production techniques (Transformación de Aditivos, 1998) and are shown in Figure 4.2.

There are many patents describing new techniques for industrially processing pectin and its application in foodstuffs, cosmetics, and pharmaceuticals. Techniques that reduce the environmental impact include the following: Buchholt and Vinter (1991) developed a process that diminishes the peel prewash, in a similar way to a proposal by Lobanok et al. (1993) that used enzymes and a slightly acidic treatment to reduce the volume of water needed in the extraction process. Suprunchuck et al. (1991) reduced the volume of acid used in the extraction; and Ehrlich (1997) reached the point of being able to extract pectin without using acid. Christensen (2003) used a prewash treatment of the peel with an acidic solution to deactivate degradative enzymes and so reduce the volume of water required. Campillo et al. (1995) started with humid peel and used a light wash treatment to obtain pectin with a strong gel factor. Golubev (2004) proposed obtaining pectin using a process of ultrasonic cavitation. Karpovich et al. (1989) reduced the volume of alcohol used in the extraction; and Ezhov et al. (1993) described a process to obtain pectin without residues in de-esterification.

Various techniques have been proposed for the extraction of pectin. The use of microwaves increases the extraction and reduces the time (Wang et al., 2007). A system of cultivating vegetable cells to produce high-molecular-weight pectin has also been proposed (Kato, 2005).

The industrial production of pectin has the following stages (Figure 4.2). In the first phase, the citrus peels must be washed fully to eliminate as many of the soluble impurities as possible, as these could jeopardize the further purification process. The peels then undergo a drying process, which inactivates the enzyme pectinesterase and decreases the moisture content, enabling stabilization of the peel for storage and reducing the cost of transport. These stages are usually performed in facilities close to the production plants of citrus juices.

The previous treatment of the raw material constitutes a crucial step that will strongly affect the quality of the pectin, both by the residual enzyme activity in the peel and by the drying process.

The enzyme pectin esterase (PE) is very active in citrus peel, and together with polygalacturonase (PG) activity it can degrade the pectin's degree of esterification and molecular weight to a commercially unacceptable gelling capacity. For this reason, in the process of traditional extraction, the peel must be subjected to the process of enzyme inactivation as rapidly as possible.

The basic characteristics of the raw material are the anticipated gelling ability (°SAG), the percentage of monogalacturonic acid (min. 65%), and the degree of esterification (a value as high as possible).

Pectin extraction is carried out at high temperature and in an acid medium, which achieves practical liquefaction of the totality of the citrus peel. Subsequently, a centrifugal separation is performed that obtains a very fluid and turbid liquid, which is filtered to obtain a clarified liquid that is concentrated. Ethanol is added to this concentrate, causing flocculation of pectin. Then, in a new separation process, the floc is pressed in a belt press, obtaining the pectin soaked in ethanol. This consistent material is subjected to drying, milling and refining, leaving a white powder that is commercial pectin.

This scheme of production has the following drawbacks: (a) the need for intense treatment of the raw material that involves the generation of a great amount of polluting waste, (b) a process of extraction in an acid medium at high temperature, and (c) a purification stage in alcohol that incurs expensive installation and production costs and also generates a large amount of polluting waste.

Therefore, alternative procedures are needed to stabilize the citrus peels without drying, using other extraction processes such as cavitation or ultrasound to soften above the processing temperature and pH at this stage; and to purify and dry the peel, leading to a white powder of commercially viable pectin, without flocculation in ethanol. Future developments in the industrial production of pectin will have these objectives.

4.2.2   Fruit Fiber from the Citrus Industry

Dietary fiber has been known for over 2000 years in different forms (bran, fodder, etc.). However, the term "fiber" first appeared in 1953, referring to hemicellulose, cellulose, and lignin.

Dietary fiber is defined by the Association of Official Analytical Chemists (AOAC, 2000) as the polysaccharides and plant waste materials that are resistant to hydrolysis (digestion) by human digestive enzymes. They lack caloric value, as they cannot be metabolized or absorbed. This is why they do not provide energy. In this way, dietary fiber is seen as a natural component of food without other criteria (Cho et al., 1997).

The fibers traditionally used in food technology come from cereals. However, fibers from vegetables and fruits, although less studied, are generally considered to have greater nutritional and technological qualities. Recently, studies of extraction and composition of fibers of diverse origins have been conducted.

In the case of dietary fibers from fruits, they are gaining greater importance than those of cereals because they present a more balanced ratio of soluble dietary fiber to total dietary fiber (TDF), and therefore better fulfill consumer health recommendations (Borroto et al., 1995).

The TDF content of a food varies depending on the characteristics of the plant: where it is obtained, origin, variety, harvest, time to maturity, growth conditions, crop irrigation, and so on. Food fiber content is also affected by the method of extraction. In general, most fruits and vegetables have values between 1% and 2.2% of TDF, vegetables have intermediate values of approximately 4% of TDF, and grains have widely diverging values: between 1% and 2.2% of TDF for corn kernels and between 15% and 15.8% for bran.

The dietary fiber content of food is also heavily influenced by the moisture content. Thus, the TDF values of cereals are high because in this type of food the moisture content is low, having a maximum of about 10%, whereas fruits and vegetables contain 80%–90% moisture. The values normally are given in percentage of food weight (Mongeau et al., 2001).

Dietary fiber intake in developed countries is deficient, and several studies on dietary guidelines recommend an increase in consumption of fiber-rich products such as fruits and vegetables (Gibney, 2000; Akoh, 1998; Thebaudin et al., 1997; Kaefersein and Clugston, 1995; Johnson and Southgate, 1994; Iyengar and Gross, 1991). In this sense, the fiber obtained from citrus peel constitutes a valuable alternative to the fiber from cereals.

4.2.2.1   Industrial Production of Fiber from Oranges and Lemons

The process of obtaining dietary fiber from citrus peel is described in Figure 4.3. The premix of core, peel, and frit is homogenized and then crushed. Water is added to this homogeneous mixture in a proportion varying from 1:3 to 1:10; it is then subjected to chemical and enzymatic treatment at a controlled temperature, which will determine the final characteristics of the fiber obtained. Then the treated mass is dried in a rotary dryer, the resulting sheets being fragmented into dry flakes. These flakes are milled and the resulting powder is sieved to the required mean particle size (MPS).

The type of fiber obtained depends on the source of fiber, the phase of treatment with water and the MPS. It is clear that the method used determines the quality of the dietary fiber. A procedure with less heat gives fiber without degradation, with good water-holding capacity (WHC; expressed in grams of water held by fiber per gram of fiber), balanced oil-holding capacity (OHC; expressed similar to WHC but with oil), the appropriate color, and higher productivity.

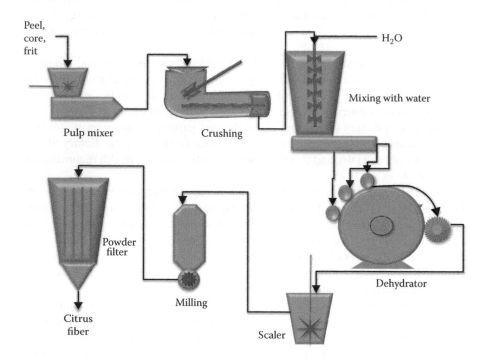

FIGURE 4.3   Flow chart of citrus fiber production.

Fiber holds water by adsorption and absorption and some is outside the fiber matrix (free water). Of course, MPS, chemical composition, and structure of dietary fiber influence the WHC. In spite of that, the *in vitro* WHC cannot be used to predict the impact of highly fermentable fiber on colonic function. Although fiber from lettuce and various other foods (0.3–1.3 g), wheat bran fiber (4.5 g), and carrot fiber (2.1 g) retains much water, from our experience the WHC has been found to be higher for citrus fiber.

WHC values between 0.8 and 1.18 g are obtained with fiber obtained from the core of Valencia Late variety oranges from Murcia (Spain). When the origin of the variety of orange is a more arid area, this value reaches 6.96 g. In the case of oranges of the variety Lane's Late Navel from Murcia (Spain), WHC values are greater than those of Valencia Late oranges of the same origin, varying between 0.5 and 4.4 g. The values for Fino variety lemons from Murcia (Spain) are higher and reach 5.5–7.1 g.

When the fiber is obtained from the frit, which comes from the small remainder of peels that accompanies the EO emulsion, WHC values are higher than those obtained for the core. Higher values occur in fiber from Lane's Late Navel from Murcia (Spain), between 7.50 and 9.05 g. Valencia Late oranges of the same origin have lower values: 6.00–8.70 g. When this variety comes from Almeria (Spain), the values are in the range of 5.70–7.40 g. Fiber from frit of lemon (Fino var.) obtained values ranging from 7.6 to 7.9 g.

Fiber with better WHC is obtained from the peel. The fiber from lemon (Fino var.) has very high values, between 10.62 and 6.5 g. Values for Lane's Late Navel oranges vary between 10.5 and 7.5 g and those for Valencia Late are between 7.4 and 7.6 g. For this same variety but from Almeria (Spain), values are between 8.7 and 7.3 g.

This shows that the best source of dietary fiber with good WHC is the peel of Lane's Late Navel variety oranges and Fino variety lemons. This could be a result of the method used to obtain the fiber and may relate to the mechanical effect of breaking the fibrous particles and the disintegration of globular particles. These give the fiber a specific structure, which is a key factor in the interaction of soluble and insoluble components with water, both of which contribute to the degree of viscosity, which is discussed below.

On the other hand, WHC values of 2.26 g (Figuerola et al., 2005), 9.20 g (Griguelmo and Belloso, 1999), and 12.4 g fiber (Larrauri et al., 1995) have been found for fiber from oranges and lemons. Others report values of WHC in fiber from peel of citrus fruits ranging between 15.5 and 16.7 g (Chau and Huang, 2003).

Apparently, the WHC of fiber from bran in ready-to-eat breakfast cereals is directly related to its MPS: the WHC of smaller wheat bran fibers was 59% of those with larger MPS. In fact, a great portion of the water held by this type of fiber appears to be free water. This is important from a physiological point of view because the WHC has an important effect on stool hardness and fecal output, and is an important factor that contributes significantly to laxative effects (Monro, 2000, 2002).

In fact, the desired WHC can be achieved by mixing citrus fibers with different MPS and choosing both the source of the raw material and the treatment as appropriate.

All this behavior is related to the fact that it is possible to separate TDF into soluble and insoluble components based on solubility in water. The problem is the quantification of the amount of soluble fiber. This is because the conditions differ among laboratories. Moreover, the differentiation between soluble and insoluble fibers is difficult to correlate and does little to predict the actual fiber solubility in the gastrointestinal tract.

Some years ago, it was generally accepted that soluble fiber was not commonly found in foods, even in those with a higher fiber content. But when studies describing guar gum, pectin, and fiber in legumes and oat bran in the 1960s lead to current estimates that about one-third of the daily TDF intake is soluble fiber. Pectic substances are the major soluble dietary fiber components of fruits, but the exact composition changes according to the fruit and variety. It is clear that when measuring dietary fiber, one must also take into account the method of fiber preparation because, as mentioned above, the soluble fiber content of a fiber source is influenced by the method of preparation. In fact, some pectic substances are susceptible to depolymerization at the high temperatures used to obtain some fibers. And similarly, some insoluble fibers are depolymerized at higher temperatures and then could be found in the soluble fiber fraction.

According to the results of the investigation with different procedures to obtain pectin from citrus wastes (Bailen et al., 2011), dietary fibers can be divided into two groups. In the first group, the content of insoluble pectin fraction is approximately equal to fruit's content of insoluble pectin fraction and in the second group, it is significantly lower. The citrus fibers obtained with low-temperature technology corresponded to the first group, having a relatively high content of insoluble pectin fraction. In our work, the content of insoluble pectin fraction in the dietary fibers was studied and compared with the content of water-soluble pectin fraction. The citrus fiber samples obtained by high-temperature technology correspond to the second group. The selected samples contain 18.3%–37.1% of the water-soluble pectin fraction and 10.7%–23.1% of the insoluble pectin fraction.

Regarding the OHC, the results show that in the fiber obtained from the core of Valencia Late oranges from Almeria (Spain), the values are between 0.9 and 1.3 g, while for the same variety from Murcia (Spain), values are lower: 0.8–1.1 g. In the other variety of orange studied, Lane's Late Navel, the fiber has a significantly higher OHC, which varies between 1.2 and 1.7 g. The lemon values are the highest among those studied, between 1.4 and 2.2 g. The OHC values of fiber from the frit are higher in general terms: for Almeria Valencia Late values vary between 1.4 and 1.1 g, greater than for fiber from the core. When evaluating the fiber for the some orange variety but from the other geographical origin studied, Murcia, the values are lower, between 1.2 and 0.7 g, but larger than those for fiber from the core of oranges of the same origin. For the fiber of Lane's Late Navel variety oranges, the OHC value is greater than that of Valencia Late oranges of the same origin, 0.7–1.4 g. For lemons, OHC values vary between 1.1 and 1.5 g, lower than those for the core.

OHC values for lemon peel fiber are lower than those of fiber from the other fractions, between 1.3 and 0.9 g, while orange peel fiber (var. Valencia Late) are have greater OHC values than other fractions of the fruit. As usual, those from Almeria have greater OHC values (1.56–1.00 g) than those from Murcia (1.39–0.69 g). In the case of fiber from Lane's Late Navel oranges, OHC values are higher than those of frit but lower than those of core (1.50–0.60 g).

It is important to highlight the case of the fiber from Valencia Late oranges from Murcia. In this case, we obtained the lowest values for OHC, 0.98 g for the core,

TABLE 4.1

Viscosity of Citrus Fiber at 5% Depending on Fruit Fraction and Variety

Citrus Variety	Fraction of Fruit	Fiber Viscosity (mPa·s)
Orange Valencia Late (Almeria)	Core	10.7–13.7
	Frit	14.0–28.4
	Peel	31.0–38.0
Orange Valencia Late (Murcia)	Core	6.5–9.6
	Frit	15.3–9.0
	Peel	14.3–14.8
Orange Lane's Late Navel	Core	63.7–12.7
	Frit	20.7–14.6
	Peel	70.7–14.7
Lemon Fino	Core	31.6–21.3
	Frit	95.3–13.2
	Peel	107.7–91.3

0.82 g for the frit, and 0.85 g for the peel. These values are low for a fiber for dairy, but make it suitable for use in meat products.

Table 4.1 shows the viscosity of various citrus fiber fractions according to the fruit used and the variety. As shown, the fiber suspension in the case of lemon peel has the highest viscosity values (107.7–91.3 mPa·s for Fino lemon), therefore lemon peel fiber has greater thickening power. This behavior could be due to the higher average molecular size of the soluble and insoluble solids present in the fiber.

This confirms the already-mentioned higher thickening power of lemon fiber but also the greater difficulty in controlling it, since very small variations in the concentration result in significant changes in the viscosity of the suspension.

Meanwhile, the lowest consistency was reached in fiber suspensions of Valencia Late oranges from Murcia and Almeria, with 6.5 mPa s, being the lowest value, in the fiber from the core of Valencia Late oranges from Murcia.

Several authors have pointed out the possibility of using exponential and potential models to describe the relationship between viscosity and concentration (Grigelmo et al., 1999).

The high viscosity that fiber from lemon provides makes it ideal for system stabilization against sedimentation or creaming. However, if the added products will be experiencing high shear rates, orange fiber would be a better option because it allows easy control of the viscosity but at higher added concentrations.

According to our experience (Figure 4.4), the fiber extraction performance is affected by the species, variety, and origin of citrus fruit. Orange peel produces more fiber than lemons. In terms of varieties, the orange variety Valencia Late is more productive than Lane Late Navel. Regarding the origin of the fruits, those from arid regions (Valencia Late of Almeria) have a higher productivity than the same variety from less arid regions (Valencia Late of Murcia).

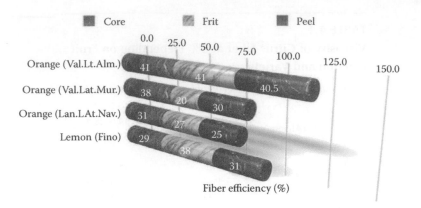

FIGURE 4.4   Fiber efficiency extraction from citrus fruits.

4.2.2.2   Industrial Fiber from Tangerines

The four main tangerine varieties (Oroval, Hernandina, Fortuna, and Clemenville) industrially processed in the Mediterranean region were analyzed for fiber content: crude fiber (CF), neutral detergent fiber (NDF), and acid detergent fiber (ADF), from the by-products (peel, core, and frit) obtained in tangerine processing in pilot plant tests (Martí et al., 2011). In this work, it was possible to correlate the configuration (understood as the adaptation of machinery to the different sizes of fruit) and characteristics of the fiber obtained from the by-products. The variety Hernandina has the highest juice content and therefore has less peel, core, and frit. The Oroval variety has more frit content, twice as much as Hernandina and Clemenville, and three times more than Fortuna (Martí, 2004). With respect to CF results, it is clearly significant that the Oroval variety has a higher content than the other varieties. Regarding the components, core has the lowest fiber content and frit the highest (Figure 4.5).

Figure 4.5 shows that the Oroval variety has higher fiber content (CF, NDF, and ADF) in the peel than in the core. The fiber content of the Hernandina variety was higher in the frit than in the peel, with the lowest content in the core. For fiber from the Fortuna variety, the same results were obtained as for the Oroval variety: CF content was higher in the peel and frit than in the core.

From the data (Figure 4.5) for the edible portion of the tangerine, we can conclude that the content was significantly lower than in the data provided by the U.S. Department of Agriculture (USDA, 2002). Regarding the results obtained, it can be concluded that the Oroval variety has higher CF, NDF, and ADF content. The Clemenville variety presented lower fiber content, with a significant difference. It can be said that the highest CF content was in the peel, not in the core or frit. Also, total fiber content was higher in the frit than in the peel and core. CF content is higher in tangerines than in oranges, but total fiber content is higher in oranges (Martí et al., 2011).

4.2.3   Industrial Citrus Pulp Production

Pulp is the solid edible part of citrus fruit present in juice, including fruit vesicles or their parts, with an irregular shape, that can be separated from the juice by filtration or centrifugation.

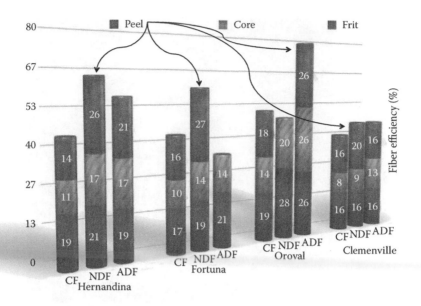

FIGURE 4.5 Fiber efficiency extraction from tangerines. CF, crude fiber; NDF, natural detergent fiber; ADF, acid detergent fiber. (Data from Martí, N., Saura, D., Fuentes, E., Lizama, V., García, E., Mico-Ballester, M.J., and Lorente, J. *Industrial Crops and Products* 33, 94, 2011.)

After the extraction process, juice composed of a liquid and a solid fraction is obtained. The solid fraction includes floating and bottom pulp:

- Floating pulp: in suspension in the juice
- Bottom pulp: recovered in a centrifuge and gives turbidity to the juice

From the point of view of industrial production, the term pulp refers only to floating pulp.

Commercial juice has variable quantity and quality of floating pulp, ranging from 6% to 8% in oranges, 5% to 7% in lemons, and 4% to 6% in tangerines. These values depend on the perforation diameter of the strainer tube of the citrus juices, a JBT in-line extractor or similar (Figure 4.6).

During recent years, there has been growing demand from consumers for natural and fresh juices. This demand will continue to grow in the future. Consumers want healthy products, with characteristics close to those of the raw fruit and a high fiber content.

The pulp quantity of a citrus juice can be regulated after extraction by regulating the hole diameter of the strainer tube and the opening diameter of the finisher screen. Pulp content can also be increased by the addition of supplementary pulp. This supplementary pulp is recovered from pulp that is discarded from the finisher.

The objective of the recovery process is to obtain a high-quality pulp. Commercially, this pulp should have following characteristics:

- Free of defects
- High integrity
- Floatability

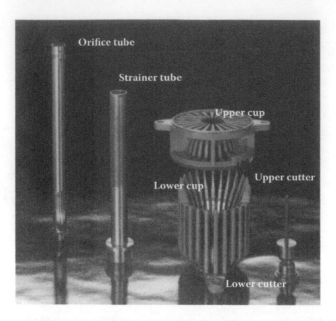

FIGURE 4.6   In-line extractor juicing components.

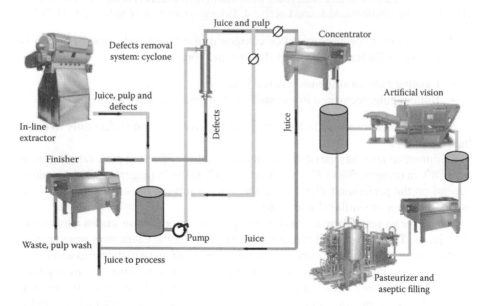

FIGURE 4.7   Flow chart of citrus pulp recovery process.

The process for obtaining pulp uses the standard juice extraction system and introduces some new steps that do not affect the final quality of the juice. Figure 4.7 is a flow chart of the process.

In the extraction step, the in-line extractors should be set with 0.062 or 0.040 in. strainer tubes. If the existence of insect larvae is suspected, 0.040 in. strainer tubes are needed. The change from 0.040 to 0.062 in. increases the pulp yield by about 1%–2% with respect to the total weight of fruit, and the cells are bigger and have better floatability properties.

Related transport systems and pumps should be fed using a Mono pump due to the density and consistency of the fluid that carries the pulp. Mono pumps are recommended in order to reduce the impact of the impulsion on the integrity of the pulp.

The juice with pulp and defects is then passed through a cyclone. The use of cyclones decreases the total defects. Figure 4.8 shows the relationship between flow rate (which must be constant), apex size, and percentage of defect removal. Table 4.2 shows the operational standards of the different types of apex.

Figure 4.9 shows the changing output flow rate of the cyclone as pressure increases by reducing the apex diameter and increasing the time of residence in the interior of the cyclone. It is clear that the flow rate increases as the residence time decreases and pressure increases (Figure 4.9).

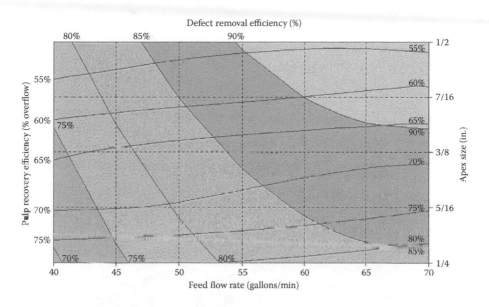

FIGURE 4.8   Cyclone efficiency chart.

TABLE 4.2

Standards of Cyclone Apex

Apex Type	Diameter (mm)	Theoretical Discharge (%)
A	5.6	
B	6.4	
C	9.55	20–80
D	11.2	30–70
E (free output)	12.7	50–50

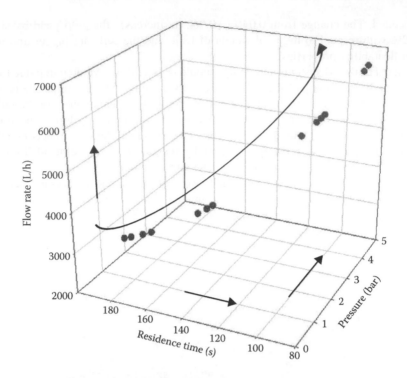

FIGURE 4.9   Cyclone flow rate versus residence time and pressure.

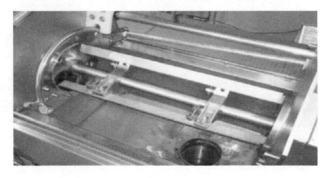

FIGURE 4.10   Inside view of JBT paddle finisher.

Cyclone outflow is then passed through a finisher to adjust the homogeneity and level of pulp. There are different types of finishers, but the one most indicated for pulp recovery is the paddle model (Figure 4.10). This design was planned to preserve pulp integrity. The optimum operational conditions are a constant flow rate. This continuous flow rate can be achieved by installing a buffer tank. This equipment has pumps with a variable-frequency drive to adjust the concentration of the outlet pulp, which is quantified by "Quick Fiber," an analytical procedure that provides fast determination of pulp humidity.

The screen of the finisher can have different opening diameters, thus influencing the quantity of small cells. This also affects the quantity of bottom pulp in the juice.

Sometimes defects cannot be easily avoided, even with a well-adjusted cyclone and finisher. In this case, an artificial vision system is needed. This equipment is recommended in cases with a high number of black specks. As the black specks have a similar density to the pulpy juice, their separation using a cyclone is difficult, increasing the quantity of pulp lost in the waste flow. Due to the characteristics of this equipment, for it to be effective the inlet pulp flow must have a low density in order to make a thin pulp layer (3 mm max.), so a second finisher is needed to achieve the final pulp concentration.

The next important aspect to consider is the pasteurization of a fluid so dense, viscous, and particulate. The characteristics of this material make the method of pasteurization critical to achieve an appropriate final product. An improper temperature of treatment or maintenance time can easily ruin all previous efforts.

Obviously, to obtain aseptic pulp a sterilization process is needed. There are some pasteurizers on the market able to sterilize citrus pulp properly. They are high pulp density pasteurizers (with pulps of density 850 g/L) that are able to operate up to a pressure of 150 bar. They include expansion joints to reduce the thermal impact and steam barrier flanges to guarantee sterility of the final cooled product. To avoid different temperatures inside the tubes, they are equipped with static mixers, such as dimple tubes, that lead to a high Reynolds number and, thus, turbulent flow inside the tubes.

The thermal treatment can be fixed using data from Figures 4.11. These conditions vary depending on the type of citrus pulp being handled, lemon pulp being softer due to its lower pH (Figures 4.11).

The pasteurization equipment must include a piston pump, which provides a constant pressure to the inlet flow, and it is recommended to make flowing high-density fluids without damaging their integrity.

Once an aseptic product is obtained, its sterility must be maintained to guarantee a commercial sterile product, whether in small (5 L) or large (1000 L) bags. This product can be added aseptically to beverages and juices to leverage its texture (Figure 4.12)

4.2.4 CITRUS ESSENTIAL OIL RECOVERY: NEW APPROACH

The recovery of essential oil (EO) consists of separating, by centrifugation, the aqueous phase (heavy phase) from oil (light phase). Currently, the system most used for this process is the system with two centrifuges in a series, which is explained below. However, Alfa Laval, jointly with JBT FoodTech, has developed a centrifuge capable of separating oil emulsion in one operation.

This emulsion comes mostly from interdigital cup extractors, although a significant proportion may come from a system of peel scrapping of the type of Peel Shaver Brown, Moscato, Speciale, and JBT MORE.

4.2.4.1 Comparison of Extraction Systems with One and Two Centrifuges

4.2.4.1.1 System with Two Centrifuges

Heavy oily suspension (slurry) that comes from a paddle finisher with small screen openings is separated by a centrifugal unit in a desludger disc centrifuge with an operational range from 8,000 to 10,000 rpm into an oil-rich emulsion, an aqueous fraction, and a sludge semisolid. The aqueous fraction is generally filtered and recycled as wash water for the production of more oily suspension in the extractor so as

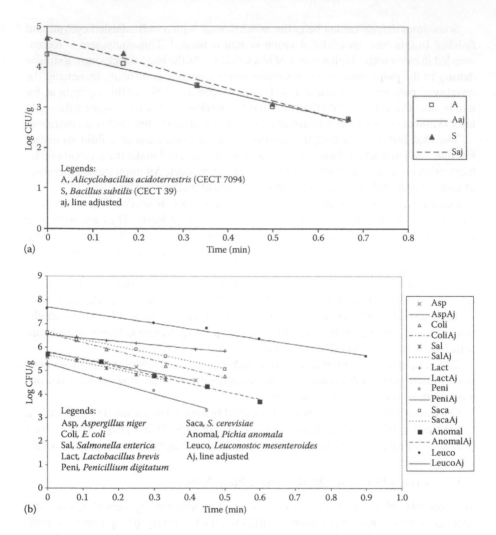

FIGURE 4.11 (a,b) Thermal treatment of citrus pulp for different microorganisms from CECT, Colección Española de Cultivos Tipo, Valencia.

to recover residual amounts of oil that may remain in the water separated from the suspension (Nagy et al., 1977; Kimball, 1999). The sludge is usually discarded and contains about 2%–6% of the oil initially present in the fruit.

The oil-rich emulsion can be subjected to an enzymatic treatment with concentrations and treatment times that depend on the enzyme used, but can be several hours. Then, the emulsion is centrifuged (16,000–18,000 rpm) in a centrifugal separator for polishing oil (polisher centrifuge), separating the emulsion into a heavy phase that is discarded (water) and a light phase consisting of clean citrus EO. The heavy phase contains about 2% of the oil initially present in the fruit and can be recycled to the extractor for increased oil recovery.

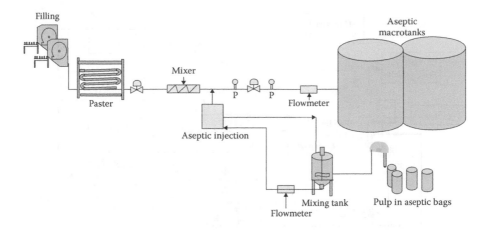

FIGURE 4.12 Flow diagram of industrial production of fruit juices and beverages with added pulp.

Depending on maturity, from 0.2% to 0.5% of whole citrus fruit is EO. Yield of extraction of EO increases with maturity of the fruit. Rain decreases the quantities of oil and because fruit softening makes it difficult to break the EO glands properly, this softening causes a decrease in yield also. Figure 4.13 summarizes the EO process with two centrifuges.

Figure 4.13 shows the EO recovery efficiency of the different equipment in the production line. The combined efficiency of the extractor and the finisher is between 70% and 84% in the best case, resulting in an emulsion with EO richness of about 1% with proper operation of the desludger. The emulsion-enriched output from the desludger should be in the range 70%–95% and the aqueous discharge (heavy phase) in the range 0.1%–0.5%. This phase is returned to the extraction with an addition of 25% fresh water. The efficiency of this centrifuge is between 53% and 86%. The effectiveness of the second centrifuge is very high, at 94%–99%. The heavy discharge is recycled to the tank from the scarifier because despite its low volume, its EO concentration is relatively high (2%–3%).

4.2.4.1.2 System with One Centrifuge

An alternative system that has been designed and developed jointly by JBT FoodTech and Alfa Laval companies and is currently under industrial implementation is a prototype system consisting of the More Oil Recovery Extraction (MORE) scarifier from JBT FoodTech together with the UPVX 507 AGT 14 centrifuge manufactured by Alfa Laval. In one single operation it is capable of separating oil emulsion into clear EO. Thus, there is no need for two centrifuges; a good-quality EO can be produced in one operation, without a polishing centrifuge, thus saving time and money.

Figure 4.14 is a diagram of the system for lemons. Comparison of both schemes shows that there is an appreciable difference in equipment needs. In this system, two tanks are removed, a finisher and a polisher, while a scarifier is introduced. Furthermore, based on lemons, EO recovery performance of MORE should be

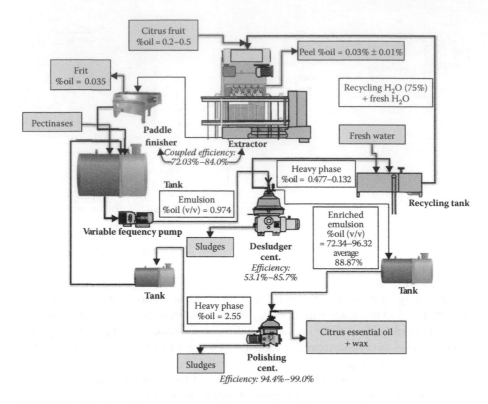

FIGURE 4.13   Flow diagram of citrus EO production with two centrifuges.

between 80% and 92%. Under these conditions, the efficiency of the centrifuge is between 98% and 99%. On the other hand, the introduction of a scarifier represents a decrease of juice extraction yield (Figure 4.15), probably because the extractors are designed to work with fruit of higher consistency and lose effectiveness when fruit is scraped. In fact, the amount of peel, core, and frit obtained during the extraction process is greater with scraped fruit than with intact fruit (Figure 4.15), 60% versus 55%, and consequently, the juice yield has an inverse behavior: 45.17% in intact fruit compared with 40.08% in scraped fruit. This is even more pronounced in tangerines (Figure 4.16), where the consistency of the skin is even lower than in lemons. In fact, EO recovery yields in tangerine are 62.37%, and the difference in juice yield is 52% in intact fruit compared with 37% in scraped fruit.

4.2.5   OTHER BY-PRODUCTS FROM THE CITRUS INDUSTRY

Currently, other by-products of the citrus industry are becoming relevant, such as d-limonene and bioethanol.

4.2.5.1   Limonene

Limonene is a monocyclic monoterpene that is very abundant in nature and has a characteristic odor of citrus and some herbs. Due to a chiral carbon in its structure,

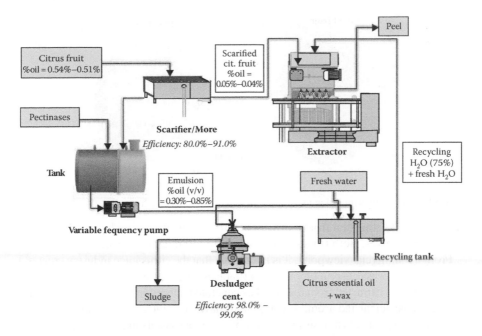

FIGURE 4.14 Flow diagram of citrus EO production with one centrifuge.

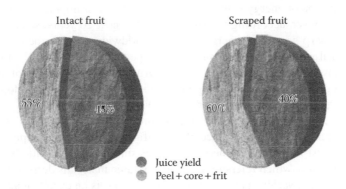

FIGURE 4.15 Lemon juice yield with intact versus scraped fruits.

there are two enantiomers with specific properties and uses. The two enantiomers of limonene are (S)-(–)-limonene, mainly from *Mentha spicata*, and (R)-(+)-limonene, which is the main component (up to 95%) of the EO obtained from citrus fruits (orange, lemon, tangerine, grapefruit) and caraway (*Carum carvi*). It is used as a biodegradable solvent for resins, pigments, inks, and so on, and as an aromatic component in the synthesis of new compounds.

Currently, there are three ways to obtain limonene as a citrus by-product: (a) recovery with a waste heat evaporator from the molasses that comes from the peel-drying process; this is a "technical-grade limonene"; (b) application of steam

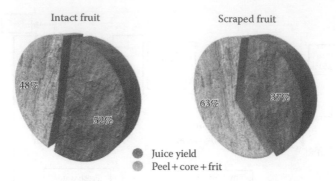

Intact fruit · Scraped fruit

● Juice yield
◐ Peel + core + frit

FIGURE 4.16   Tangerine juice yield with intact versus scraped fruits.

stripping on EO emulsion from extractors, without centrifuges; and (c) distillation of the EOs themselves. Both (b) and (c) produce "food-grade limonene."

From a commercial viewpoint, it is interesting that the citrus juice industry creates a large amount of waste, useful for obtaining limonene. The low cost of enantiopure limonene (€2–€7/kg) extracted from residues has generated interest in the chemical industry. A series of medicinal and aromatic compounds have the same carbon skeleton as limonene, suggesting large synthesis potential. For these reasons, its market is expanding.

4.2.5.2   Bioethanol from Citrus By-Products

Among all the major energy sources, crude oil is the most important for developed countries. Moreover, according to estimates for the next 20 years, scientists project a continued sharp growth in energy demand worldwide through the period 2004–2030, and total world energy consumption is expected to grow by 57%. In addition, burning of fossil fuels contributes to global warming and degradation of air quality, since it is a disadvantage from the point of view of sustainable development and generates health problems in the entire world population.

Environmental concerns, the uncertain future availability of fossil fuels, and the growing awareness of the importance of self-sufficiency of energy supply have led to extensive interest in renewable energy resources since the late twentieth century. In this sense, biomass, which refers to renewable organic materials derived from plants or animals through various natural or human activities, is an excellent alternative to petroleum products.

The significant advantage of the process of converting biomass into biofuel is lower net emission of carbon dioxide. Since the carbon dioxide generated during use of biofuels is recaptured primarily by photosynthesis during the growth of new plants harvested, and that settle a new carbon loop nearly closed with great potential to become possible (Wyman, 1999; Fatsikostas et al., 2002). Although it is a difficult time for the world economy, the reports of the various agencies that are dedicated to the rational and sustainable use of energy suggest that it is now possible to produce enough biofuel to replace 30% of that used for all global transport (Perlack et al., 2005). It would be impossible to reach this objective using cereal-based ethanol alone. In this sense, the use of citrus peel as a source of fermentable biomass for bioethanol is a very interesting option (Choi et al., 2013). Pectin-rich biomass fermentation of these materials is problematic because *Saccharomyces cerevisiae* cannot naturally ferment galacturonic acid or pentose sugars but is the only microorganism that has a homoethanol pathway; and other microorganisms, *Escherichia coli*, *Erwinia chrysanthemi*, and *Klebsiella oxytoca*, can metabolize a diverse array of sugars and are capable of degrading many of the cell wall components of pectin-rich materials, including pectin (Edwards and Doran-Peterson, 2012), but during fermentation they produce side products such as acetic acid that prevent the use of these microorganisms (Grohmann et al., 1996).

Tools and enzymatic pretreatments have been developed that are capable of achieving 80%–90% liquefaction of orange peel bark and resulting in 20°Brix liquids ready to ferment. The problem is that only a small proportion of these are soluble solids that are monosaccharide fermentable by *Saccharomyces*, the remainder being various substances derived from pectin.

4.3 BY-PRODUCTS FROM THE GRAPE JUICE INDUSTRY AND WINERIES

The wine industry contributes substantially to the national economies of many countries. The European Union produces almost 70% of the world's wine and the main European wine-producing countries are Italy, France, and Spain (OIV, 2011). The main by-products generated by the wine-making industry are grape pomace and stalks (10%–20% and 2%–8% of processed material, respectively) (González-Centeno et al., 2010). After extraction in the distilleries of a wide range of products (ethanol, grape seed oil, anthocyanins, and tartrate), the remaining pomace is currently not upgraded but used for composting or discarded in open areas, potentially causing environmental problems (Rondeau et al., 2013).

Grape marc is 20%–25% of the weight of grapes crushed for wine production and its utilization has an important environmental impact by reducing waste and permitting the production of value-added products (Buil et al., 2008; Spigno et al., 2008; Ping et al., 2011a,c; Prozil et al., 2012b). Grape marc has also been evaluated as a source of antioxidants because of its high polyphenol content (Negro et al., 2003; Saura-Calixto, 1998).

There are a lot of nutraceutical ingredients and phytochemical extracts obtained from grapes on the world market, the main ones being seeds, grape skin extracts, and vines. Their qualities include the amount of anthocyanins, expressed in purity on dry weight basis, between 2% and 25%; and the amount of total polyphenols, varying from 20% to 80%.

4.3.1 GRAPE SKIN

Grape (*Vitis vinifera*) skins are used mainly in animal feeds and for obtaining wine alcohol, but due to the high content of phenolic compounds it is widely used for the production of food additives and dietary supplements. They are a good source of flavonols, flavonol glycosides, anthocyanins, phenolic acids, resveratrol (another important polyphenol) (Lafka et al., 2007; Mildner-Szkudlarz et al., 2010), and dietary fiber (Lizarraga et al., 2011).

The phenolic content of grape skin ranges from 285 to 550 mg phenols/kg of raw material, depending on the grape variety and type of industrial processing (Pinelo et al., 2005a). Among this group, anthocyanins are the main interesting compound for recovery. Furthermore, for several years, the anthocyanins have attracted interest from the food, cosmetics, and pharmaceutical industries. The reason for this interest is that these natural compounds can be the perfect substitutes for antioxidants and synthetic dyes currently used in these industries, and they have health benefits (Burns et al., 2000; Hertog, 1993). For example, anthocyanins from grapes and berries are used as food colorants (Shahidi and Naczk, 2004) in food products fortified with plant extracts, which contain polyphenols. These are beverages including water- or tea-based drinks, dairy products such as yoghurt, and special formulations such as "smoothies" (Buchwald-Werner et al., 2009). A significant effort has been made over the past decade to explore the potential of grape pomace to produce functional ingredients. Grape pomace extracts have been granted Generally Recognized As Safe (GRAS) status and can be used as color additives in fruit juice and as antioxidants in flavored beverages (FDA, 2003).

Anthocyanins are probably the most valuable components and many extraction methods have been reported. The aim of an extraction process should be to provide the maximum yield of substances of the highest quality (concentration of target compounds and antioxidant power of the extracts) (Spigno and De Faveri, 2007). Solid–liquid extraction is usually used for extraction of phenolic compounds from grapes, but there are many factors that can influence the extraction efficacy such as extraction method, particle size, solvent type, solvent concentration, solvent-to-solid ratio, extraction temperature, extraction time, and pH (Pinelo et al., 2005a; Spigno et al., 2007). The solid particle size and its primary microstructure are very important aspects for the extraction process. The extraction solvent is often ethanol, methanol, acetone, or formic acid and water in different ratios. Although the solvent extraction offers a high recovery of phenolic compounds from grapes, the use of large amounts of organic solvents poses health and safety risks to researchers, and is unfriendly to the environment. Thus, several methods have been developed to extract phenolic compounds from grape by-products that could eliminate or reduce the use of organic solvents. These methods include microwave-assisted extraction (Hong et al., 2001), ultrasound-assisted extraction (Cárcel et al., 2010), supercritical fluid extraction (Fiori et al., 2009), subcritical water extraction (Ju and Howard, 2005), and even the use of green technologies for degradation of the plant tissue structure like Instant Controlled Pressure Drop or DIC (Detente Instantanee Controle) (treatment of high and low pressure) and flash expansion. This new industrial equipment is based on the application of vacuum and high pressure to increase the performance of extraction. After these processes, it would be recommended to apply different adsorption resins and methods of liquid–liquid extraction in order to purify the anthocyanin concentration in the final extract. High extraction efficiency is necessary for an industrial process to be economically feasible.

Benlloch (2006) compared anthocyanin and total phenol purity for some grape skin extraction methods. Among the tested solvents, methanol and ethanol have different extraction yields, but the solvent used must be based on the price and destination of the final product. Using methanol:water in a 50:50 (v:v) or 60:40 (v:v) proportion for anthocyanin solvent extraction increased the concentration of the resulting extract, comparable to concentrations obtained by Cacace and Mazza

(2003). Formic acid or hydrochloric acid used to acidify the solvent revealed results similar to pH 3.5 and pH 2.5, but eventually resulted in extraction at lower pH due to the increase anthocyanin stability (Giusti et al., 1999; Monagas et al., 2006). Another important factor in any solid–liquid extraction is the reaction time and the quantity of solvent with respect to the initial solid matrix. The optimal extraction time is between 1.5 and 3 h with 10 and 20 times solvent quantity per weight of solid fraction. The extraction yield is 50% higher with the latter.

It is known that plant cells are covered by a cell wall composed mostly of cellulose (Pauly et al., 1999), which makes it more difficult to extract these compounds by conventional techniques such as hydroalcoholic extraction and enzymatic treatments. Because the natural structure of plants offers resistance to penetration by any liquid, the solvent extraction process is very slow. To improve the technological aptitude, intensify solvent extraction, and ensure the expansion of the grain structure, we propose treatment of stem powder with (APIB) high and low pressure. APIB treatment consists of thermomechanical processing induced by subjecting the material to an abrupt transition from high steam pressure to close to a vacuum (Amor and Allaf, 2009). This expansion provokes porous structures in the treated material (Kamal et al., 2008; Kristiawan et al., 2011). Similar to the APIB technique, flash expansion is a technique that allows the destructuring of the tissues, but unlike the previous technique, where the expansion is produced under controlled conditions, in this case, the expansion is drastic and produces total rupture of tissues and cells. Thus, compounds, in our case anthocyanins, located in vacuoles inside the cells are extracted without applying a solvent. In this sense, the process of flash extraction causes a deep degradation of cellular structures. This green technology has been oriented toward increasing the yield of phenolic compound extraction from must in the vinification industry (Moutonet and Escudier, 2000), and recently extraction by means of this technology has been considered interesting for its use in the production of extracts with bioactive substances. (Morel-Salmi et al., 2006).

Although initial investment in these technologies is relatively expensive, their use has increased the concentration of anthocyanins and polyphenols by 15% compared with classical techniques of extraction. Furthermore, the extracts could present added value due to the absence of solvents during the extraction process, a decisive factor in the final quality of the product and its end use in the pharmaceutical, cosmetics, and food industries.

4.3.2 Grape Seed

Grape (*V. vinifera*) seeds can provide oil and a subsequent raw material rich in phenolic compounds. Since grape seeds are usually discarded as part of the wine-making process, the extraction and sale of grape seed oil and grape seed extract can be a profitable sideline (Da Porto et al., 2013). They are rich in extractable phenolic antioxidants such as phenolic acid, flavonoids, procyanidins, and resveratrol, and furthermore, they contain 13%–19% oil, which is rich in essential fatty acids, about 11% protein, 60%–70% nondigestible carbohydrates, and nonphenolic antioxidants such as tocopherols and beta-carotene (Bravi et al., 2007). Some research highlights the nutritional properties of oil extracted from grape seeds. Its peculiar fatty acid composition; unsaturated fatty acid mass fraction: mainly linoleic acid (C18:2)

>70%, oleic acid (C18:1) 17.0%, palmitic acid (C16:0) 6.6%, stearic acid (C18:0) 4.1%, other acids 1.1%; high concentration of polyphenols, and high smoke point (about 190°C–230°C) make it suitable for cooking (Bail et al., 2008). Furthermore, grape seed oil is a preferred cosmetics ingredient. The regenerative and restructuring qualities of grape seed oil are most likely due to its high antioxidant and sterol contents, which may make it an attractive product for direct food consumption and skin care.

Grape seed extract is usually obtained by solid–liquid extraction with different solvents from defatted seeds. The conventional extraction methods of oil and polyphenols from grape seeds have some limitations regarding the high solvent consumption and the long extraction time required. When solid–liquid extraction is assisted by ultrasound, the possible benefits of their application in extraction are an intensification of mass transfer, improved solvent penetration into the plant tissue, and capillary effects. Ultrasound-assisted extraction carried out at 20 kHz, 150 W for 30 min gave grape seed oil yield (14% w/w) similar to Soxhlet extraction for 6 h. Grape seed extracts obtained from seeds defatted by ultrasound and then extracted by maceration had the highest polyphenol concentration (105.20 mg GAE/g flour) and antioxidant activity (109 Eq aToc/g flour) (Da Porto et al., 2013).

Passos et al. (2009) investigated the possibility of using supercritical CO_2 fluid extraction to produce high-quality grape seed oil. Dos Santos Freitas et al. (2008) found that the best solvent for grape seed oil extraction is propane because oil samples extracted with propane present smaller amounts of free fatty acids in the oil than samples extracted with carbon dioxide. However, owing to the high cost of supercritical fluid extraction, commercial grape seed oil is mainly produced by traditional oil extraction methods such as hydraulic cold press and solvent extraction.

The press residues of grape seed oil production are still a rich source of polyphenolics with strong antioxidant activity. Ethyl acetate was reported as one of the best solvents for extraction of polyphenols from grape seeds (it is capable of selectively extracting proanthocyanidins) and water addition up to a certain level (10%) increased proanthocyanidin yield because of increased permeability of grape seeds; but beyond this level, significant amounts of concomitant substances were extracted.

4.3.3 LEES

This by-product is a solid substance obtained in the process of settling which comes after the fermentation of the must. Lees consist mainly of dead yeast remains, tartrates, and high-molecular-weight materials that are initially present in the grape juice and finally accumulate at the bottom of the wine tanks. Currently, this by-product is distilled for the production of wine alcohol. However, the high content of proteins and tartrates of this material suggests potential uses that currently are not sufficiently exploited.

4.3.4 STALKS

The stalk is the woody part of the grape cluster and represents between 3% and 6% of its weight. A typical chemical composition of stalks is 70%–80% water, 1% potassium bitartrate, 2%–3.5% tannic substances, 2%–2.5% mineral matter, 1%–1.5%

nitrogenous substances, and 1% sugar (Oreglia, 1979). Most of the research has focused on the exploitation of grape stalks as a biosorbent material for the removal of toxic compounds and as a bulking agent in composting processes, but knowledge of their chemical composition is crucial to defining their possible areas of utilization. In recent years, researchers have started working on use of grape stalks as a potential source of high value-added compounds, such as phenolic compounds with antioxidant activity, lignin, and cellulose. The high tannin content makes grape stalks a potentially rich source of antioxidants, and the quite high hemicellulose content (mainly composed of xyloglucans) (Prozil et al., 2012a) makes it a potential source of fermentable sugars. Utilization of grape stalks as lignocellulose biomass resource has been described in the literature. Spigno et al. (2008) studied a mild chemical fractionation procedure consisting of hemicellulose acid hydrolysis followed by an alkaline/oxidative step for lignin solubilization and Ping et al. (2011b) applied three pretreatment steps for ethanol production from grape stalks: dilute sulfuric acid, ethanol organic-solvent process with sulfuric acid as catalyst, and wet oxidation.

To improve the technological aptitude and intensify solvent extraction, Sánchez-Valdepeñas (2006) quantified the impact of APIB pretreatment prior to conventional solvent processes on the yields of six phenolic compounds extracted from grape stalk powder of the Monastrell variety (*V. vinifera* L.). Results indicate that APIB treatment had a positive and significant effect on the concentration of these compounds. Mainly, the APIB treatment increased the availability of gallic acid, quercetin, ellagic acid, and resveratrol by up to 25% in 50% (v/v) aqueous ethanol, ethyl acetate, or propanol extracts. It had a much greater effect than the solvent used in the extraction process. More polar solvents (ethanol and propanol) were efficient to extract phenolic acids (gallic, caffeic, and ellagic acids) and stilbenes (resveratrol), while a moderately polar solvent (ethyl acetate) was better for flavonoids ((+)-catechin and quercetin).

REFERENCES

Akoh, C.C. (1998). Fat replacers. *Food Technology* 52: 47–53.
Alastalo, H., Räikkönen, K., Pesonen, A., Osmond, C., Barker, D.J.P., Heinonen, K., Kajantie, E., and Eriksson, J.G. (2013). Early life stress and blood pressure levels in late adulthood. *Journal of Human Hypertension* 27(2): 90–94.
Alemzadeh, I. (2010). A study on plant polymer: Pectin production and modification. *International Journal of Engineering, Transactions B: Applications* 23(2): 107–114.
Amor, B. and Allaf, K. (2009). Impact of texturing using instant pressure drop treatment prior to solvent extraction of anthocyanins from Malaysian roselle (*Hibiscus sabdariffa*). *Food Chemistry* 115(3): 820–825.
AOAC. (2000). AOAC official method 962.09. Fiber (crude) in animal feed and pet food. In W. Horwitz (ed.), *Official Methods of Analysis of AOAC International*, section 4.6.01, Gaithersburg, MD: AOAC International.
Bail, S., Stuebiger, G., Krist, S., Unterweger, H., and Buchbauer, G. (2008). Characterisation of various grapeseed oils by volatile compounds, triacylglycerol composition, total phenols and antioxidant capacity. *Food Chemistry* 108(3): 1122–1132.
Bailén, L., Martí, N., and Ignatieva, G. (2011). Caracterización de fibras dietéticas procedentes de subproductos de la industria de transformación de zumos cítricos. Thesis. Universidad Miguel Hernández de Elche. Elche. Alicante, Spain.

Bailey, D.G. (2010). Fruit juice inhibition of uptake transport: A new type of food–drug interaction. *British Journal of Clinical Pharmacology* 70(5): 645–655.

Bailey, D.G., Arnold, J.M.O., and Spence, J.D. (1994). Grapefruit juice and drugs: How significant is the interaction? *Clinical Pharmacokinetics* 26(2): 91–98.

Bailey, D.G. and Dresser, G.K. (2004). Natural products and adverse drug interactions. *Canadian Medical Association Journal* 170(10): 1531–1532.

Bailey, D.G., Dresser, G., and Arnold, J.M.A. (2012). Grapefruit and medication interactions: Forbidden fruit or avoidable consequences? *Canadian Medical Association Journal* 185: 309–316.

Bailey, D.G., Spence, J.D., Munoz, C., and Arnold, J.M.O. (1991). Interaction of citrus juices with felodipine and nifedipine. *Lancet* 337(8736): 268–269.

Barker, D.J.P. (1999). The fetal origins of type 2 diabetes mellitus. *Annals of Internal Medicine* 130(4 I): 322–324.

Barker, D.J.P. (2012). Developmental origins of chronic disease. *Public Health* 126(3): 185–189.

Barker, D.J.P., Gelow, J., Thornburg, K., Osmond, C., Kajantie, E., and Eriksson, J.G. (2010a). The early origins of chronic heart failure: Impaired placental growth and initiation of insulin resistance in childhood. *European Journal of Heart Failure* 12(8): 819–825.

Barker, D.J.P., Larsen, G., Osmond, C., Thornburg, K.L., Kajantie, E., and Eriksson, J.G. (2012). The placental origins of sudden cardiac death. *International Journal of Epidemiology* 41(5): 1394–1399.

Barker, D.J.P., Osmond, C., Thornburg, K.L., Kajantie, E., and Eriksson, J.G. (2013). The intrauterine origins of Hodgkin's lymphoma. *Cancer Epidemiology* 15: 23–34.

Barker, D.J.P., Thornburg, K.L., Osmond, C., Kajantie, E., and Eriksson, J.G. (2010b). The prenatal origins of lung cancer. II. The placenta. *American Journal of Human Biology* 22(4): 512–516.

Benlloch, M.J. (2006). Extracción de antocianos a partir de orujos de vinificación de uva tinta (*Vitis vinifera* L.). Trabajo Final de Carrerra. Escuela Politécnica Superior de Orihuela. Universidad Miguel Hernández de Elche, Spain.

Berardini, N., Knödler, M., Schieber, A., and Carle, R. (2005). Utilization of mango peels as a source of pectin and polyphenolics. *Innovative Food Science and Emerging Technologies* 6(4–1): 442–452.

Bidlack, W.R., Omaye, S.T., Meskin, M.S., and Topham, D.K.W. (2000). *Phytochemicals as Bioactive Agents*. Boca Raton, FL: CRC Press.

Borroto, B., Larrauri, J.A., and Cribeiro, A. (1995). Influencia del tamaño de partículas sobre la capacidad de retención de agua de la fibra obtenida a partir de cítricos y piña. *Alimentaria* 3: 89–90.

Braddock, R.J. (1999). *Handbook of Citrus By-Products and Processing Technology*. New York: John Wiley & Sons.

Braddock, R.J. (2004). Importance of by-products to citrus juice processing. *Fruit Processing* 14(5): 310–313.

Bravi, M., Spinoglio, F., Verdone, N., Adami, M., Aliboni, A., D'Andrea, A., De Santis, A., and Ferri, D. (2007). Improving the extraction of a-tocopherol-enriched oil from grape seeds by super-critical CO_2. Optimisation of the extraction conditions. *Journal of Food Engineering* 78: 488–493.

Buchholt, H.C., and Vinter, H. (1991). Pectin-containing product and method for producing same. Patent WO91/15571.

Buchwald-Werner, S., Gartner, C., Horlacher, P., and Schwarz, G. (2009). Fortification with substances other than vitamins and minerals (polyphenols, carotenoids, fatty acids and phytosterols). In: P.B. Ottaway (ed.), *Food Fortification and Supplementation Technology*, pp. 41–59. Boca Raton, FL: CRC Press.

Burns, J., Gardner, P.T., O'Neil, J., Crawford, S., Morecroft, I., McPhail, D.B., Lister, C., et al. (2000). Relationship among antioxidant activity, vasodilation capacity and phenolic content of red wines. *Journal of Agricultural and Food Chemistry* 48: 220–230.

Cacace, J.E. and Mazza, G. (2003). Optimization of extraction of anthocyanins from black currants with aqueous ethanol. *Journal of Food Science* 68(1): 240–248.

Campillo, J.S., Dolisnki, A., Proteychine, B., Valynberg, R., Bogdanov, S., Bouskii, N., and Poliakov, M. (1995). Método de producción de pectina de alto y bajo metoxilo a base de cítricos. Patent 95-108736/13.

Cárcel, J.A., García-Pérez, J.V., Mulet, A., Rodrígueza, L., and Riera, E. (2010). Ultrasonically assisted antioxidant extraction from grape stalks and olive leaves. *Physics Procedia* 3: 147–152.

Chakravarty, T.K. (1997). Pectin from citrus wastes. Report Pub. of National Research Development Corporations. (A Government of India Enterprise).

Chau, C.F. and Huang, Y.L. (2003). Comparison of the chemical composition and physico-chemical properties of different fibers prepared from the peel of *Citrus sinensis* L. Cv. Liucheng. *Journal of Agricultural and Food Chemistry* 51: 2615–2618.

Cho, S., DeVries, J., and Prosky, L., (1997). *Dietary Fiber Analysis and Applications.* Gaithersburg, MD: AOAC International.

Choi, I.S., Kim, J., Wi, S.G., Kim, K.H., and Bae, H. (2013). Bioethanol production from mandarin (*Citrus unshiu*) peel waste using popping pretreatment. *Applied Energy* 102: 204–210.

Christensen, J.A. (2003). Improved process for treating pectin containing plant material. Patent CO8B37/06.

Crandall, P.G., Braddock, R.J., and Rouse, A.H. (1978a). Effect of drying on pectin made from lime and lemon pomace. *Journal of Food Science* 43(76): 1680–1682.

Crandall, P.G., Braddock, R.J., and Rouse, A.H. (1978b). Determining the yield and quality of pectin from fresh peel and pectin pomace. *Proceedings of the Florida State Horticultural Society.* 91: 109–111.

D'Amico, E. (2005). Cargill acquires Citrico's worldwide pectin business. *Chemical Week.* 167(19): 39.

Da Porto, C., Porretto, E., and Decorti, D. (2013). Comparison of ultrasound-assisted extraction with conventional extraction methods of oil and polyphenols from grape (*Vitis vinifera* L.) seeds. *Ultrasonics Sonochemistry* 20: 1076–1080.

dos Santos Freitas, L., de Oliveira, J.V., Dariva, P., Jacques, R.A., and Caramão, E.B. (2008). Extraction of grape seed oil using compressed carbon dioxide and propane, extraction yields and characterization of free glycerol compounds. *Journal of Agricultural and Food Chemistry* 58: 2558–2564.

Edwards, M.C. and Doran-Peterson, J. (2012). Pectin-rich biomass as feedstock for fuel ethanol production. *Applied Microbiology and Biotechnology* 95(3): 565–575.

Ehrlich, R.M. (1997). Methods for making pectin and pectocellulosic products. Patent US5656734.

El-Nawawi, S.A. and Heikal, Y.A. (1995a). Factors affecting the production of low-ester pectin gels. *Carbohydrate Polymers* 26: 189–193.

El-Nawawi, S.A. and Heikal, Y.A. (1995b). Production of a low ester pectin by de-esterification of high ester citrus pectin. *Carbohydrate Polymers* 27: 191–195.

Eriksson, J.G., Kajantie, E., Lampl, M., Osmond, C., and Barker, D.J.P. (2013). Markers of biological fitness as predictors of all-cause mortality, *Annals of Medicine* 45(2): 156–161.

Eriksson, J.G., Kajantie, E., Thornburg, K.L., Osmond, C., and Barker, D.J.P. (2011). Mothers body size and placental size predict coronary heart disease in men. *European Heart Journal* 32(18): 2297–2303.

Eriksson, J.G., Thornburg, K.L., Osmond, C., Kajantie, E., and Barker, D.J.P. (2010). The prenatal origins of lung cancer. I. The fetus. *American Journal of Human Biology* 22(4): 508–511.

Ezhov, V.N., Lebedev, V.V., Lukanin, A.S. Petrushevskii, V.V., and Romanovskaya, T.I. (1993). Wasteless processing of apple pressings. Patent SU1785639.

Fatsikostas, A.N., Kondarides, D.I., and Verykios, X.E. (2002). Production of hydrogen for fuel cells by reformation of biomass-derived ethanol. *Catalysis Today* 75(1–4): 145–155.

FDA (Food and Drug Administration). (2003). Agency response letter GRAS Notice No. GRN 000125. CFSAN/Office of Food Additive Safety, August 18.

Figuerola, F., Hurtado, M.L., Estevez, A.M., Chiffelle, I., and Asenjo, F. (2005). Fibre concentrates from apple pomace and citrus peel as potential fibre sources for food enrichment. *Food Chemistry* 91: 395–401.

Fiori, L., de Faveri, D., Casazza, A.A., and Perego, P. (2009). Grape by-products: Extraction of polyphenolic compounds using supercritical CO_2 and liquid organic solvent, a preliminary investigation. *CyTA—Journal of Food Science* 7(3): 163–171.

Gibney, M.J. (2000). Nutrition and diet for healthy lifestyles in Europe. In: B.V. McCleary, L. Prosky (eds), *Advanced Dietary Fibre Technology*, pp. 3–11. Oxford: Blackwell Publishig.

Gibson, G.R. and Williams, C.M. (2003). *Functional Foods. Concept to Product*. Abington, UK: Woodhead.

Gilbert, J. and Şenyuva, H.Z. (2008). *Bioactive Compounds in Foods*. Oxford, UK: Blackwell Publishing.

Giusti, M.M., Rodriguez-Saona, L.E., and Wrolstad, R.E. (1999). Molar absorptivity and color characteristics of acylated and non-acylated pelargonidin-based anthocyanins. *Journal of Agricultural and Food Chemistry* 47(11): 4631–4637.

Godfrey, K.M. and Barker, D.J.P. (2000). Fetal nutrition and adult disease. *American Journal of Clinical Nutrition* 71(5 Suppl.): 1344S–1352S.

Golubev, V.N. (2004). Procedure is for obtaining pectin and uses vegetal raw material for use in food industry, implicating hydraulic extraction. Patent no. ES2216722.

González-Centeno, M.R., Rosselló, C., Simal, S., Garau, M.C., López, F., and Femenia, A. (2010). Physico-chemical properties of cell wall materials obtained from ten grape varieties and their byproducts: grape pomaces and stems. *Food Science and Technology-Lebensmittel-Wissenschaft & Technologie* 43(10): 1580–1586.

Grigelmo, N., Ibarz, A., and Belloso, O. (1999). Flow properties of orange dietary fiber suspensions. *Journal of Texture Studies* 30: 245–257.

Griguelmo-Miguel, N. and Martin-Belloso, O. (1999). Comparison of dietary fibre from by-product of processing fruit and greens and from cereals. *Lebensmittel-Wissenschaft & Technologie* 32: 503–508.

Grohmann, K., Cameron, R.G., and Buslig, B.S. (1996). Fermentation of orange peel hydrolysates by ethanologenic *Escherichia coli* effects of nutritional supplements. *Applied Biochemistry and Biotechnology—Part A Enzyme Engineering and Biotechnology* 57–58: 383–388.

Hertog, M.G.L., Feskens, E.J.M., Hollman, P., Katan, M.B., and Kromhout, D. (1993). Dietary antioxidant flavonoids and risk of coronary heart disease: The Zutphen elderly study. *The Lancet* 342: 1007–1011.

Hong, N., Yaylayan, V.A., Raghavan, G.S.V., Paré, J.R.J., and Bélanger, J.M.R. (2001). Microwave assisted extraction of phenolic compounds from grape seed. *Natural Product Letters* 15(3): 197–204.

Iyengar, R. and Gross, A. (1991). Fat substitutes. In: I. Goldberg and R. Williams, (eds.), *Biotechnology and Food Ingredients,* pp. 287–313, New York: Van Nostrand Reinhold.

Javaid, M.K., Eriksson, J.G., Kajantie, E., Forsén, T., Osmond, C., Barker, D.J.P., and Cooper, C. (2011). Growth in childhood predicts hip fracture risk in later life. *Osteoporosis International* 22(1): 69–73.

Johnson, I.T. and Southgate, D.A.T. (1994). Dietary fiber and related substances. In: J. Edelman and S. Miller, (eds.), *Food Safety Series*, pp. 39–65, London, England: Chapman & Hall.

Johnson, I. and Williamson, G. (2003). *Phytochemical Functional Foods*. Abington, UK: Woodhead.

Johnston, R.B. (2002). Confidential report on existing pectin plant. Report on pectin peel. FMC (Australia).

Ju, Z. and Howard, L.R. (2005). Subcritical water and sulfured water extraction of anthocyanins and other phenolics from dried red grape skin. *Journal of Food Science* 70(4): S270–S276.

Kajantie, E., Osmond, C., Barker, D.J.P., and Eriksson, J.G. (2010). Preterm birth—A risk factor for type 2 diabetes? The Helsinki Birth Cohort study. *Diabetes Care* 33(12): 2623–2625.

Kamal, I.M., Sobolik, V., Kristiawan, M., Mounir, S.M., and Allaf, K. (2008). Structure expansion of green coffee beans using instantaneous controlled pressure drop process. *Innovative Food Science and Emerging Technologies* 9(4): 534–541.

Karpovich, N.S., Suprunchuk, V.K., and Kioresku, E.N. (1989). Manufacturing of pectin from sugar beet pulp—Involving extraction, neutralisation and centrifuging with specified to increase yield and quality. UKRPISHCHEPROEKTMEK (UKRP-Soviet Institute). Patent no SU1507293-A.

Kato, Y. (2005). Pectin originating in plant cell. Patent PCT/JP2005/002706.

Kaeferstein, F.K. and Clugston, G.A. (1995). Human health problems related to meat production and consumption. *Fleischwirtschaft* 75: 889–892.

Kertesz, Z.L. (1951). *The Pectic Substances*. New York: Interscience Publisher.

Kimball, J. (1999). *Procesado de cítricos*. ACRIBIA (ed.), Zaragoza, Spain.

Kristiawan, M., Sobolik, V., Klíma, L., and Allaf, K. (2011). Effect of expansion by instantaneous controlled pressure drop on dielectric properties of fruits and vegetables. *Journal of Food Engineering* 102(4): 361–368.

Lafka, T.I., Sinanoglou, V., and Lazos, E.S. (2007). On the extraction and antioxidant activity of phenolic compounds from winery waste. *Food Chemistry* 104: 1206–1214.

Larrauri, J.A., Perdomo, U., Fernández, M., and Borroto, B. (1995). Selección de método más apropiado para la elaboración de tabletas de fibra dietética. *Alimentaria* 265: 67–70.

Li, Y., Lu, J., and Paxton, J.W. (2012). The role of ABC and SLC transporters in the pharmacokinetics of dietary and herbal phytochemicals and their interactions with xenobiotics. *Current Drug Metabolism* 13(5): 624–639.

Li, Y. and Paxton, J.W. (2013). The effects of flavonoids on the ABC transporters: Consequences for the pharmacokinetics of substrate drugs. *Expert Opinion on Drug Metabolism and Toxicology* 9(3): 267–285.

Li, Y., Revalde, J.L., Reid, G., and Paxton, J.W. (2010). Interactions of dietary phytochemicals with ABC transporters: Possible implications for drug disposition and multidrug resistance in cancer. *Drug Metabolism Reviews* 42(4): 590–611.

Liang, R.H., Chen, J., Liu, W., Liu, C.M., Yu, W., Yuan, M., and Zhou, X.Q. (2012). Extraction, characterization and spontaneous gel-forming property of pectin from creeping fig (*Ficus pumila* Linn.) seeds. *Carbohydrate Polymers* 87(1): 76–83.

Lizarraga, D., Vinardell, M.P., Noe, V., van Delft, J.H., Alcarraz-Vizán, G., van Breda, S.G., Staal, Y., et al. (2011). A lyophilized red grape pomace containing proanthocyanidin-rich dietary fiber induces genetic and metabolic alterations in colon mucosa of female C57BL/6J mice. *Journal of Nutrition* 141(9): 1597–1604.

Lobanok, A.G., Mikhailova, R.V., Sapunova, L.I., Selivanova N.Y., Simkhovich R.G., and Nosachevskii, P.N. (1993). Manufacture of pectin. Patent SU1791455.

Martí, N. (2004). Calidad y rendimientos de extracción de zumos cítricos mediterráneos. PhD. Thesis. Universidad Miguel Hernández de Elche, Elche, Alicante, Spain.

Martí, N., Saura, D., Fuentes, E., Lizama, V., García, E., Mico-Ballester, M.J., and Lorente, J. (2011). Fiber from tangerine juice industry. *Industrial Crops and Products* 33(1): 94–98.

May, C.D. (1990). Industrial pectins: Sources, production and applications. *Carbohydrate Polymers* 12: 79–99.

May, C.D. (1994). Pectins. In: A. Imeson (ed.), *Thickening and Gelling Agents for Food*, pp.124–152, Chapter 6. Glasgow, UK: Blackie Academic and Professional.

Mazi-Kotwal, N. and Seshadri, M. (2013). Drug interactions with grapefruit juice. *British Journal of Medical Practitioners* 5(4): 76–83.

Mazza, G. (1998). *Functional Foods*. Lancaster, PA: Technomic.

Mildner-Szkudlarz, S., Zawirska-Wojtasiak, R., and Goslinski, M. (2010). Phenolic compounds from winemaking waste and its antioxidant activity towards oxidation of rapeseed oil. *International Journal of Food Science and Technology* 45: 2272–2280.

Monagas, M., Hernández-Ledesma, B., Gómez-Cordovés, C., and Bartolomé, B. (2006). Commercial dietary ingredients from *Vitis vinifera* L. leaves and grape skins: antioxidant and chemical characterization. *Journal of Agricultural and Food Chemistry* 54(2):319–327.

Mongeau, R., Brassard, R., Deeks, J.R., Laffey, P.J., Nguyen, L., and Brooks, S.P.J. (2001). Comparison of dietary fiber contents of selected baby foods from two major brands in Canada using three methods. *Journal of Agricultural and Food Chemistry* 49(8): 3782–3786.

Monro, J.A. (2000). Faecal bulking index: A physiological basis for dietary management of bulk in the distal colon. *Asia Pacific Journal of Clinical Nutrition* 9(2): 74–81.

Monro, J.A. (2002). Faecal bulking efficacy of Australasian breakfast cereals. *Asia Pacific Journal of Clinical Nutrition* 11(3): 176–185.

Morel-Salmi, C., Souquet, J.M., Bes, M., and Cheynier, V. (2006). Effect of flash treatment on phenolic extraction and wine composition. *Journal of Agricultural and Food Chemistry* 54: 4270–4276.

Moutonet, M. and Escudier, J.L. (2000). Prétreatement des raisins par Flash-détente sous vide. Incidence surla qualité des vins. *Le Bulletin de L'OIV—Organisation Internationale du la VIgne et du Vin*. 73: 5–19.

Nagy, S., Shaw, P.E., and Veldhuis, M.K. (1977). *Citrus Science and Technology*. Vol. 2. *Fruit Production, Processing Practices, Derived Products and Personnel Management*. Westport, CT: AVI.

Negro, C., Tommasi, L., and Miceli, A. (2003). Phenolic compounds and antioxidant activity from red grape marc extracts. *Bioresource Technology* 87: 41–44.

Norsker, M., Jensen, M., and Adler-Nissen, J. (2000). Enzymatic gelation of sugar beet pectin in food products. *Food Hydrocolloids* 14(3): 237–243.

OIV (Organisation Internationale de la Vigne et du Vin). (2011). State of the vitiviniculture world market March 2011. OVI. www.oiv.int/oiv/info/enconjoncture.

O'Neill, M., Albersheim, P., and Darvill, A. (1990). The pectic polysaccharides of primary cell walls. In: P.M. Dey and J.B. Harborne (eds), *Methods in Plant Biochemistry*, vol. 2, pp. 415–441. London: Academic Press.

Oreglia, F. (1979). *Enología Teórico-Práctica*. Buenos Aires: Instituto Salesiano de Artes Gráficas.

Passos, C.P., Silva, R.M., Da Silva, F.A., Coimbra, M.A., and Silva, C.M. (2009). Enhancement of the supercritical fluid extraction of grape seed oil by using enzymatically pre-treated seed. *The Journal of Supercritical Fluids* 48: 225–229.

Pauly, M., Albersheim, P., Darvill, A., and York, W.S. (1999). Molecular domains of the cellulose/xyloglucan network in the cell walls of higher plants. *Plant Journal* 20(6): 629–639.

Perälä, M.-M., Männistö, S., Kaartinen, N.E., Kajantie, E., Osmond, C., Barker, D.J.P., Valstra, L.M., and Eriksson, J.G. (2012), Body size at birth is associated with food and nutrient intake in adulthood. *PLoS ONE* 7(9): e46139: 1–6.

Perälä, M.-M., Moltchanova, E., Kaartinen, N.E., Männistö, S., Kajantie, E., Osmond, C., Barker, D.J.P., Valsta, L.M., and Eriksson, J.G. (2011). The association between salt intake and adult systolic blood pressure is modified by birth weight. *American Journal of Clinical Nutrition* 93(2): 422–426.

Perlack, R.D., Wright, L.L., Turhollow, A.F., Graham, R.L., Strokes, B.J., and Erbach, D.C. (2005). Biomass as feedstock for a bioenergy and bioproducts industry: The technical feasibility of a billion-ton annual supply. U.S. Department of Agriculture. DOE/GO-102005-2135, Oak Ridge National Laboratory, Oak Ridge, Tennessee (http://feedstockreview.ornl.gov/pdf/billion_ton_vision.pdf). (accessed November 7, 2012).

Pesonen, A.-K., Räikkönen, K., Feldt, K., Heinonen, K., Osmond, C., Phillips, D.I.W., Barker, D.J.P., Eriksson, J.G., and Kajantie, E. (2010). Childhood separation experience predicts HPA axis hormonal responses in late adulthood: A natural experiment of World War II. *Psychoneuroendocrinology* 35(5): 758–767.

Pinelo, M., Fabbro, P.D., Manzocco, L., Nuñez, J.M., and Nicoli, M.C. (2005a). Optimization of continuous phenol extraction from *Vitis vinifera* by-products. *Food Chemistry* 92(1): 109–117.

Pinelo, M., Rubilar, M., Jerez, M., Sineiro, J., and Nunez, M.J. (2005b). Effect of solvent, temperature, and solvent-to-solid ratio on the total phenolic content and antiradical activity of extracts from different compounds of grape pomace. *Journal of Agricultural and Food Chemistry* 53: 2111–2117.

Piñera, R.M., Vicente, I., Núñez, J.M., and Figueroa, C. (1996). Evaluación de dos métodos d extracción parala extracción de pectina a partir de residuos del procesamiento de la Lima Persa. *Alimentaria* 3: 28–34.

Ping, L., Brosse, N., Chrusciel, L., Navarrete, P., and Pizzi, A. (2011a). Extraction of condensed tannins from grape pomace for use as wood adhesives. *Industrial Crops and Products* 33: 253–257.

Ping, L., Brosse, N., Sannigrahi, P., and Ragauskas, A. (2011b). Evaluation of grape stalks as a bioresource. *Industrial Crops and Products* 33: 200–204.

Ping, L., Pizzi, A., Guo, Z.D., and Brosse, N. (2011c). Condensed tannins extraction from grape pomace: Characterization and utilization as wood adhesives for wood particleboard. *Industrial Crops and Products* 34: 907–914.

Prozil, S.O., Costa, E.V., Evtuguin, D.V., Lopes, L.P., and Domingues, M.R. (2012a). Structural characterization of polysaccharides isolated from grape stalks of Vitis vinifera L. *Carbohydrate Research* 356: 252–259.

Prozil, S.O., Evtuguin, D.V., and Lopes, L.P.C. (2012b). Chemical composition of grape stalks of *Vitis vinifera* L. from red grape pomaces. *Industrial Crops and Products* 35: 178–184.

Rabin, R.C. (2012). Grapefruit is a culprit in more drug reactions. *New York Times*, December 17.

Raghupathy, P., Antonisamy, B., Geethanjali, F.S., Saperia, J., Leary, S.D., Priya, G., Richard, J., Barker, D.J.P., and Fall, C.H.D. (2010). Glucose tolerance, insulin resistance and insulin secretion in young south Indian adults: Relationships to parental size, neonatal size and childhood body mass index. *Diabetes Research and Clinical Practice* 87(2): 283–292.

Ravelli, A.C.J., Van Der Meulen, J.H.P., Osmond, C., Barker, D.J.P., and Bleker, O.P. (1999). Obesity at the age of 50 y in men and women exposed to famine prenatally. *American Journal of Clinical Nutrition* 70(5): 811–816.

Rondeau, P., Gambier, F., Jolibert, F., and Brosse, N. (2013). Compositions and chemical variability of grape pomaces from French vineyard. *Industrial Crops and Products* 43: 251–254.

Ros, J.M., Schols, H.A., and Voragen, A.G.J. (1995). Extraction, characterisation, and enzymatic degradation of lemon peel pectins. *Carbohydrate Research* 282: 271–284.

Roseboom, T.J., Van Der Meulen, J.H.P., Ravelli, A.C.J., Van Montfrans, G.A., Osmond, C., Barker, D.J.P., and Bleker, O.P. (1999). Blood pressure in adults after prenatal exposure to famine. *Journal of hypertension* 17(3): 325–330.

Rouilly, A., Jorda, J., and Rigal, L. (2006). Thermo-mechanical processing of sugar beet pulp. I. Twin-screw extrusion process. *Carbohydrate Polymer* 66: 81–87.

Rouse, A.H. and Crandall, P.G. (1976). Nitric acid extraction of pectin from citrus peel. *Proceedings of the Florida State Horticultural Society* 89: 166–168.

Rouse, A.H. and Crandall, P.G. (1979). Pectin content of lime and lemon peel as extracted by nitric acid. *Journal of Food Science* 43: 72–75.

Sachdev, H.P.S., Osmond, C., Fall, C.H.D., Lakshmy, R., Ramji, S., Dey Biswas, S.K., Prabhakaran, D., et al. (2009). Predicting adult metabolic syndrome from childhood body mass index: Follow-up of the New Delhi birth cohort. *Archives of Disease in Childhood* 94(10): 768–774.

Sánchez-Valdepeñas, V. (2006). Extracción y recuperación de compuestos con actividad biológica a partir de raspón de uva de vinificación. Trabajo Final de Carrerra, Escuela Politécnica Superior de Orihuela, Universidad Miguel Hernández de Elche.

Saura-Calixto, F. (1998). Antioxidant dietary fiber product: A new concept and a potential food ingredient. *Journal of Agricultural and Food Chemistry* 46(10): 4303–4306.

Shahidi, F. and Naczk, M. (2004). *Phenolics in Food and Nutraceuticals*, pp. 443–482. Boca Raton, FL: CRC Press.

Spigno, G. and De Faveri, D.M. (2007). Antioxidants from grape stalks and marc: Influence of extraction procedure on yield, purity and antioxidant power of the extracts. *Journal of Food Engineering* 78(3): 793–801.

Spigno, G., Pizzorno, T., and De Faveri, D.M. (2008). Cellulose and hemicelluloses recovery from grape stalks. *Bioresource Technology* 99: 4329–4337.

Spigno, G., Tramelli, L., and De Faveri, D.M. (2007). Effects of extraction time, temperature and solvent on concentration and antioxidant activity of grape marc phenolics. *Journal of Food Engineering* 81(1): 200–208.

Suprunchuck, V.K., Karpovich, N.S., Romenskii, N.P., Kioresku, E.N., Zharik, B.N., Slobodyan, O.P., and Telichuck, L.K. (1991). Manufacture of food grade pectin from dried sugar beet pulp. Patent SU 1650064A1.

Thebaudin, J.Y., Lefebvre, A.C., Harrington, M., and Bourgeois, C.M. (1997). Dietary 4 fibers: Nutritional and technological interest. *Trends Food Science Technology* 8: 41–48.

The Copenhagen Pectin Factory (1998). Pectin. Industrial oriented booklets.

Transformación de aditivos (1998). *Métodos de Análisis de Pectinas*. Company documentation. Restricted.

USDA (U.S. Department of Agriculture). (2002). Nutritive value of foods. http://www.ars.usda.gov/SP2UserFiles/Place/12354500/Data/hg72/hg72_2002.pdf (accessed November 7, 2012).

Viser J. and Voragen, A.G.J. (eds), (1996). *Pectins and Pectinases*. Amsterdam: Elsevier Science.

Wang, S., Chen, F., Wu, J., Wang, Z., Liao, X., and Hu, X. (2007). Optimization of pectin extraction assisted by microwave from apple pomace using response surface methodology. *Journal of Food Engineering* 78: 693–700.

Watson, R.R. (2003). *Functional Foods and Nutraceuticals in Cancer Prevention*. Ames: Iowa State Press.

Wesfalia Separator, I.B. (1996). Report on types and capacities of clarifiers used in pectin production. GEA/ Westfalia Pectin Extraction Brochure. Restricted.

Wildman, R.E.C. (2007). *Nutraceuticals and Functional Foods*, 2nd edn. Boca Raton, FL: CRC Press.

Wyman, C.E. (1999). Biomass ethanol: Technical progress, opportunities, and commercial challenges. *Annual Review of Energy and the Environment* 24: 189–226.

5 Assessing Juice Quality
Measuring Quality and Authenticity

Núria Rafel, Xavier Costa, and Carlos Berdún

CONTENTS

5.1 Introduction 75
5.2 History 76
5.3 Legislation 76
5.4 Contaminants 76
5.5 Sugar 77
5.6 Juice/Concentrate 77
5.7 Chemical Markers 78
5.8 Orange 78
5.9 Lemon 79
5.10 Apple 79
5.11 Pomegranate 79
5.12 Berries 79
5.13 New Analytical Trends 80
References 80

5.1 INTRODUCTION

Fruit juice adulteration, like any other food adulteration, is an economic issue. This means that any such process should generate an economic profit, which must not be forgotten. The market prices of the different products are a good starting point for an analysis. The main substances used for adulteration must be cheaper than the more expensive juices, starting with water and sugar, and, more recently, cheaper fruits.

Due to the high level of analytical resources, some manufacturers have added substances, some dangerous, in an attempt to achieve compliance with the reference parameters for the prepared "fruit juice" to avoid detection of the adulteration and, in this way, to generate a high economic profit.

It is also clear that the fruit market is very active and a long way ahead of research; in order to avoid mistakes, scientific bodies wait 4–5 years to include variances due to the seasons and their conditions, such as rain, temperature, wind, or sun (AIJN 2001); then, new fruit varieties are not fully included in their findings. Sometimes, values appear that must be explained by experts who must always be able to trace the product fully, and have, of course, a good knowledge of the fruit industry.

In a few cases, some unidentified juice mixtures may be found, but in such low quantities that they are due to a problem during the manufacturing process; they can be recognized by their low concentration, and are a long way from making a real economic profit.

5.2 HISTORY

Initially, the easiest way to make a quick profit was just to add water. The final form of the drink does not change very much when a quantity of water is added; but, of course, all the nutritional properties of the fruit juice are decreased by the same proportion as that of the water added. Once it became easy to measure the concentration of the juice quickly, manufacturers started to add sugar. Using this method, the sugar concentration was almost the same as before; but with less sugar, the taste was sweeter, so then some acid was also needed. Finally, a nectar or soft drink was sold as a pure juice, deceiving the consumer. In this way, the "race" started between the analytical chemist and the adulterator.

5.3 LEGISLATION

The main problem here is usually a defect with the product labeling. The general philosophy of any labeling legislation is that it must not introduce an error, meaning that the label must not lie to the consumer: if a manufacturer declares a juice to have 80% fruit content and the drink has this content, the labeling is accurate and there is no problem. Problems start when this same manufacturer wants to declare it as a 100% pure juice.

In this case, it is clearly stated in legislation that a juice must contain 100% fruit; even if it comes from a juice concentrate, the quality of the water used must be potable and the maximum quantity to be added back is also fixed. If it is declared to be nectar, the minimum fruit content is fixed for each fruit, but this must also be reflected on the label.

Analytical parameters for each fruit have been determined and published by the Food and Agriculture Organization (FAO) in the Codex Alimentarius and by the European Union in the Code of Practice issued by the International Association of Fruit Juice and Nectar Producers (AIJN 2001); both codes are voluntary but usually some aspects of them are transposed into official legislation.

As fruit juice is considered a food, health claims on the packaging are clearly regulated and some claims are prohibited. Legislation concerning fruit juices will be thoroughly reviewed in Chapter 17.

5.4 CONTAMINANTS

More and more different chemical substances have been recognized as harmful to health, and new legislation has been issued, limiting the radioactive content of the juice or the use of heavy metals. In the past, the fruits used in the industry were sometimes poorly stored or controlled, making the growth of mold possible. This produced some strains of mycotoxins. The amounts of these allowed in juice according to European regulations are limited: patulin has a maximum limit of 50 µg/L in grape juice, but ochratoxin A only has a limit of 2 µg/L.

For such kinds of analysis, sophisticated equipment is required and only a limited number of laboratories can achieve reliable results.

5.5 SUGAR

In the past, sucrose was added, but once the definitions of sugar profiles were determined, it was easy to detect this addition. If one wanted to avoid this situation, the sucrose could be decomposed in glucose and fructose using an invertase. However, the origin of the sugar (i.e., beet or cane) can be detected by using mass spectrometry, identifying the metabolic pathway. It is also possible to detect if pineapple has been used in the preparation by this method.

Another kind of analysis emerges when sugars are produced from starch; oligosaccharides are produced and can be detected by gas chromatography after derivatization (or liquid chromatography). It is only a qualitative analysis; if these kinds of products are appearing it means that foreign liquid sugar has been added at levels below 5%.

Also, the sugar alcohol *sorbitol* is a component in apples, pears, or stone fruits, but not in citrus fruits. This means that if sorbitol is found in analysis in high enough amounts, this is due to a mixture of citrus and pip fruits; if the amount is low, this can be due to a cross-contamination or the use of some kinds of enzymes that use sorbitol to protect against an increase in the percentage of soluble solids. Lastly, in some berries, sorbitol can originate from microbiological damage, which means that the raw material used is not of sufficient quality.

5.6 JUICE/CONCENTRATE

The main increase in fruit juice consumption is through single-strength juice (not from concentrate [NFC] juices). The quality of such juices is better because the thermal treatment is shorter (seconds rather than minutes). Such a process causes the aroma and flavor notes to remain in the juice, resulting in more fruity notes and freshness, and also avoiding some cooked notes and browning.

In the past, the analysis was based on the detection of the minerals present in the water (Holemann 1984), but due to the increase of reverse-osmosis plants producing low-mineral water, other kinds of analysis must be used, such as isotopic analysis. This compares the ratio between different isotopes of the oxygen in the water. If it originates from rainfall, the ratio is lower (more negative) than the water from a fruit. This method always uses ocean water as a standard, and is based on a nuclear magnetic resonance (NMR) analysis that then requires very sophisticated and expensive equipment, but it always needs interpretation by an expert who must be able to trace the product fully.

This method is very useful but has some limitations. For example, if an orange juice is manufactured from fruits that are grown during a rainy season (Attaway et al. 1972) or are not fully ripe, or even if there is some process where the juice is passed through water—for example, pasteurization, debittering, or loading, including cooling—such analysis must always be studied by an expert, taking into account not only one sole analysis value but a combination of them.

5.7   CHEMICAL MARKERS

Some substances occur in only one kind of fruit, helping its detection in a mixture of fruits. Some of them are typical:

- Arbutin appears in pears; if arbutin occurs in an apple juice, some pear juice has been mixed with it during its production or filling. In the past, pear juice concentrate was much cheaper than apple.
- Eriocitrin only appears in lemons; if one wishes to acidify another juice with lemon juice, this substance will be present. Conversely, if lemon juice concentrate is bought then eriocitrin must be present and if the concentrate is made only with citric acid it will not be present.
- Naringin appears in grapefruit; if present in an orange juice then some grapefruit juice has been added to it. As grapefruit juice is cheaper than orange juice, this adulteration is known in the juice world.
- Amino acids: The ratio of different acids is unique for each fruit, so it is easy to detect a mixture of juices when the ratio is outside the correct range. It is also possible to detect whether the juice has been squeezed recently or in the past, because the glutamine content decomposes quickly during storage.

5.8   ORANGE

Orange juice comprises almost 50% of the juice market; therefore, one can understand why it is the juice that is studied most, with more research references available, and, of course, it is the juice that is adulterated most often (Navarro et al. 1984).

Besides the typical adulterations—the addition of water and sugar—there are others such as mixing with cheaper fruits: grapefruit, which is easily detected by the presence of naringin (Greiner and Wallrauch 1984) and mandarin. The latter case is a special one, because U.S. legislation allows orange juice to contain 10% mandarin juice, but European legislation does not allow any quantity that is not declared on the label.

The classical analytical method was based on the carotenoid content and ratios (Sholten 1984, IFU 2001), but the reference standard values did not include oranges from Mediterranean countries. Now, new analytical methods based on DNA profiles allow the detection of mandarin adulteration in orange juice.

Other products that can be mixed into the orange concentrate are lower-quality products such as pulp wash (Petrus and Attaway 1986). This can usually be easily detected through its ultraviolet (UV) absorbance spectra, but if it comes from the same fruit, it is very difficult to identify except by more sophisticated analysis.

Another possible situation is if the juice is declared as an NFC juice (i.e., squeezed) but instead comes from a concentrate with added water; this fact could be easily detected by NMR spectroscopy, through the ratio of oxygen-18 to oxygen-16.

Other kinds of analysis have been undertaken in order to discover the origin of particular fruits. If a certain place of origin is declared on the labeling, it can also be discovered whether this is correct through the particular ratio of rubidium isotopes in the juice or through statistics, or whether another juice from a different place of origin has been used, which is probably cheaper and, in the worst cases, comes from an area close to pollution.

5.9 LEMON

The main adulteration to this juice is the addition of citric acid. The easiest way to detect it is by analyzing the isocitric acid content. This isomer of citric acid is identified in the fruits with a relation that is well established. Then, in a laboratory with a spectrophotometer this adulteration can be easily, cheaply, and quickly detected.

Another aspect to take into account is that lemon juice must have a very light color and is usually preserved with sulfur dioxide. This substance forms sulfites in the juice that must be declared on the labeling, because they are considered allergenic at levels above 10 mg/L.

5.10 APPLE

The main adulteration is mixture with pear juice (Elkin et al. 1996, Spanos and Wrolstad 1992, Awad et al. 2000); as a cheaper juice, it is easily detected by the amounts of citric acid and sorbitol (Bielig et al. 1977). There are some other substances, such as arbutin, which can also be used to detect such adulteration. The other, more important one is the addition of foreign sugar, which can be easily detected by the determination of sucrose and its ratio against other sugars such as glucose or fructose, or even liquid sugar (syrup); it is possible to detect this through the oligosaccharide fingerprint (Low method; Low 1996).

5.11 POMEGRANATE

This fruit is very important due to its high content of polyphenols, which can be claimed as a healthy product on the labeling. The main production areas are Turkey and Iran, and sometimes there may be shortages in European markets; then, in order to obtain a similar product, some sugars, berry juices (to give the dark and strong color), and acids are mixed together. This adulteration may be easily detected through the polyphenol profile, which is unique for each fruit.

The Food and Drug Administration (FDA) detected products in the United States with colorants, sweeteners, and cheaper juices such as cherry, blackcurrant, pear, and apple, and issued a corresponding alert at the end of 2012.

5.12 BERRIES

Cheaper berry juices are used in order to change the color, and then the mixture is declared as containing 100% of the most expensive juice. This can be detected easily by chromatography to obtain the polyphenol profile or fingerprint; also, new technologies allowing the acquisition of many analytical values can detect if any mixing has occurred.

5.13 NEW ANALYTICAL TRENDS

Analytical methods to prevent adulteration are based on a larger number of analyses of the same sample, including all changes that can affect health and safety, and, of course, decrease cost. To assess these three characteristics, profile analysis is preferred; if only one characteristic is examined (e.g., a decreased cost), many different values are obtained in analysis, which makes it much more difficult to check all the parameters that are required in an authentic fruit juice. The last technique is based on NMR (Rinke and Spraul 2008), also allowing analysis of whether the juice is NFC or comes from concentrate. This method is based on statistics: the whole data bank used must be very well checked and accurately obtained, requiring a big effort to achieve traceability on all samples in order to understand and explain possible abnormal values.

The interpretations of the results are very important; acquiring authentic analysis parameters is a slower process than the pace of the fresh fruit market (AIJN 2001). Sometimes the "new" fruit is already growing in orchards and then some quantity of it is used in the industry, while the analysis parameters are not yet issued.

From the point of view of health and safety, the analytical trend is to try to obtain a full screening of residues using chromatographic techniques that have a better resolution, using mass spectrometer detectors and triple quadrupole mass spectrometry; the same equipment is also used to analyze other residues such as mycotoxins. In microbiology, reverse transcription polymerase chain reaction (RT-PCR) technology is already on the market and allows very sensitive, quick, and accurate identification of any pathogenic or allergenic microorganism.

In the near future, it will be very important to label all health claims on the packaging; then, it will also be very important to use all analytical methods to obtain the correct values in order to guarantee an exact labeling of each product.

REFERENCES

AIJN (2001). *Code of Practice for Evaluation of Fruit and Vegetable Juices*. Brussels: AIJN.
Attaway, J.A., Barron, R.W., Blair, J.G., Buslig, B.S., Carter, R.D., Dougherty, M.H., Fellers, P.J., et al. (1972). Some new analytical indicators of processed orange juice. *Proc. Fla. State Hort. Soc.* 85: 191–203.
Awad, M.A., De Jager, A., and Westing, M. (2000). Flavonoid and chlorogenic acid levels in apple fruit: Characterisation of variation. *Sci. Hort.* 83: 249–263.
Bielig, H., Faethe, W., Koch, J., Wallrauch, S., and Wucherpfennig, K. (1977). Richtwerte und Schwankungsbreiten Bestimmter Kennzahlen (RSK-Wert) für Apfelsaft, Traubensaft und Orangensaft. *Die ind. Obst-u. Gemüseverwertung* 62: 209.
Elkin, R.E., Matthys, A., Lyon, R., and Huang, C.J. (1996). Characterisation of commercial apple juice concentrate. *J. Food Compos. Anal.* 9: 43–56.
Greiner, G. and Wallrauch, S. (1984). Naringin as evidence for blending grapefruit juice with orange and tangerine juice. *Fluss. Obst.* 12: 626–628.
Holemann, E.H. (1984). Food adulteration detection: 100 years of progress in AOAC methodology. *J. Assoc. Off. Anal. Chem.* 67: 1029–1034.

IFU (Internationale Fruchtsaftunion) (2001). *Analytical Methods.*

Low, N.H. (1996). Food authenticity analysis via oligosaccharide fingerprinting. In *Book of Abstracts 212th ACS National Meeting.* Orlando, FL: American Chemical Society.

Navarro, J.L., Aristoy, M., and Izquierdo, L. (1984). El análisis estadístico en la detección de adulteraciones en zumos de cítricos. *Rev. Agroquim. Tecnol.* 24 (1): 48–58.

Petrus, D.R. and Attaway, J.A. (1986). Visible and ultraviolet absorption and fluorescence and emission characteristics of Florida orange juice and orange pulp wash: Detection of adulteration. *J. Assoc. Off. Anal. Chem.* 63: 1317–1331.

Rinke, P. and Spraul, M. (2008). Successful application of SGF-profiling. *New Food* (1): 18–23.

Sholten, G. (1984). Determination of bioflavonoids in citrus juices by high pressure liquid chromatography. *Fluss. Obst.* 51: 519–522.

Spanos, G.A. and Wrolstad, R.E. (1992). Phenolics of apple, pear and white grape juices and their changer with processing and storage: A review. *J. Agric. Food Chem.* 40: 1478–1487.

6 Assessing Juice Quality
Advances in the Determination of Rheological Properties of Fruit Juices and Derivatives

Pedro E. D. Augusto and Alfredo A. Vitali

CONTENTS

6.1 Introduction 83
6.2 Principles of Rheology 84
    6.2.1 Fluid Flow: Steady-State Shear Properties.....................................84
    6.2.2 Time-Dependent Flow Properties..90
    6.2.3 Viscoelastic Properties 92
6.3 Assessing Fruit Juices and Derivatives Rheological Properties....................94
    6.3.1 Fluid Flow: Steady-State Shear Properties.....................................95
    6.3.2 Time-Dependent Flow Properties..97
    6.3.3 Viscoelastic Properties 97
        6.3.3.1 Viscoelastic Properties: Dynamic Oscillatory Procedure 97
        6.3.3.2 Viscoelastic Properties: Creep and Recovery Procedure 102
6.4 Effect of Product Composition and Processing Conditions on
the Rheological Properties of Fruit Juices and Derivatives 104
    6.4.1 Effect of Processing Conditions: Temperature 104
    6.4.2 Effect of Product Properties: Concentration...................................110
    6.4.3 Effect of Product Properties: Composition.....................................116
    6.4.4 Effect of Unit Operations and Processing 120
6.5 Conclusions...128
6.6 Nomenclature...130
References..132

6.1 INTRODUCTION

Consumer demand for fruit products is growing, creating the need for a better understanding of their processing and properties. Rheology is the science that studies the flow and deformation of solids and fluids under the influence of mechanical forces. The rheological characterization of food is important for the design of unit operations, process optimization, and high-quality product assurance (Ibarz and Barbosa-Cánovas, 2003; Rao, 1999).

Rheological properties are used to design equipment and processing plants, as well as food packages, and even to determine shelf life. These properties influence the transference of mass (such as the diffusion of ingredients during processing or pulp sedimentation during storage), momentum (such as the velocity profile in pipes or the propeller requirements during mixing), and energy (such as the heating rate in heat exchangers and vessels). Therefore, not only are the process conditions and dimensions (such as the pump power, pipes, evaporators, and heat exchangers dimensions or the temperature profile during the thermal process) defined based on the rheology of the product, but also the product's behavior during storage (such as the phase separation or gelation). The rheological properties are also important for food quality control, as they are used to guarantee the desirable standards. Finally, the rheological properties are directly related to the consumer's sensorial perception of fruit products, as they are essential to their acceptance.

Fruit juices are composed of an insoluble phase (the pulp) dispersed in a viscous solution (the serum). The dispersed phase, or pulp, is composed of fruit tissue cells and their fragments, cell walls, and insoluble polymer clusters and chains. The serum is an aqueous solution of soluble polysaccharides, sugars, salts, and acids. The rheological properties of fruit juices are thus defined by the interactions within and between each phase (Augusto et al., 2012b). Therefore, fruit juices show a complex rheology, described by non-Newtonian behavior, with time-dependent, shear-thinning, and viscoelastic (either viscous or solid) properties.

The rheology of fruit juice is a function of its composition, processing, and condition. Moreover, the study of the rheology of fruit juices, as well as the effect of the products and the processing conditions on their properties, is fundamental to guaranteeing high-quality products.

This chapter describes the main principles of the rheology of fruit products, as well as the most important methods to evaluate them in order to assess the quality of fruit juices.

6.2 PRINCIPLES OF RHEOLOGY

6.2.1 FLUID FLOW: STEADY-STATE SHEAR PROPERTIES

The rheological properties of a fluid flow can be understood by the following experiment. Consider two parallel plates separated by a fluid (Figure 6.1a). Each plate has an area A in contact with the fluid separated by a distance dy. Suppose that there are no border effects (which could be true for a long, wide plate). If the upper plate is moved by a force F, applied in the z direction (Figure 6.1b), then, after a short transient period, the upper plate will keep moving with velocity v by the force F, while the lower plate will remain at rest. In this scenario, the fluid layer just below the plate will follow it, moving in the z direction with the same velocity v. On the other hand, the fluid layer just above the lower plate will remain

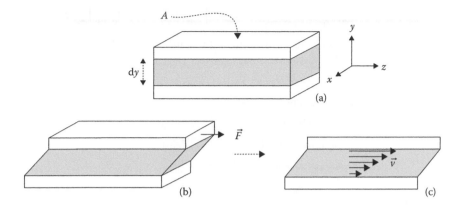

FIGURE 6.1 A fluid (in gray) between two parallel plates (in white) at rest. Each plate has an area A in contact with the fluid, and the distance between the plates is dy (a); a force F is applied to the upper plate, which is moved in the z direction (b); a cross section in the yz plane, showing the velocity vectors v on the fluid (c).

at rest. Therefore, the fluid between these two layers will move in the z direction with a velocity profile (Figure 6.1c), as each fluid layer will drag the layer immediately below it.

Thus, with this procedure we can define two important properties of fluid flow. The first is the shear stress (σ, Equation 6.1), which relates the force F with the applied area A, tangent to the F direction (in the experiment, the area A is on the xy plane, while the force F is in the z direction; Figure 6.1).

Then, we can define the shear rate ($\dot{\gamma}$, Equation 6.2), that is, the fluid velocity gradient across the plates. Some typical shear rate ($\dot{\gamma}$) values in food processing are shown in Figure 6.2.

$$\sigma = \frac{F}{A} \tag{6.1}$$

$$\dot{\gamma} = \frac{dv}{dy} \tag{6.2}$$

If a perfect fluid is placed between the plates, the shear rate will be linearly proportional to the applied shear stress (Figure 6.3). Thus, the constant of proportionality is called viscosity (η, Equation 6.3: Newton's law; Ibarz and Barbosa-Cánovas, 2003; Rao, 1999; Steffe, 1996), and represents the fluid resistance to flow. Such fluids are called Newtonian fluids, examples of which are water, gases, oils, milk, clarified juices, solutions of sugars, and other dilute solutions.

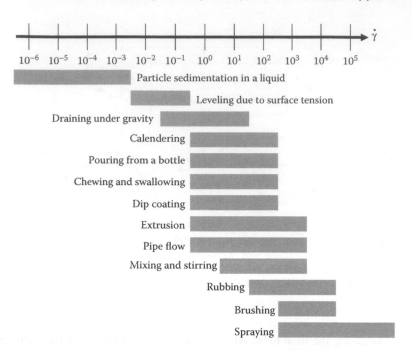

FIGURE 6.2 Some typical shear rate ($\dot{\gamma}$) values in food processing. (Adapted from Steffe, J.F., *Rheological Methods in Food Process Engineering*, 2nd edn., Freeman Press, East Lansing, MI, 1996.)

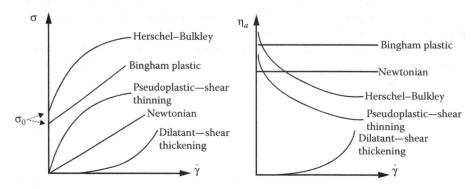

FIGURE 6.3 Flow behavior of fluids. Shear stress versus shear rate (left) and the variation on the apparent viscosity as a function of the shear rate (right).

$$\sigma = \eta \cdot \dot{\gamma} \tag{6.3}$$

However, most foods behave differently under flow. Fluids whose behavior deviates from Newton's law are called non-Newtonian fluids, and are defined by some different structural changes during flow.

Figure 6.4 shows three common explanations for non-Newtonian behavior in foods. When the product is composed of irregular-shaped suspended particles

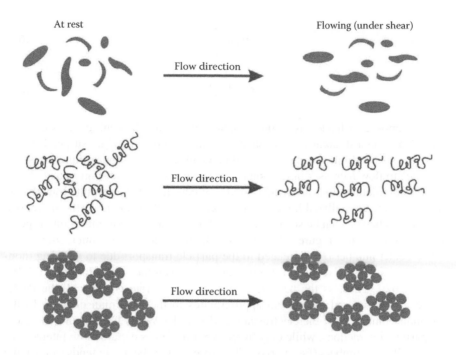

At rest   Flowing (under shear)

Flow direction

Flow direction

Flow direction

FIGURE 6.4   Explanation of pseudoplastic (shear-thinning) behavior.

(such as the pulp in fruit products, which is composed of fruit tissue cells and their fragments, cell walls, and insoluble polymer clusters and chains), the spatial distribution of three-dimensional polymer clusters and chains (such as polysaccharides and proteins) and nonregular aggregates (such as particle clusters and flocks) at rest is random (Figure 6.4, left) and there is a higher resistance to flow. However, when sheared, those suspended structures tend to align in the flow direction, reducing the overall resistance. Thus, this kind of fluid, where the resistance to flow decreases as the shear rate increases, is called pseudoplastic or shear-thinning fluid.

Pseudoplastic fluid cannot be described by Newton's law (Equation 6.3) as its "viscosity" is not a constant property, but a decreasing function of the shear rate. Therefore, the resistance to flow will be characterized by the apparent viscosity (η_a), defined in Equation 6.4, and a new model must be used.

The Ostwald–de Waele model (Equation 6.5; Ibarz and Barbosa-Cánovas, 2003; Rao, 1999; Steffe, 1996), which is also called the power law model, describes the fluid flow behavior using two parameters. The parameter k, known as the consistency coefficient, is related to the fluid consistency and its resistance to flow. The parameter n, known as the flow behavior index, describes the flow behavior under shear. For Newtonian fluids, $n = 1$ and Equation 6.5 is reduced to Newton's law. For pseudoplastic fluids, $n < 1$, which describes the power-decreasing behavior of η_a in relation to the shear rate. The Ostwald–de Waele model is commonly used to describe the rheological properties of food products, especially fruit juices and derivatives, and provides a good explanation of the pseudoplastic behavior shown in Figure 6.4.

$$\eta_a = \frac{\sigma}{\dot{\gamma}} \qquad (6.4)$$

$$\sigma = k \cdot \dot{\gamma}^n \qquad (6.5)$$

The opposite behavior is called dilatant or shear thickening, as shown in Figure 6.5. When dilatant fluid is sheared, many collisions of its suspended particles are observed, increasing its overall resistance. In this kind of fluid, thus, the resistance to flow increases in relation to the shear rate increase (Figure 6.3). A few examples of dilatant fluids are special food products, highly concentrated starch suspensions, some crystallized honey, and suspended sand in water. Furthermore, two other flow behaviors can be seen in food products because of an important property called yield stress (σ_0, Figure 6.3), which is related to interparticle interactions.

The Peclet number (*Pe*) is related to the particle transport due to shearing (non-Brownian system) and diffusion (Brownian system) (Fischer et al., 2009; Rao, 1999; Equation 6.6). Thus, as the particle size or the shear rate is reduced, the Peclet number decreases and the system approximates to the Brownian domain. In the Brownian domain, both the electrostatic and van der Waals forces can dictate the interparticle interactions, while only hydrodynamic forces dictate those interactions at higher Peclet numbers (Figure 6.6). Therefore, as the shear rate tends to zero, the

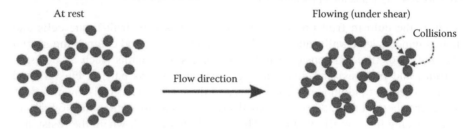

FIGURE 6.5 Explanation of dilatant (shear thickening) behavior.

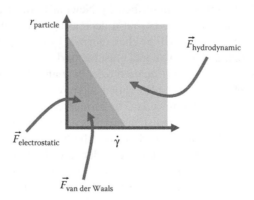

FIGURE 6.6 The forces involved in interparticle interactions at different Peclet numbers.

fluid is under the Brownian domain, and both the electrostatic and van der Waals forces act in order to maintain the stability of the suspended particles, forming an internal structure similar to a network.

$$Pe = \frac{\eta_{continuous\_phase} \cdot \bar{r}_{particle}^{3} \cdot \dot{\gamma}}{k_B \cdot T} \qquad (6.6)$$

The yield stress is the minimum shear stress required to initiate product flow, which is related to the material's internal structure, which must be broken to allow flow (Genovese and Rao, 2005; Tabilo-Munizaga and Barbosa-Cánovas, 2005). Below the yield stress, the material deforms elastically, behaving like an elastic solid; above the yield stress, the material starts flowing, behaving like a viscous liquid (Bayod et al., 2007). The presence of a yield stress is a typical characteristic of multiphase materials (Sun and Gunasekaran, 2009), such as fruit pulps and juices, which are formed by the dispersion of insoluble components (materials of cellular walls) in a water solution (a serum containing sugars, minerals, proteins, and soluble polysaccharides).

Both the Bingham model (Equation 6.6; Ibarz and Barbosa-Cánovas, 2003; Rao, 1999; Steffe, 1996) and the Herschel–Bulkley (HB) model (Equation 6.7; Ibarz and Barbosa-Cánovas, 2003; Rao, 1999; Steffe, 1996) describe a fluid with a yield stress (Figure 6.3).

A Bingham fluid, also called Bingham plastic, requires a stress above its yield stress to start flowing; thus, it behaves as a Newtonian fluid, with constant apparent viscosity (called plastic viscosity in the Bingham model—η_p; Figure 6.3). Some sauces such as mayonnaise can be classified as a Bingham fluid. An HB fluid also requires a stress above its yield stress to start flowing; then, it behaves as a pseudoplastic fluid, with decreasing apparent viscosity in relation to the shear rate (Figure 6.3). Fruit pulps, juices, and derivatives can be classified as HB fluids.

It is also important to observe that the amount of dispersed phase in the suspension can change the rheological classification of the fluid. Fruit juices, for example, can behave as pseudoplastic or HB fluids in relation to the amount of pulp and to its nature, which define the interactive forces among them. Another example is mayonnaise, an emulsion of oil-in-water, which is classically described as a Bingham fluid. However, due to the addition of hydrocolloids (e.g., to reduce its fat content), it behaves as an HB fluid.

It is also interesting to observe that the HB model (Equation 6.7) comprises the Newton, Bingham, and Ostwald–de Waele (power law) models.

$$\sigma = \sigma_0 + \eta_p \cdot \dot{\gamma} \qquad (6.7)$$

$$\sigma = \sigma_0 + k \cdot \dot{\gamma}^n \qquad (6.8)$$

Other mathematical models have been proposed to describe the rheological behavior of fluids, such as the Casson, Mizrahi–Berk, Sisko, Ellis, and Vocadlo models, which describe the shear stress as a function of the shear rate, or the Cross and Carreau model, which describes the apparent viscosity as a function of the shear rate (Rao, 1999; Steffe, 1996). However, most fluids can be described using the HB model, as it is widely used to characterize food products.

We highlight the recently proposed Falguera–Ibarz model (Falguera and Ibarz, 2010; Equation 6.9), which describes the apparent viscosity as a function of the shear rate. In the Falguera–Ibarz model, the variation of the apparent viscosity (η_a) with the shear rate is described by a power decay function from an initial value (η_0) to an equilibrium value (η_∞), and the parameter k_{FI} of the decay constant. It was successfully used to describe the flow behavior of some fruit juices such as orange, mandarin, and tomato juices. Although there are other mathematical expressions fitting the evolution of viscosity with shear rate, these models are mathematically complex, with four or five parameters related in different ways. The Falguera–Ibarz model, however, is an easy, intuitive equation to describe the apparent viscosity change with the shear rate of non-Newtonian fluids, with only three parameters that can be easily interpreted (Falguera and Ibarz, 2010).

$$\eta_a = \eta_\infty + \left(\eta_0 - \eta_\infty\right) \cdot \gamma^{\left(-k_{FI}\right)} \tag{6.9}$$

Some examples of the rheological behavior of fruit juices and derivatives are show in Figure 6.7.

6.2.2 Time-Dependent Flow Properties

The rheological properties of some materials change during the flow time. The consistency of these materials can increase or decrease with time under the same conditions (shear rate).

Time dependence is related to the structural change due to shear (Ramos and Ibarz, 1998), that is, the destruction (Cepeda et al., 1999) and reaggregation of the internal structure during flow. Thus, both behaviors are attributed to the continuous change of the material's internal structure, which can be reversible or irreversible. Consequently, time-dependent rheological characterization is extremely important for understanding the changes that occur in products during the process.

A fluid that shows an increase in consistency (apparent viscosity) is called rheopectic; a fluid that shows a decrease in apparent viscosity is called thixotropic. The factors that contribute to thixotropy also contribute to pseudoplasticity, and the factors that cause rheopecticity also cause shear thickening (Ibarz and Barbosa-Cánovas, 2003).

Rheopectic behavior is related to the formation or reorganization of the internal structure, with a consequent increase in the resistance to flow. It is a rare phenomenon in food products. On the other hand, thixotropic behavior is very common in dispersions and suspensions in many food products. Fruit juices, pulps, and derivatives are classic examples of thixotropic materials. Figure 6.8 shows the thixotropic behavior of foods such as fruit juices. In the original product, the internal structure formed by the insoluble pulp that is dispersed in the serum has a higher resistance to deformation due to its interparticle interactions (and also aggregation), resulting in a

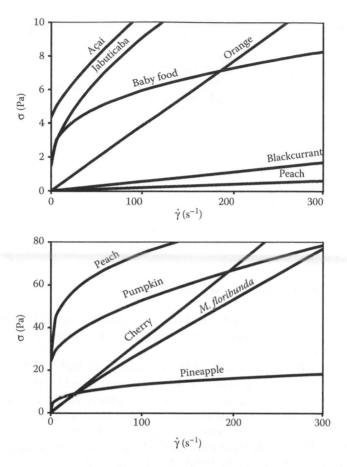

FIGURE 6.7 Some examples of the rheological behavior of fruit juices and derivatives: açaí pulp (14% solids, 25°C; data from Tonon, R.V., et al., *Journal of Food Engineering*, 92, 425–431, 2009); jabuticaba pulp (14% solids, 25°C; data from Sato, A.C.K., Cunha, R.L., *Journal of Food Engineering*, 91, 566–570, 2009); sweet potato baby food (20°C; data from Ahmed, J., and Ramaswamy, H.S., *Journal of Food Process Engineering*, 29, 219–233, 2006); clarified concentrated orange juice (66°Brix, 25°C; data from Ibarz, R., et al., *Journal of Texture Studies*, 40, 445–456, 2009); clarified concentrated blackcurrant juice (35°Brix, 25°C; data from Ibarz, A., et al., *Journal of Food Engineering*, 15, 63–73, 1992); clarified concentrated peach juice (12°Brix, 20°C; data from Augusto, P.E.D., et al., *International Journal of Food Science and Technology*, 46, 1086–1092, 2011a); peach puree (25°C, 21°Brix; data from Massa, A., et al., *Journal of Texture Studies*, 41, 532–548, 2010); pumpkin puree (60°C; data from Dutta, D., et al., *Journal of Food Engineering*, 76, 538–546, 2006); clarified concentrated cherry juice (66°Brix, 20°C; data from Giner et al., *Journal of Food Engineering*, 30, 147–154, 1996); *Malus floribunda* juice (68°Brix, 25°C; data from Cepeda et al., *Journal of Texture Studies*, 30, 481–491, 1999); and pineapple pulp (11.2°Brix; data from Silva et al., *International Journal of Food Science and Technology*, 45, 2127–2133, 2010).

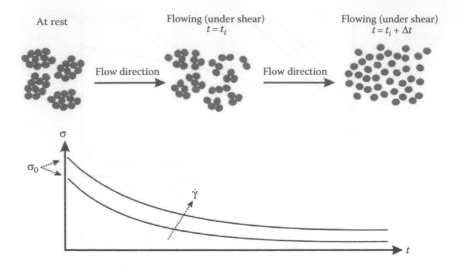

FIGURE 6.8 Explanation of thixotropic behavior.

higher shear stress. When shearing is carried out, this structure is broken down, as can be noted by the stress decay. Thus, for this type of fluid, the resistance to flow decreases over time.

The models of Figoni–Shoemaker (1983; Equation 6.10), Weltman (1943; Equation 6.11), and Hahn–Ree–Eyring (Hahn et al., 1959; Equation 6.12) are widely used to describe thixotropy in foods (Ibarz and Barbosa-Cánovas, 2003). The three models describe the shear stress decay at an imposed shear rate over time. It is important to observe that both the Figoni–Shoemaker and the Hahn–Ree–Eyring models are essentially similar, with the same mathematical expression (if the exponential function is applied to both sides of the Hahn–Ree–Eyring model).

$$\sigma = \sigma_e + \left(\sigma_0 - \sigma_e\right) \cdot \exp\left(-k_{FS} \cdot t\right) \tag{6.10}$$

$$\sigma = A_W - B_W \cdot \ln t \tag{6.11}$$

$$\ln\left(\sigma - \sigma_e\right) = A_{HRE} - B_{HRE} \cdot t \tag{6.12}$$

Some examples of the thixotropic behavior of fruit juices and derivatives are show in Figure 6.9.

6.2.3 VISCOELASTIC PROPERTIES

As previously described, some food products behave as perfect fluids, with a Newtonian rheological behavior, such as water, gases, oils, milk, clarified juices, solutions of sugars, and other dilute solutions. However, most food products, particularly those derived from fruits, show a rheological behavior between a perfect

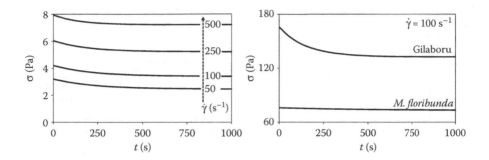

FIGURE 6.9 Examples of the thixotropic behavior of fruit juices and derivatives. Left: Tomato juice at 5°Brix, 25°C. (From Augusto, P.E.D., Falguera, V., Cristianini, M., and Ibarz, A., *Food and Bioprocess Technology*, 5, 1715–1723, 2012d. With permission.) Right: Gilaboru juice at 60°Brix, 20°C (Data from Altan, A., Kus, S., and Kaya, A., *Food Science and Technology International*, 11, 129–137, 2005. With permission.); *M. floribunda* juice at 72°Brix, 20°C (Data from Cepeda, E., Villarán, M.C., and Ibarz, A., *Journal of Texture Studies*, 30, 481–491, 1999. With permission.).

fluid (i.e., with purely viscous behavior) and a perfect solid (i.e., with purely elastic behavior), which are classified as viscoelastic materials.

Ideal solids respond by deforming finitely and instantaneously when a load is applied, and immediately recovering that deformation upon removal of the load. The energy involved in this deformation is stored as potential energy, and it is completely recovered when the material is unloaded. This is called elastic behavior and is described by Hooke's law (Equation 6.13; Ibarz and Barbosa-Cánovas, 2003, Rao, 1999; Steffe, 1996).

$$\sigma = \frac{G}{\gamma} \tag{6.13}$$

Ideal fluids (liquids and gases) respond by deforming continually while the load is applied, and the material does not recover its deformation when the load is removed. The energy involved is dissipated during the deformation (flow), and cannot be recovered. This is the called viscous behavior and is described by Newton's law (Equation 6.3).

Viscoelastic material, therefore, shows both a viscous and a solid component, simultaneously, when deformed. Moreover, its behavior can be described by combining both components, obtained by using oscillatory shear and creep compliance experiments. Figure 6.10 shows the elastic, viscous, and viscoelastic behaviors during the creep and recovery procedure.

From an engineering standpoint, the steady flow curve is the most effective way to characterize the rheological behavior of fluids. However, many phenomena cannot be described by their viscosity function alone and their elastic behavior must be taken into consideration (Steffe, 1996). The microstructure of a product can be correlated with its rheological behavior; and viscoelastic properties are very useful in the design and prediction of the stability of stored samples

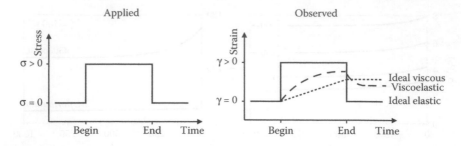

FIGURE 6.10 Elastic, viscous, and viscoelastic behaviors during the creep and recovery procedure. (Adapted from Rao, M.A., *Rheology of Fluid and Semisolid Foods: Principles and Applications*, Aspen, Gaithersburg, MD, 1999; Steffe, J.F., *Rheological Methods in Food Process Engineering*, 2nd edn., Freeman Press, East Lansing, MI, 1996.)

(Ibarz and Barbosa-Cánovas, 2003). Moreover, viscoelastic products may exhibit some interesting behavior, such as the Weissenberg and the Barus effects (Ibarz and Barbosa-Cánovas, 2003; Steffe, 1996). Therefore, the study and description of the viscoelastic properties of foods are important to better understand the product's behavior during processing, storing, and consumption.

6.3 ASSESSING FRUIT JUICES AND DERIVATIVES RHEOLOGICAL PROPERTIES

The main rheological procedures are based on fundamental methods using rotational viscometers (with different operational procedures and geometries), pressure-driven flow viscometers (such as tube viscometers), and extensional flow viscometers (Ibarz and Barbosa-Cánovas, 2003; Rao, 1999; Steffe, 1996). By using fundamental procedures, a mathematical description of the rheological phenomenon is obtained. Therefore, the product properties can be suitably described, as well as their behavior during processing, storing, and consumption.

However, other empirical procedures and equipment are often used in the food industry, such as the Adams consistometer and the Bostwick consistometer, as well as procedures whose designs only allow one-condition experiments, such as the falling ball viscometer and the glass capillary viscometer. In these situations, a mathematical analysis is difficult or impossible, and the information obtained is poor and inadequate.

Rotational viscometers, also called rheometers, are the most versatile and complete equipment that can be used to determine all the rheological properties of foods (such as the steady-state shear and the time-dependent and viscoelastic properties).

In the rotational viscometers, the sample is placed between a geometry, which is connected to a motor to be rotationally moved, and a stationary basis. The motor can apply a shear stress (σ), a shear rate ($\dot{\gamma}$), or a specific strain (γ) to the sample, in a continuous or an oscillating way. In this way, the response of the samples to the deformation or flow (the correspondent shear stress, shear rate, or strain) can be quantified by a sensor. Finally, a quantitative analysis can be carried out, based on the mathematical description of the physical phenomenon, in order to obtain the rheological behavior of the product. Rotational viscometers can thus be used to obtain the steady-state shear and the time-dependent and viscoelastic properties of different materials.

It is important to highlight that food products are very complex materials, with complex rheological behavior. Therefore, rheological procedures must be carried out with extreme care, as many sources of error can compromise the obtained results. Thus, the limitations of the technique, sample, equipment, and accessories must be known and evaluated (in fact, it is not uncommon for specialists to be unable to measure some properties of the evaluated material due to limitations of one or more of the aforementioned issues).

Consequently, each procedure and parameter must be preevaluated for each sample before the final evaluation. The main issues to be evaluated are the type, dimensions, material, and surface of the geometry to be used, the range of shear rate, shear stress, strain, temperature, and time to be used, the procedure to load the sample, and the calculation of the properties and sample reactions during the procedure (such as drying, separating, chemical reactions, gelling, among others).

Figure 6.11 shows the most common geometries that are used on rotational viscometers (rheometers) in order to access the rheological properties of fruit juices and derivatives. See Ibarz and Barbosa-Cánovas (2003), Rao (1999), and Steffe (1996) for a mathematical description of the rheological phenomenon, as well as more information related to the rheological procedure.

The following sections describe the main issues in assessing the rheological properties of fruit juices and derivatives (steady-state shear, time-dependent and viscoelastic properties) using rotational viscometers.

6.3.1 FLUID FLOW: STEADY-STATE SHEAR PROPERTIES

To obtain steady-state shear properties (fluid flow properties), procedures are carried out to obtain product flow curves (Figure 6.3), which are evaluated using the different models described in Section 6.2.1.

For this, once the sample has reached the desired temperature, it is continuously rotated between the geometry and the stationary basis, after a preshearing period to guarantee the steady-state condition (i.e., to reach equilibrium and avoid measuring the time-dependent behavior; Figures 6.8 and 6.9). The rotational process can be carried out by imposing a shear stress (σ) and measuring the corresponding shear rate ($\dot{\gamma}$) or vice versa, which is a function of the equipment design. The shear stress is related to the torque at the geometry axis and its contact area, while the shear rate is related to the velocity gradient of the product through the gap between the geometry and the stationary basis. In fact, the procedure is similar to that shown in Figure 6.1, but considering a circular movement instead of a linear one.

From an engineering standpoint, the steady flow curve is the best way to characterize the rheological behavior of fluids (Steffe, 1996), as the flow properties are directly related to the behavior of the product as it flows through pipes, the temperature profile in heat exchangers, the pump and impeller design, among others.

The main limitations of the steady-state shear procedures are related to the product's slip, separation, and the shear rate range that can be evaluated. The product slip in the geometry walls can be avoided using rough surface geometries, while

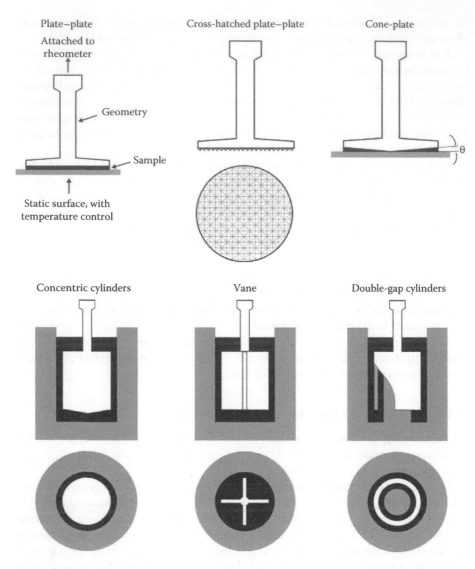

FIGURE 6.11 Main geometries (in white) used on rotational viscometers (rheometer) to access the rheological properties of fruit juices and derivatives. The sample is colored in black and the static surface, with temperature control, in gray.

the product separation can be prevented by using the correct geometries and shear ranges.

The shear rate range is limited in this type of procedure, as it is a function of the equipment, geometries, and samples. The lower values of the shear rate are of the order of 10^{-2} s^{-1} (Rao, 1999), which can compromise the yield stress (σ_0) value determination, but it is a good representation of most of the unit operations involved in processing food products (Figure 6.3). On the other hand, the higher values of the shear rate are of the order of 10^2 s^{-1}, which is a function of the evaluated product. At higher shear rates, Taylor's vortex can occur (Steffe, 1996), whose turbulence avoids rheological analysis, or the sample can be squeezed from the geometry.

Once the rheological experimental procedure has been carried out, the rheological model parameters are determined by linear or nonlinear regression, and the obtained parameters are used to describe the properties of the product.

6.3.2 TIME-DEPENDENT FLOW PROPERTIES

The time-dependent flow properties must be obtained using samples of the highest integrity possible. The procedure is similar to the one described in Section 6.2.1. The sample is placed on the rheometer and is kept at rest not only to guarantee the equilibrium of the temperature, but also to allow the recovery of the sample's internal structure. The time needed to obtain this equilibrium is, in general, from 5 to 20 min, and must be preevaluated. Then, the sample is sheared at a constant shear rate, which is the stress decay measured over time. As only one shear rate can be evaluated for each sample, it should be well defined (based on Figure 6.3), or multiple experiments must be conducted.

6.3.3 VISCOELASTIC PROPERTIES

Although the steady-state flow procedure is the most used method to evaluate the rheological behavior of food products (Steffe, 1996), it has limitations related to slippage and the migration of sample constituents (Gunasekaran and Ak, 2000), which is particularly true in some food products such as fruit juices. Moreover, in these experiments, the internal structure of the sample is broken, limiting the understanding of the product's behavior in low-shear situations, as in particle sedimentation. Dynamic rheological experiments can then be used to characterize those products, focusing on the properties of the product at small deformations.

Therefore, once more, these procedures must be conducted using samples of the highest integrity possible, and the resting time in the rheometer must be evaluated. After stabilization, two main procedures can be used to characterize the viscoelastic properties of the material: the dynamic oscillatory shear and the creep and recovery. Both procedures must be carried out in the linear viscoelastic range of the product (the range within which the stress is proportional to the applied strain and the theory described here is applied; Gunasekaran and Ak, 2000; Steffe, 1996); therefore, pretests must be conducted in order to determine the parameters of analysis.

6.3.3.1 Viscoelastic Properties: Dynamic Oscillatory Procedure

The dynamic oscillatory shear procedure is conducted by imposing a small amplitude (<5%; Gunasekaran and Ak, 2000) oscillatory movement on the sample. Three parameters are involved in this movement: the strain (γ), the shear stress (σ), and the oscillatory frequency (ω). During this procedure, one of these parameters is kept constant, another is varied, and the third is measured. Further, other variables can be varied, such as the temperature (e.g., for melting evaluation) or time (e.g., for gelling evaluation).

The main oscillatory procedure that is used to describe the properties of a food product is the frequency sweep, where the strain (γ) or the shear stress (σ) is kept constant, and its response is evaluated as a function of the oscillatory frequency (ω) (these are the three variables within the linear viscoelastic range of the product).

In this experiment, a sinusoidal oscillating movement is applied to the material, and the phase difference between the oscillating stress and strain is measured (Rao, 1999). Thus, the strain over time can be obtained using Equation 6.14 (where $\gamma_{amplitude}$ is the strain amplitude; Rao, 1999; Steffe, 1996).

$$\gamma(t) = \gamma_{amplitude} \cdot \sin(\omega \cdot t) \tag{6.14}$$

The applied sinusoidal strain input results in a periodic shear stress (σ), which is related to the consequent shear rate (Equation 6.15; obtained by deriving Equation 6.14; Rao, 1999; Steffe, 1996), and this is expressed by Equation 6.16 (where $\sigma_{amplitude}$ is the stress amplitude and δ is the phase lag between the stress and strain curves; Steffe, 1996).

$$\frac{d\gamma(t)}{dt} = \dot{\gamma}(t) = \gamma_{amplitude} \cdot \cos(\omega \cdot t) \tag{6.15}$$

$$\sigma(t) = \sigma_{amplitude} \cdot \sin(\omega \cdot t + \delta) \tag{6.16}$$

Figure 6.12 shows the stress and the strain responses of an ideal fluid (Newtonian), an ideal solid (Hookean), and a viscoelastic material during dynamic oscillatory procedures.

For ideal solids (i.e., those with pure elastic behavior, described by Hook's law), the stress and the strain curves are aligned (i.e., $\delta = 0$). For ideal liquids (i.e., those with pure viscous behavior, described by Newton's law), the stress and the strain curves are perfectly $\pi/2$ (90°) out of phase. Therefore, for a viscoelastic material, the phase lag between the stress and the strain curves is between these two values ($0 < \delta < \pi/2$), and the obtained shear stress can be described using Equation 6.17 (Rao, 1999).

$$\sigma(t) = \gamma_{amplitude} \cdot G' \cdot \sin(\omega \cdot t) + \gamma_{amplitude} \cdot G'' \cdot \cos(\omega \cdot t) \tag{6.17}$$

The storage modulus (G') is defined by Equation 6.18, and describes the elastic (solid) behavior of the product and, consequently, the energy stored and released at each oscillatory cycle; while the loss modulus (G'') is defined by Equation 6.19, and describes the viscous (fluid) behavior of the product and, consequently, the energy dissipated at each oscillatory cycle (Gunasekaran and Ak, 2000; Steffe, 1996).

$$G' = \left(\frac{\sigma_{amplitude}}{\gamma_{amplitude}} \right) \cdot \cos(\delta) \tag{6.18}$$

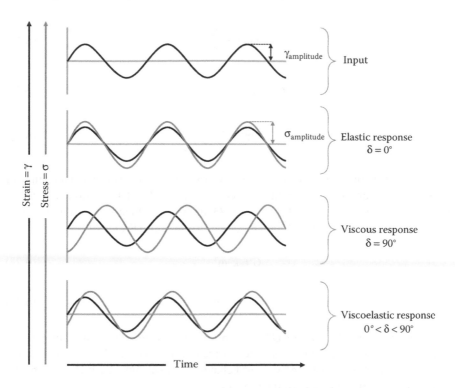

FIGURE 6.12 Stress and strain response of an ideal fluid (Newtonian), an ideal solid (Hookean), and a viscoelastic material during dynamic oscillatory procedures. (Adapted from Dogan, H. and Kokini, J.L., *Handbook of Food Engineering*, 2nd edn., Taylor & Francis, Boca Raton, FL, 2007; Rao, M.A., *Rheology of Fluid and Semisolid Foods: Principles and Applications*, Aspen, Gaithersburg, MD, 1999; Steffe, J.F., *Rheological Methods in Food Process Engineering*, 2nd edn., Freeman Press, East Lansing, MI, 1996.)

$$G'' = \left(\frac{\sigma_{amplitude}}{\gamma_{amplitude}} \right) \cdot \sin(\delta) \qquad (6.19)$$

Both the storage (G') and loss (G'') modules are not constant properties, but functions of the strain (γ), oscillatory frequency (ω), and temperature (T). Therefore, the dynamic oscillatory procedures can be carried out considering the strain, frequency, or temperature sweeps, with different results and interpretations from each one.

Moreover, based on the G' and G'' values, three other important rheological functions can be obtained: the loss tangent (tan δ, Equation 6.20), which describes the ratio between the energy dissipated and stored at each deformation cycle; and the complex modulus (G^*, Equation 6.21) and the complex viscosity (η^*; Equation 6.22), which describe the overall resistance of the material to deformation, regardless of whether that deformation is recoverable (elastic, solid) or nonrecoverable (viscous, fluid) (Rao, 1999; Steffe, 1996).

$$\tan \delta = \frac{G''}{G'} \tag{6.20}$$

$$G^* = \sqrt{(G')^2 + (G'')^2} \tag{6.21}$$

$$\eta^* = \frac{G^*}{\omega} \tag{6.22}$$

Typical frequency sweep results are shown in Figure 6.13. The rising tendency of the storage (G') and loss (G'') modules is commonly modeled as a power function of the oscillatory frequency (ω) (Equations 6.23 and 6.24), which is useful for describing the viscoelastic behavior of food and food dispersions (Rao, 1999).

$$G' = k' \cdot \omega^{n'} \tag{6.23}$$

$$G'' = k'' \cdot \omega^{n''} \tag{6.24}$$

Therefore, as neither G' nor G'' are constant properties, the elastic and viscous behaviors of the product can be evaluated by the parameters k' and k'', which describe the magnitude of the elastic and viscous behaviors, and n' and n'', which describe the elastic and viscous behaviors of the product.

In general, the elastic properties of fruit juices and derivatives are more dominant than the viscous properties, as the k' values are higher than the k'' values

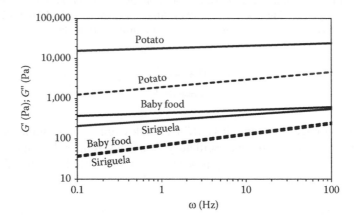

FIGURE 6.13 Some examples of typical frequency sweep results for fruit juices and derivatives: storage (G', continuous lines) and loss (G'', dashed lines) modules of potato puree (20°C; data from Alvarez, M.D., Fernández, C., and Canet, W., *European Food Research Technology*, 218, 544–553, 2004); apple baby food (20°C; data from Ahmed, J. and Ramaswamy, H.S., *Journal of Food Science and Technology*, 44, 579–585, 2007); and siriguela pulp (20°C; data from Augusto, P.E.D., Cristianini, M., and Ibarz, A., *Journal of Food Engineering*, 108, 283–289, 2012a).

(i.e., demonstrating that $G' > G''$), with the exception of clarified and diluted juices (Newtonian products). Moreover, in general, the n' values are lower than the n'' values, demonstrating that in comparison with the elastic behavior, the viscous behavior is more affected by the oscillatory frequency (ω). Therefore, at lower frequencies, representing the product at rest or at very low deformation conditions (as in sedimentation), the product behaves as a solid, while at higher frequencies, representing the flowing condition, it behaves as a fluid. In fact, it well describes the behavior of fruit juices and derivatives.

Dynamic rheological tests are generally conducted using small-amplitude oscillatory measurements, which are nondestructive experiments (Rao, 2005; Dogan and Kokini, 2007). Thus, it is possible to conduct multiple tests on the same sample under different test conditions (Dogan and Kokini, 2007). However, small-amplitude oscillatory measurements have the limitation of not being appropriate in practical processing situations due to their low rates and the strain at which the test is applied (Dogan and Kokini, 2007; Steffe, 1996). For this characterization, steady-state shear experiments must be conducted (Gunasekaran and Ak, 2000). However, steady-state shear experiments have limitations related to slippage and the migration of sample constituents (Gunasekaran and Ak, 2000), which is particularly true in some food products such as fruit juices. Moreover, in these experiments, the internal structure of the sample is broken, limiting the understanding of the product's behavior in low-shear situations, as in particle sedimentation. Dynamic rheological experiments can then be used to characterize those products. Therefore, it is interesting to establish a correlation between steady-state shear and dynamic oscillatory experiments using the so-called Cox–Merz rule.

The Cox–Merz rule states that the apparent viscosity (η_a) at a specific shear rate ($\dot{\gamma}$) is equal to the complex viscosity (η^*) at a specific oscillatory frequency (ω), when $\dot{\gamma} = \omega$ (Equation 6.25; Rao, 1999). Based on the validity of this rule, the rheological properties of food can be determined by oscillatory or steady-state shear experiments (Gunasekaran and Ak, 2000). It is particularly useful due to the characteristics and limitations of each type of experiment.

However, the Cox–Merz rule cannot be directly applied to food products, whose complex viscosity (η^*) magnitudes are, in general, higher than the apparent viscosity (η_a) magnitudes, in the whole oscillatory frequency (ω) and shear rate ($\dot{\gamma}$) ranges. Although the Cox–Merz rule has been confirmed experimentally for several polymeric dispersions and solutions, in complex systems such as food products it is generally necessary to modify the original rule (Gunasekaran and Ak, 2000; Rao, 1999). The nonfitting of the Cox–Merz rule for complex dispersions is attributed to structural decay due to the extensive strain applied (Ahmed and Ramaswamy, 2006), the presence of high-density entanglements, or the development of structure and intermolecular aggregation in a solution (Da Silva and Rao, 1992). Therefore, the rheological oscillatory and steady-state shear properties of foods are generally correlated by linear or nonlinear modifications of the Cox–Merz rule (Gunasekaran and Ak, 2000; Rao, 1999), such as those described in Equations 6.26 and 6.27.

$$\eta^*(\omega) = \eta_a(\dot{\gamma})\big|_{\dot{\gamma}=\omega} \qquad (6.25)$$

$$\eta * (\omega) = \alpha \left[\eta_a(\dot{\gamma}) \right] \Big|_{\dot{\gamma}=\omega} \tag{6.26}$$

$$\eta * (\omega) = \alpha \left[\eta_a(\dot{\gamma}) \right]^{\beta} \Big|_{\dot{\gamma}=\omega} \tag{6.27}$$

6.3.3.2 Viscoelastic Properties: Creep and Recovery Procedure

The creep and recovery experiment is a valuable tool to characterize the behavior of food products. By carrying out creep and recovery experiments, it is possible to describe the rheological behavior of the product using mechanical models and constitutive equations, combining Newton's viscosity equation and Hooke's elasticity equation.

In this experiment, an instantaneous stress (σ—in the sample linear viscoelastic range) is applied to the sample and the change in strain (γ) is measured over time. Then, the stress is instantaneously released and the recovery behavior of the sample is observed (Steffe, 1996). The results are expressed according to the compliance function of time ($J(t)$; Equation 6.28). The elastic, viscous, and viscoelastic behaviors during the creep and recovery procedure are shown in Figure 6.10. Also, Figure 6.14 shows some examples of the typical creep and recovery results for fruit juices and derivatives.

$$J(t) = \frac{\gamma(t)}{\sigma_{\text{applied}}} \tag{6.28}$$

An ideal fluid shows only viscous behavior, which is described by Newton's law (Equation 6.3) and is represented by a dashpot. Thus, its compliance at each instant of

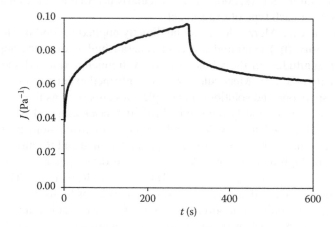

FIGURE 6.14 Example of a typical creep and recovery result for fruit juices and derivatives: tomato juice (4.5°Brix, 25°C). (Data from Augusto, P.E.D., Ibarz, A., and Cristianini, M., *Food Research International*, 54, 169–176, 2013.)

time is described by Equation 6.29. On the other hand, an ideal solid shows only elastic behavior, which is described by Hooke's law (Equation 6.13) and is represented by a spring. Its compliance at each instant of time is described by Equation 6.30.

$$J(t)_{viscous} = \frac{t}{\eta} \tag{6.29}$$

$$J(t)_{elastic} = \frac{1}{G} \tag{6.30}$$

Based on these two fundamental mechanical models (dashpot = ideal fluid = viscous behavior = Newton's law; spring = ideal solid = elastic behavior = Hooke's law), viscoelastic materials can be evaluated and modeled by combining dashpots and springs in a series or in parallel (Figure 6.15). The most used mechanical models are those of Kelvin–Voigt (a Hookean spring and a Newtonian dashpot placed in parallel),

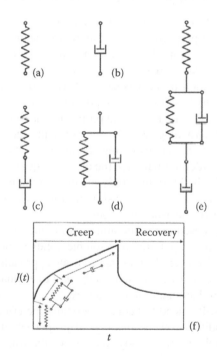

FIGURE 6.15 Mechanical models used to describe the viscoelastic properties of foods: (a) the Hookean spring, (b) the Newtonian dashpot, (c) the Maxwell model, (d) the Kelvin–Voigt model, (e) the Burger model, and (f) a typical creep and recovery plot described by the Burger model. (Adapted from Ibarz, A. and Barbosa-Cánovas, G.V., *Unit Operations in Food Engineering*, CRC Press, Boca Raton, FL, 2003; Rao, M.A., *Rheology of Fluid and Semisolid Foods: Principles and Applications*, Aspen, Gaithersburg, MD, 1999; Steffe, J.F., *Rheological Methods in Food Process Engineering*, 2nd edn., Freeman Press, East Lansing, MI, 1996.)

Maxwell (a Hookean spring and a Newtonian dashpot placed in a series), and Burger (a Kelvin–Voigt model and a Maxwell model placed in a series). Due to the complexity of the product, the Burger model better describes the viscoelasticity of food, and is expressed by Equation 6.31 (Steffe, 1996).

$$J(t)_{\text{Burger}} = \frac{1}{G_0} + \frac{1}{G_1}\left(1 - \exp\left(\frac{-G_1 t}{\eta_1}\right)\right) + \frac{t}{\eta_0} \qquad (6.31)$$

Therefore, by using creep and recovery experiments it is possible to isolate and evaluate the viscous and elastic behaviors of a material, which is an important tool in the evaluation of fruit products.

6.4 EFFECT OF PRODUCT COMPOSITION AND PROCESSING CONDITIONS ON THE RHEOLOGICAL PROPERTIES OF FRUIT JUICES AND DERIVATIVES

As previously described, the parameters that define the rheological behavior of a material are not constant properties, but a function of some processing conditions such as $\dot{\gamma}$, ω, T, and t. Therefore, by selecting the most appropriate procedure, it is possible to characterize and evaluate the properties of the product at the conditions that represent the evaluation process (such as thermal processing, pumping, flow, storage, and consumption). Moreover, it is important to understand how the composition of the product can affect its rheological properties, as well as how a specific unit operation can change the rheological behavior of the product. Therefore, the effect of the product's composition and processing conditions on its rheological properties must be well known in order to guarantee the desirable quality and optimization.

Most of the works in the literature study the effect of some of those parameters on the steady-state shear properties of food, with a few works describing the time-dependent flow and the viscoelastic properties.

The general approach used in the literature is to model the viscosity or apparent viscosity as a function of temperature and soluble solids or pulp contents, even for non-Newtonian fluids. However, the most appropriate approach is to evaluate each of the fundamental parameters (σ_0, k, n) separately, and to evaluate the thixotropy and viscoelasticity of the product in an integrated way.

Therefore, there is still a need to better understand the effect of product composition and process conditions on the rheological properties of food products, with integrated studies correlating the steady-state shear, the time-dependent flow, and the viscoelastic properties with the structure and functions of the product.

The following sections describe the main product composition and the processing effects on the rheological behavior of fruit juices and derivatives.

6.4.1 EFFECT OF PROCESSING CONDITIONS: TEMPERATURE

Temperature is an indirect measure of the internal energy of a product, greatly affecting its rheological properties. Higher temperatures represent a higher level of internal energy, with a greater distance between molecules, which facilitates molecular movement and vibration, leading to less consistency.

This decrease in consistency follows, in general, an exponential function, which is well described by the Arrhenius equation (Equation 6.32, where each parameter A is modeled by a preexponential factor [A_0] and the activation energy [Ea]; R is the constant of the ideal gases; and T is the absolute temperature; Rao, 1999). This mathematical model is successfully used to describe the viscosity (η), apparent viscosity (η_a), yield stress (σ_0), consistency coefficient (k), and the consistency coefficients related to the viscoelastic properties k' and k'' of food products. Figures 6.16 through 6.20 show

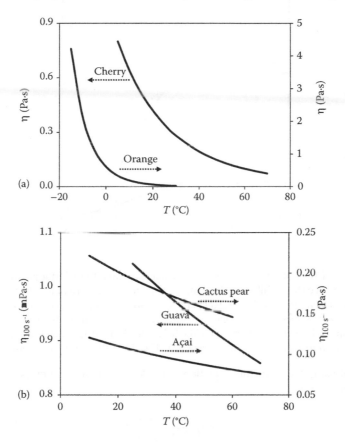

FIGURE 6.16 Effect of temperature on the viscosity (η) or apparent viscosity $\left(\eta_{100\,s^{-1}}\right)$ of fruit juices and derivatives: mathematical description by the Arrhenius equation. (a) Concentrated clarified juices (66°Brix): cherry (data from Giner, J., Ibarz, A., Garza, S., and Xhian-Quan, S., *Journal of Food Engineering*, 30, 147–154, 1996); and orange (data from Ibarz, R., Falguera, V., Garvín, A., Garza, S., Pagan, J., and Ibarz, A., *Journal of Texture Studies*, 40, 445–456, 2009). (b) Pulps and purees: guava (9.8°Brix; data from Vitali, A.A., and Rao, M.A., *Journal of Texture Studies*, 13, 275–289, 1982); cactus pear (16°Brix; data from Augusto, P.E.D., Cristianini, M., and Ibarz, A., *International Journal of Food Engineering*, 7, 14, 2011b); and açai (14% solids; data from Tonon, R.V., Alexandre, D., Hubinger, M.D., and Cunha, R.L., *Journal of Food Engineering*, 92, 425–431, 2009).

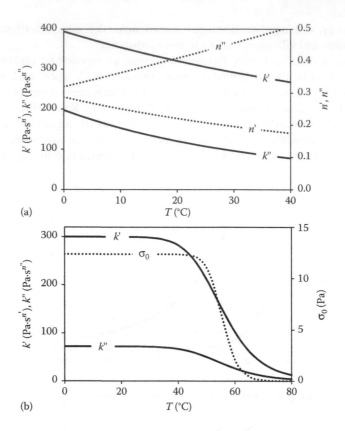

FIGURE 6.17 Effect of temperature on the rheological properties of fruit juices and derivatives. (a) Peach juice (10% of fiber) k', k'', n', and n'' mathematical description using the Arrhenius equation. (Data from Augusto, P.E.D., Falguera, V., Cristianini, M., and Ibarz, A., *International Journal of Food Science and Technology*, 46, 1086–1092, 2011a. With permission.) (b) Siriguela pulp (11°Brix) k', k'', and σ_0 sigmoidal behavior. (From Augusto, P.E.D., Ibarz, A., and Cristianini, M., *Journal of Food Engineering*, 111, 474–477, 2012a. With permission.)

examples of using the Arrhenius equation to model the rheological properties of fruit juices and derivatives.

$$A = A_T \cdot \exp\left(\frac{Ea}{R \cdot T}\right) \tag{6.32}$$

The effect of temperature on the viscoelastic properties of peach juice (clarified + 10% of peach fiber) is shown in Figure 6.17. The parameters k', k'', n', and n'' could be well described by the Arrhenius equation. Moreover, it is interesting to observe that while the values of n' decrease with temperature, the values of n'' show the opposite behavior. These tendencies clearly show that the viscous behavior of the product becomes more important when it is heated.

Figures 6.16a and 6.18b show the rheological behavior of concentrated citrus juices at low temperatures. Citrus juices are concentrated to 60°Brix–66°Brix and

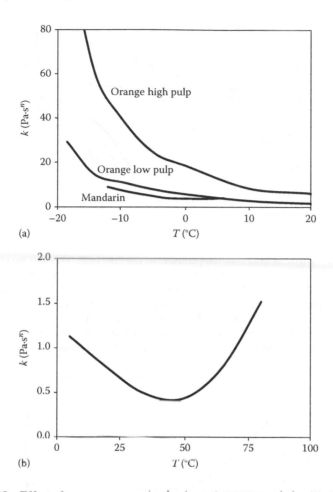

FIGURE 6.18 Effect of temperature on the rheological consistency index (k) of fruit juices and derivatives. (a) Concentrated citrus juice (63°Brix–65°Brix) described by the Arrhenius equation: orange with high pulp content (21%; data from Vitali, A.A., and Rao, M.A., *Journal of Texture Studies*, 13(3), 275–289, 1984); orange with low pulp content (7%; data from Rao, M.A., Cooley, H.J., and Vitali, A.A., *Food Technology*, 38(3), 113–119, 1984); and mandarin (data from Falguera et al., 2010). (b) Sweet potato baby food, with increased consistency due to starch gelatinization. (Data from Ahmed, J., and Ramaswamy, H.S., *Journal of Food Process Engineering*, 29, 219–233, 2006.)

then "frozen" at temperatures close to −18°C for storage and distribution. Clarified orange juice shows a Newtonian behavior, whose viscosity (η) follows the Arrhenius equation (Figure 6.16a). When juice containing pulp is considered, both orange juice and mandarin juice show pseudoplastic behavior, whose consistency coefficient (k) follows the Arrhenius equation (Figure 6.18b), but whose flow behavior index (n) shows a quasi-constant trend.

The flow behavior index (n) is generally assumed to be relatively constant with the temperature (Rao, 1999). However, as the temperature increases, the

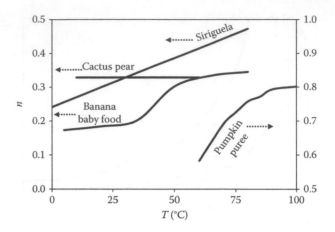

FIGURE 6.19 Different effects of temperature on the flow behavior index (n) of fruit juices and derivatives: siriguela pulp (data from Augusto, P.E.D., Cristianini, M., and Ibarz, A., *Journal of Food Engineering*, 108(2), 283–289, 2012a), cactus pear pulp (data from Augusto, P.E.D., Cristianini, M., and Ibarz, A., *International Journal of Food Engineering*, 7, 14, 2011b), banana baby food (data from Ahmed, J., and Ramaswamy, H.S., *Journal of Food Science and Technology*, 44(6), 579–585, 2007), and pumpkin puree (data from Dutta, D., Dutta, A., Raychaudhuri, U., and Chakraborty, R., *Journal of Food Engineering*, 76, 538–546, 2006).

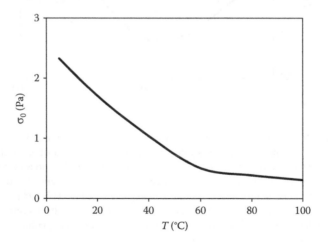

FIGURE 6.20 Effect of temperature on the goldenberry yield stress (σ_0): mathematical description using the Arrhenius equation. (Data from Sharoba, A. and Ramadan, M.F., *Journal of Food Processing and Preservation*, 35, 201–219, 2011.)

molecular mobility yields a product flow behavior index (n) close to unity, as the molecules and particles can be easily aligned (Figure 6.4) and are less susceptible to collision (Figure 6.5). In fact, it is important to observe that the property behavior in relation to the temperature is a function not only of the product itself, but also of the studied temperature range (i.e., the property value can vary slightly at the studied temperature range, which is different from being constant

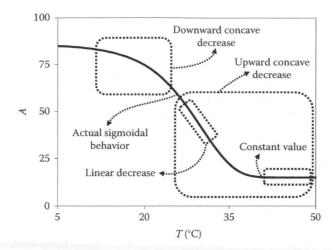

FIGURE 6.21 Effect of temperature on the rheological properties of fruit juices and derivatives. Description of the effect of the studied temperature range on the observed behavior for a generic property A.

in relation to the temperature; Figure 6.21). Thus, at higher temperatures, the shear-thinning behavior of fruit products is less pronounced and an increase in the flow behavior index (n) is observed. When this property is not assumed to be constant, its increase is modeled using the Arrhenius equation or even a linear function (Figure 6.19).

However, other behaviors different from the exponential decay of the Arrhenius equation can be observed. Firstly, due to the studied temperature range, as the observed profile only represents the product's behavior within the evaluated range. Figure 6.21 graphically represents this issue. Secondly, due to the reactions and changes in the structure of the product because of the consequent thermal processes, such as gelling (starch, other biopolymers), vaporization (sample partial drying), melting (lipids, crystals), among others.

Figures 6.17, 6.18, and 6.37 show examples of the rheological properties of fruit products whose behavior in relation to the temperature does not follow the Arrhenius equation. Figure 6.17b shows the results for siriguela (*Spondias purpurea*) pulp, a small native fruit of Central America. The yield stress shows a falling sigmoidal trend in relation to temperature, in contrast with the continuous decrease of the exponential function (Arrhenius equation). Up to 40°C, the yield stress shows quasi-constant values followed by a rapid decrease in the temperature between 40°C and 60°C. Then, it tends to remain at a constant value. This behavior can be described by a power sigmoidal function (Equation 6.33), and shows that an important transformation is carried out in siriguela pulp between 40°C and 60°C, as the changes in the yield stress value are more important at this temperature range. A viscoelastic analysis corroborates this observation, with the parameters k' and k'' showing the same behavior. Therefore, using rheology, structural changes due to thermal processing can be evaluated in this fruit pulp.

$$\sigma_0 = \frac{\alpha}{1+(\beta \cdot T)^\lambda} \qquad (6.33)$$

Figure 6.18b shows the interesting effect of temperature on the sweet potato baby food consistency coefficient (k). The k value shows a decreasing behavior until 50°C, and shows the opposite trend in temperatures higher than 50°C. This is the typical behavior of starch-rich products, such as sweet potato (Figure 6.18) and potato puree (Figure 6.37), as it is related to gelatinization and the consequent increase in consistency. Moreover, it is similar to that observed in products with other polysaccharides and proteins with gelation properties. However, it is the opposite behavior of those products that show a melting behavior related to the heating. Therefore, it reinforces the need for a better understanding of the properties of each food product, which can change during processing.

Finally, as the thermal process is one of the most used methods for food preservation, and as such processes, which are carried out at higher temperatures, are able to guarantee food safety with lower sensory changes and nutritional losses (Augusto et al., 2013b), it highlights the need to conduct more studies regarding the rheological properties of food products at higher temperatures. In fact, due to the difficulty of conducting the experiments (mainly due to water vaporization), there are only a few works in the literature with rheological evaluations at temperatures above 100°C. Rao et al. (1999) needed to place the rheometer inside a retort, while Ros-Polski (2011) developed a pressurized capillary rheometer in order to conduct her experiments. Rao et al. (1999) evaluated the apparent viscosity (η_a) of tomato puree (11°Brix) at between 76°C and 120°C, following the Arrhenius equation (Equation 6.32). On the other hand, Ros-Polski's (2011) evaluation of the apparent viscosity (η_a) of banana puree (22°Brix) deviated from the Arrhenius behavior. Therefore, there is still a need for more rheological studies at higher temperatures.

6.4.2 EFFECT OF PRODUCT PROPERTIES: CONCENTRATION

The concentration of fruit products highly affects their rheological properties. The concentration is a unit operation that is widely used in fruit processing, due to its preservation (reduction of Aw) and logistic (reduction in the product volume and mass, which are important issues for storage and transportation) objectives.

The effect of concentration on the rheological properties of fruit juices and derivatives is exponential, and it is usually described using Equation 6.34 (Ibarz and Barbosa-Cánovas, 2003; Rao, 1999). Figures 6.22 through 6.24 show some examples of using Equation 6.34 for modeling the influence of solids content on the rheological properties of fruit juices and derivatives.

$$A = A_C \cdot \exp(B \cdot C) \qquad (6.34)$$

Figure 6.22 shows the typical effect of concentration on the viscosity (η) or apparent viscosity $\left(\eta_{100\,s^{-1}}\right)$ of fruit juices and derivatives, which can be well modeled by the exponential function of Equation 6.34.

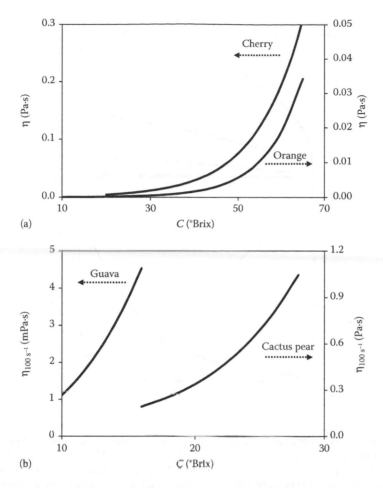

FIGURE 6.22 Effect of concentration on the viscosity (η) or apparent viscosity ($\eta_{100\ L/S}$) of fruit juices and derivatives: mathematical description using an exponential function (Equation 6.34). (a) Concentrated clarified juices (25°C): cherry (data from Giner, J., Ibarz, A., Garza, S., and Xhian-Quan, S., *Journal of Food Engineering*, 30, 147–154, 1996) and orange (data from Ibarz, R., Falguera, V., Garvín, A., Garza, S., Pagan, J., and Ibarz, A., *Journal of Texture Studies*, 40, 445–456, 2009). (b) Pulps and purees: guava (25°C; data from Vitali, A.A. and Rao, M.A., *Journal of Texture Studies*, 13, 275–289, 1982) and cactus pear (25°C; data from Augusto, P.E.D., Cristianini, M., and Ibarz, A., *International Journal of Food Engineering*, 7, 14, 2011b).

In fact, most of the works in the literature only study the effect of concentration on the viscosity or apparent viscosity of fruit products, even for non-Newtonian fluids. It is important to highlight once more that the most appropriate approach is to evaluate each of the fundamental parameters (σ_0, k, n) separately, as well as the thixotropy and viscoelasticity of the product.

Figure 6.23 shows the flow curves (shear stress as a function of shear rate) of ready-to-drink peach juice (12.3°Brix) with the addition of 0% (i.e., the clarified and depectinized peach juice) to 10% of peach fiber. It is interesting to note that not only

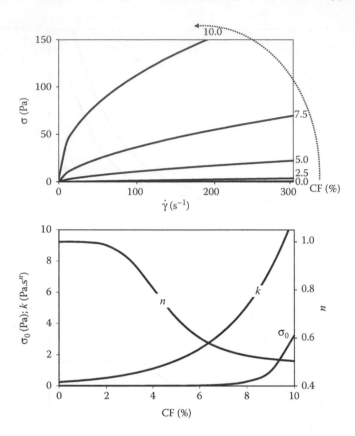

FIGURE 6.23 Effect of fiber concentration (CF in percentage) on the rheological properties of peach juice (20°C; Augusto, P.E.D., Falguera, V., Cristianini, M., Ibarz, A., *International Journal of Food Science and Technology*, 46, 1086–1092, 2011a. With permission). Flow profile and parameters of the Herschel–Bulkley model: k and σ_0 are described by an exponential function (Equation 6.34), and n is described by a sigmoidal function.

is the consistency changed but also the product flow behavior is changed due to the addition of the fiber. Juices pass from a Newtonian (CF = 0.0%) to a pseudoplastic behavior (CF = 2.5%–7.5%), and then to an HB behavior (CF = 10.0%).

The influence of the addition of peach fiber on the rheological behavior of the product can be explained by the interactions among the different polysaccharides that are present in peach fiber, as well as the interactions among polysaccharides and the natural sugars and acids of peach juice. The peach fiber composition is typical of vegetable products, reflecting the vegetable cell wall components, containing soluble and insoluble fractions with cellulose, hemicelluloses, lignin, and pectic substances. Thus, the obtained products can be described as insoluble polymer clusters and chains dispersed in a viscous medium composed of soluble polysaccharides, sugars, and acids.

This model explains the shear-thinning (Figure 6.23) and viscoelastic behaviors (Figure 6.26) of the obtained products, as well as the observed effect of the fiber concentration on the rheological properties of the products (Rao, 1999).

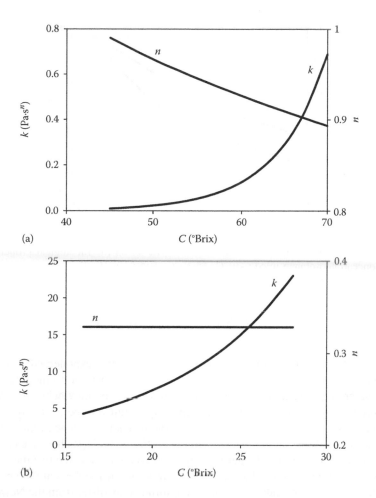

FIGURE 6.24 Effect of concentration on the rheological properties of fruit products (25°C). (a) k and n are described by an exponential function (Equation 6.34) in *M. floribunda* juice. (Data from Cepeda, E., Villarán, M.C., and Ibarz, A., *Journal of Texture Studies*, 30, 481–491, 1999.) (b) k is described by Equation 6.34 and n is a constant in cactus pear pulp. (Data from Augusto, P.E.D., Cristianini, M., and Ibarz, A., *International Journal of Food Engineering*, 7, 14, 2011b.)

In fact, the soluble and insoluble solids present in fruit products can have a different impact on the rheology of the product. Figure 6.25 shows the effect of pulp concentration on the rheological properties of frozen concentrated orange juice, considering the same soluble solids content (65°Brix). Moreover, Equation 6.35 describes the influence of the soluble solids concentration ($C_{\text{soluble\_solids}}$) and pectin ($C_{\text{pectin}}$) on the serum viscosity of tomato (Tanglertpaibul and Rao, 1987). It is interesting to note the parameters $\lambda < 1.0$ and $\psi > 1.0$ in Equation 6.35. This demonstrates that the increase in the soluble solids content results in a downward concave increase in the serum viscosity, with an asymptotic behavior (i.e., a maximum value). On the other hand, the pectin concentration results in an upward concave increase in the serum viscosity.

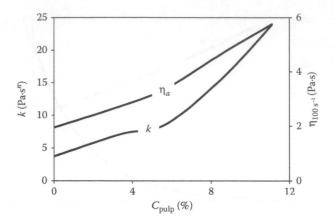

FIGURE 6.25 Effect of pulp concentration (C_{pulp} in %) on the rheological properties of frozen concentrated orange juice (−10°C, 65°Brix; data from Vitali, A.A. and Rao, M.A., *Journal of Texture Studies*, 13(3), 275–289, 1984).

$$\eta_{serum} = \alpha + \beta \cdot \left(C_{soluble\_solids} \right)^{\lambda} \cdot \left(C_{pectin} \right)^{\psi} \qquad (6.35)$$

Although the increase in the concentration of the product exponentially increases the consistency index (k) and yield stress (σ_0) of the product due to the interactions among the product constituents (Figures 6.23 and 6.24), the flow behavior index (n) once more shows a particular trend. It is generally assumed to be relatively constant with concentration (Rao, 1999), which is only true in a narrow-range evaluation (note that it is a similar discussion to that carried out on Figure 6.21), such as in cactus pear between 16°Brix and 28°Brix (Figure 6.24b). However, it is expected that the increase in the concentration of the product results in changes in the rheological fluid behavior (i.e., in the flow behavior index, n), whose magnitude may differ from the Newtonian flow. Therefore, the flow behavior index (n) tends to be reduced due to the concentration of the product, increasing the shear-thinning behavior of the fruit product.

Figure 6.23 shows the particular trend of the flow behavior index (n) when peach fiber is added to clarified peach juice. In contrast with the continuous decrease of an exponential function, it shows a sigmoidal behavior. When the fiber amount is relatively low, n shows quasi-constant values, close to the initial Newtonian behavior (i.e., $n = 1$), followed by a significant decrease in the concentrations of the intermediate fiber. Then, for relatively high amounts of fiber, the flow behavior index tends to remain constant. This behavior can be described by a power sigmoidal function (Equation 6.36).

$$n = \alpha + \frac{1 - \alpha}{1 + \left(\beta \cdot C \right)^{\lambda}} \qquad (6.36)$$

Although the expected behavior is similar to the observed behavior in the steady-state shear properties, there is still a need to better understand the effect of the

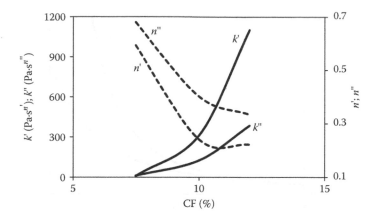

FIGURE 6.26 Effect of fiber concentration (CF in %) on the viscoelastic properties of peach juice (20°C; data from Augusto, P.E.D., Falguera, V., Cristianini, M., and Ibarz, A., *International Journal of Food Science and Technology*, 46, 1086–1092, 2011a).

concentration of the product on the viscoelastic and time-dependent properties of food products. In fact, this is partially shown by the addition of peach fiber in peach juice (Figure 6.26). However, more studies should be carried out to better describe the viscoelastic and time-dependent properties.

The effect of temperature and concentration can be modeled by combining the Arrhenius equation (Equation 6.32) with the exponential function of the concentration (Equation 6.34). The derived function is shown in Equation 6.37, which is extensively used to model the combined effect of concentration and temperature on the rheological behavior of fruit products (Ibarz and Barbosa-Cánovas, 2003; Rao, 1999).

$$\Lambda = \Lambda_{IC}\ \exp\left(B\ C + \frac{Ea}{R \cdot T}\right) \tag{6.37}$$

Fruit juices are dispersions, composed of an insoluble phase (the pulp) dispersed in a viscous solution (the serum). The dispersed phase or pulp is made up of fruit tissue cells and their fragments, cell walls, and insoluble polymer clusters and chains. The serum is an aqueous solution of soluble polysaccharides, sugars, salts, and acids. The rheological properties of fruit juices are thus defined by the interactions inside and between each phase.

The relative viscosity (η_r, Equation 6.38) of a dilute solid particle dispersed in a liquid medium is described by the Einstein equation (Equation 6.39; Genovese et al., 2007; Metzner, 1985), considering rigid noninteractive particles. Thus, the viscosity of the dispersion is affected by the continuous phase viscosity (the juice serum), the particle intrinsic viscosity ($[\eta]$—which depends on the particle shape), and the particle volume fraction (ϕ). Therefore, the concentration of fruit products results in higher volume fractions (ϕ) and, consequently, higher viscosities.

However, the linear relationship described by the Einstein equation (Equation 6.39) is only valid for dilute dispersions, which, in general, is not the case for fruit products.

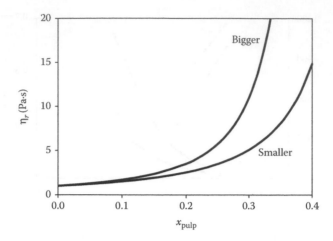

FIGURE 6.27 Effect of concentration (as the mass fraction of pulp—x_{pulp}) and particle size (Bigger and smaller) on the relative viscosity of tomato concentrate. (From Yoo, B. and Rao, M. A., *Journal of Texture Studies*, 25(4), 421–436, 1994. With permission.)

Moreover, one of the most used models derived for concentrated dispersions is the Krieger–Dougherty equation (Equation 6.40; Genovese et al., 2007), which is more appropriate to describe the rheology of fruit products. According to this equation, the viscosity of the dispersion is also affected by the particle maximum packing fraction of solids (ϕ_m), showing an abrupt increase at $\phi \approx \phi_m$. In fact, it explains the effect of concentration on the rheological properties of fruit products, which is exemplified in Figure 6.27 for tomato concentrates.

$$\eta_r = \frac{\eta_{dispersion}}{\eta_{continuous\_phase}} \tag{6.38}$$

$$\eta_r = 1 + [\eta] \cdot \phi \tag{6.39}$$

$$\eta_r = \left(1 - \frac{\phi}{\phi_m}\right)^{-[\eta] \cdot \phi_m} \tag{6.40}$$

However, it is important to highlight that the suspended particles of fruit products are not rigid and noninteractive particles, which can deviate the actual rheological behavior from those stated in Equations 6.38 through 6.40. Nevertheless, those equations are very useful in order to understand the role of solids concentration on rheological properties.

6.4.3 EFFECT OF PRODUCT PROPERTIES: COMPOSITION

The natural and industrial composition of food products highly affects their rheological properties. The cell wall and intracellular material composition define the shape and properties of the suspended particles, as well as the pH and charge of the product. Moreover, the addition of ingredients during processing can change the properties of the product. For example, the addition of hydrocolloids in fruit products is very common to minimize the pulp sedimentation and increase the sensorial acceptance of the product. Therefore, the intrinsic characteristics of the material composition and those changed due to the ingredients added during processing define the final product's behavior.

The composition and morphological characteristics of cell tissues, which are related to the intrinsic composition or changes during processing, will dictate the interparticle interactions among the suspended particles, as well as the alignment behavior under flow (Figure 6.4). Products with a broader particle size distribution (PSD), for example, show less consistency than those with a narrower distribution. This is related to the lubricant effect of small particles over larger particles, with a consequent small resistance to flow (Servais et al., 2002). Moreover, particles with smooth surfaces and more regular shapes flow more easily than those with rough surfaces and irregular shapes. However, the rheology of the final product cannot be simply described by the hydrodynamic forces and the PSD of the product.

A reduction in the size of the suspended particles can improve interparticle interaction, since the particle surface area is greatly increased. The interaction of small particles can be due to the van der Waals (Genovese et al., 2007; Tsai and Zammouri, 1988) and electrostatic forces because of the interaction between the negatively charged pectins and the positively charged proteins (Takada and Nelson, 1983; Figure 6.28). Thus, for small particles, the Peclet number (Equation 6.6) of the product is small and the system approximates to the Brownian domain. In the Brownian domain, both the electrostatic and van der Waals forces can dictate the interparticle interactions, while only the hydrodynamic forces dictate those interactions at higher Peclet numbers. Therefore, it is possible to observe higher values of consistency at intermediary particle sizes, with a less consistent product with higher and smaller particle sizes.

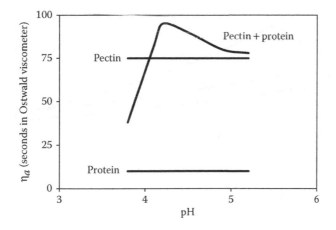

FIGURE 6.28   Effect of pH on the apparent viscosity (measured using an Ostwald viscometer) of pectins and proteins solutions. (From Takada, N. and Nelson, P.E., *Journal of Food Science*, 48(5), 1408–1411, 1983. With permission.)

For example, the effect of the particle mean size on the rheological behavior of the jabuticaba pulp is shown in Figure 6.29, which clearly shows a maximum consistency index (k) at intermediary particle sizes. Moreover, the effect of ripening on the apparent viscosity of pineapple is shown in Figure 6.30. Due to enzymatic activity during ripening, with the consequent cell disruption, breaking of clusters and polysaccharide chains, and changes to pectin charges, the consistency of the juice is decreased. This reinforces the differences in the rheology of fruit products due to their intrinsic characteristics.

Therefore, the addition of acidulants to fruit products, a widely used technique to reduce the pH, microbial growth, and enzyme activity of the product,

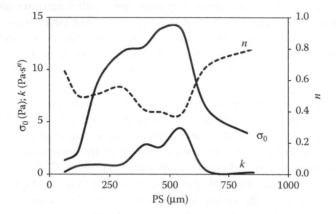

FIGURE 6.29 Effect of particle mean size (PS) on the rheological behavior of jabuticaba pulp (14% solids, 25°C). (Data from Sato, A.C.K. and Cunha, R.L., *Journal of Food Engineering*, 91, 566–570, 2009.)

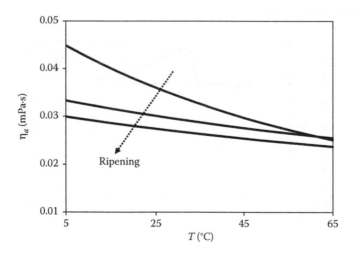

FIGURE 6.30 Effect of ripening and temperature on the apparent viscosity of pineapple. (4.3°Brix; data from Shamsudin, R., Daud, W.R.W., Takrif, M.S., Hassan, O., and Ilicali, C., *International Journal of Food Science and Technology*, 44, 757–762, 2009.)

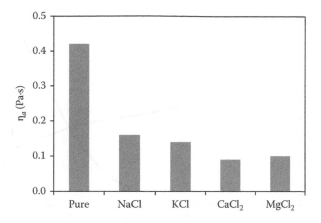

FIGURE 6.31 Effect of salt addition (1% of NaCl, KCl, CaCl$_2$, and MgCl$_2$) on the apparent viscosity of *Lepidium perfoliatum* seed gum solution (46.16 s^{-1} and 25°C; data from Koocheki, A., Taherian, A.R., and Bostan, A., *Food Research International*, 50, 446–456, 2013).

can also affect the final rheology due to the electrostatic interactions of the particle. Figure 6.28 shows the effect of pH on the apparent viscosity of pectins and proteins solutions, simulating the interactions on fruit juices. It can be seen that, although the pH has no effect on either the pectin or the protein solutions when isolated, it significantly changes the viscosity of the solution containing both molecules.

Similarly, the addition of salt, as well as the addition of ingredients with electric charge, can significantly change the rheology of the fruit products. For example, Figure 6.31 shows the effect of various salt additions on the apparent viscosity of a seed gum solution.

Similar behavior can be seen by the naturally present polysaccharides of fruit or those added as hydrocolloids. Hydrocolloids are water-soluble gums that are extensively used as thickening and gelling agents in food products.

Figure 6.32 shows the effect of the addition of starch to the steady-state shear and viscoelastic properties of grape juice concentrates. The addition of starch greatly increases the consistency of the juice (k, k', and k''), with a higher effect on the elastic behavior (k') of the product due to the gelatinization of the starch.

Figures 6.33 and 6.34 show the effects of the addition of xanthan gum, guar gum, locust bean gum (LBG), carboxymethylcellulose (CMC), and pectin on the rheology of fruit juices. Although the effect of increasing the consistency and pseudoplastic behavior of fruit juices is clear, it is interesting to note the complex behavior, which is different for each fruit product, and cannot be predicted without an entire evaluation. Moreover, due to possible interactions with other components (as in Figures 6.28 and 6.31) and different pHs (as in Figure 6.28), the addition of hydrocolloids to fruit products must be evaluated for each situation. Therefore, there is still a need for more rheological studies regarding the composition effects on the rheology of fruit products.

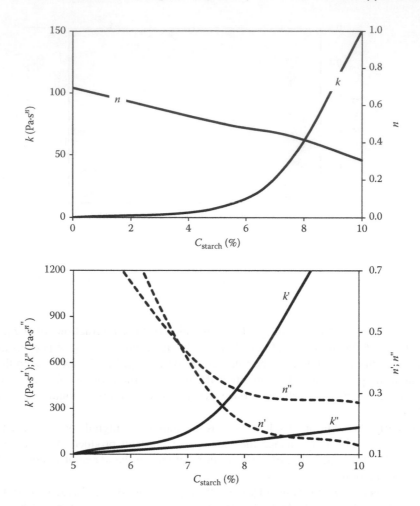

FIGURE 6.32 Effect of starch addition (C_{starch}) on the steady-state shear and viscoelastic properties of grape juice concentrates (60°C; data from Goksel, M., Dogan, M., Toker, O.S., Ozgen, S., Sarioglu, K., and Oral, R.A., *Food and Bioprocess Technology*, 6, 259–271, 2013.)

6.4.4 EFFECT OF UNIT OPERATIONS AND PROCESSING

Understanding the impact of each of the unit operations that are used in the rheology of the final product is important to guarantee optimum properties. During processing, the fruit tissues and cells are disrupted and fragmented, which not only increases the surface area of the suspended particles, but it also changes the properties of the particles and serum. Cell fragmentation exposes and releases the cell wall constituents, such as pectins and proteins, improving the particle–particle and particle–serum interactions. Moreover, the aspect ratio, shape, and other characteristics of the suspended particles are changed, as well as their mean diameter and their PSD. Once the internal constituents of the cell are released and put together, chemical and biochemical changes are also induced, due to enzyme activity and also

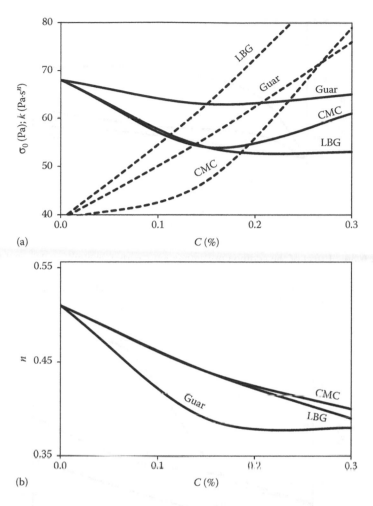

FIGURE 6.33 Effect of the addition of guar gum, carboxymethylcellulose (CMC), and locust bean gum (LBG) on the steady-state shear properties of model fruit juices (25°C): consistency index (a, dashed curves), yield stress (a, continuous curves), and flow behavior index (b). (Data from Wei, Y.P., Wang, C.S., and Wu, J.S.B., *Food Research International*, 34, 377–381, 2001).

chemical reactions catalyzed by the temperature, modifying the properties of pectins, proteins, and others. Therefore, the rheology of the product is also changed, which modifies how the product behaves during processing, storage, and consumption.

Figure 6.35 shows the effect of finisher operation parameters (rotational speed and sieve dimension) on the consistency of tomato juice. Pulping is one of the first unit operations used in fruit processing, which is conducted to eliminate skin and seeds from the product pulp. However, it not only separates these two fractions, but it also selects the shape and dimensions of the suspended particles of pulp. As consistency is one of the most important properties in tomato products, it is clear in Figure 6.35 that there are optimum values for the sieve dimension (1.0 mm) and the rotational speed (500 rpm; up to this value an asymptotic behavior is shown).

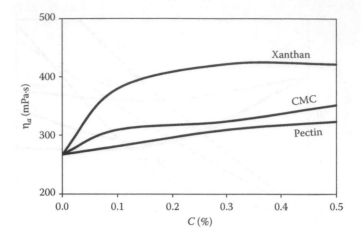

FIGURE 6.34 Effect of the addition of xanthan gum, carboxymethylcellulose (CMC), and pectin on the apparent viscosity of apple juice (437.4 s⁻¹, 25°C; data from Ibrahim, G.E., Hassan, M.I., Abd-Elrashid, A.M., El-Massry, K.F., Eh-Ghorab, A.E., Manal, M.R., and Osman, F., *Food Hydrocolloids*, 25, 91–97, 2011).

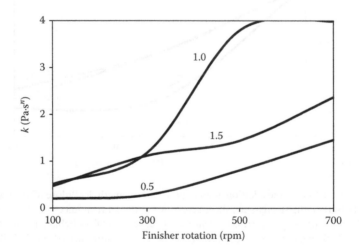

FIGURE 6.35 Effect of rotational speed and sieve dimensions (0.5–1.5 mm) on the consistency of tomato juice. (Data from Noomhorm, A. and Tansakul, A., *Journal of Food Process Engineering*, 15(4), 229–239, 1992.)

Therefore, each process step can change the rheological behavior of the final product, and even the most simple unit operation must be evaluated in order to obtain a final product with optimum characteristics.

When food products are frozen, some of their cells are disrupted due to ice crystals that form during the freezing process. This cell disruption is inversely proportional to the freezing rate. When the cells are disrupted, the cell wall fragments and the internal constituents of the cell are released, which changes the rheology of the

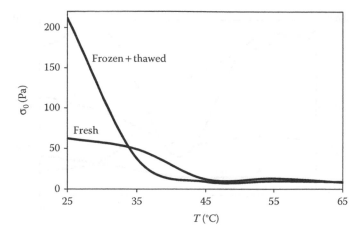

FIGURE 6.36 Effect of freezing and temperature on the yield stress of potato puree (σ_0, 18.5%–20.5% solids, 25°C; data from Canet, W., Alvarez, M.D., Fernández, C., and Luna, P., *Journal of Food Engineering*, 68, 143–153, 2005.)

product. Figures 6.36 and 6.37 show these changes to potato puree. The structures and components of the product are changed, which can be observed by the different behavior of the product when heated. The typical gelatinization profile of starch-based products (i.e., the k' behavior shown in Figure 6.37a) is lost, suggesting modifications to the starch granules. This highlights the potential for using rheology as a tool to study the microstructure and functions of food.

The thermal process can also change the rheology of a product. The consistency of the product can be improved due to gelation, but it can also be reduced due to pectin damage (as the molecules are heated at a low pH). Also, tissues and cells can be disrupted due to thermal or nonthermal effects, such as the shear stresses that the product is submitted to when pumped through heat exchangers. For example, Figure 6.38 shows the increase in the consistency of pineapple juice due to thermal processing.

The rheology of the product can also change during storage due to interactions among different components, such as the increase in the dispersion consistency of lemon fiber shown in Figure 6.39. In fact, age gelation is a well-known phenomenon in products containing soluble fibers and hydrocolloids and, in some cases, proteins.

The impact of new technologies (also called emerging technologies) must also be acknowledged. Figures 6.38, 6.40 through 6.46 show the effect of UV, PEF, high-pressure homogenization (HPH), ultrasound, and irradiation processing on the rheological properties of fruit juices and polysaccharides.

It is interesting to note that each fruit product can behave differently with the different processes. In fact, this is expected due to the particular configuration of tissues, cells, and components, which result in different resistances and reactivities. For example, Figure 6.40 shows the increase in the consistency of tomato juice due to PEF processing, the opposite behavior to strawberry juice. Moreover, Figures 6.41 through 6.43 show the increase in the viscous and elastic behaviors of tomato juice

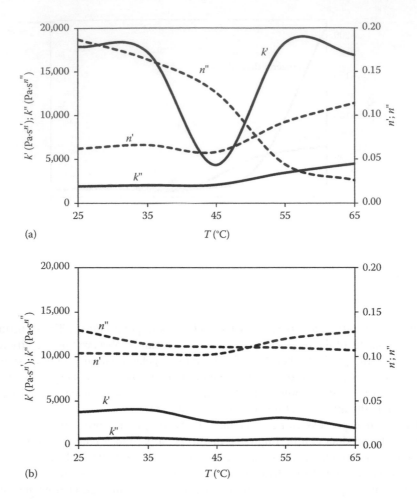

FIGURE 6.37 Effect of freezing process and temperature on the viscoelastic properties of potato puree (18.5%–20.5% solids, 25°C): (a) fresh potato puree; (b) frozen and thawed puree. (Data from Alvarez, M.D., Fernández, C., and Canet, W., *European Food Research Technology*, 218, 544–553, 2004.)

due to HPH processing, the opposite behavior to cashew apple juice. This highlights once more the need to evaluate each fruit product independently, and that it is not possible to predict a general behavior.

In HPH studies with tomato juice (Augusto et al., 2012c, 2013a; Kubo et al., 2013), it was shown that the HPH process disrupts the tomato cells and greatly changes their rheological behavior. Whereas the original juice is composed of whole cells, with intact membranes and their characteristic lycopene crystals, the homogenized samples just show a large amount of small particles, composed of cell walls and internal constituents suspended in the juice serum. As expected and confirmed by a PSD analysis, the suspended particles are smaller at higher homogenization pressure values, highlighting the effect of HPH in disrupting the fruit pulp particles

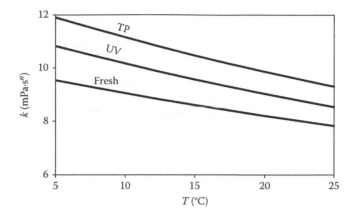

FIGURE 6.38 Effect of temperature, thermal process (TP), and ultraviolet processing (UV) on the consistency of pineapple juice (14°Brix; data from Shamsudin, R., Daud, W.R.W., Takrif, M.S., Hassan, O., and Ilicali, C., *International Journal of Food Science and Technology*, 44, 757–762, 2013).

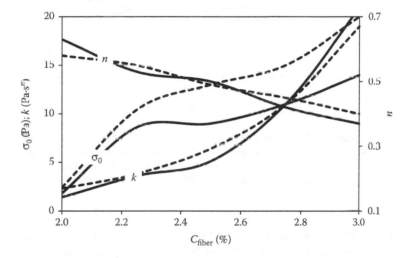

FIGURE 6.39 Effect of concentration and storage time (continuous curves: 24 h of preparation; dashed curves: after 20 days) on the steady-state shear properties of lemon fiber dispersion. (Data from Córdoba, A., Camacho, M.M., and Martínez-Navarrete, N., *Food and Bioprocess Technology*, 5, 1083–1092, 2012.)

and reducing their Peclet number (Equation 6.6). Therefore, highly interactive forces increase the viscous and elastic behaviors of the product (Figures 6.41 and 6.42), resulting in the aggregation of small particles, forming a network. When sheared, these aggregates are broken, reducing the product's resistance to deformation (thixotropic behavior; Figure 6.8). Thus, the HPH process increases the thixotropy of tomato juice (Figure 6.41). Moreover, the changes in the rheology of tomato juice

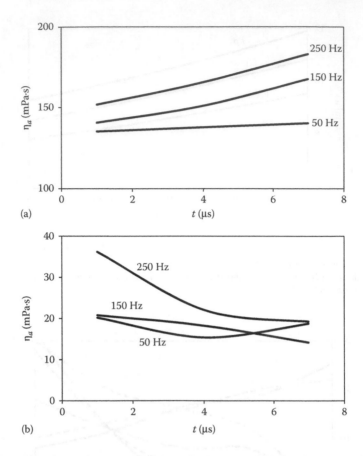

FIGURE 6.40 Effect of frequency and time of pulsed electric field (PEF) processing on the apparent viscosity of juices: (a) tomato juice (4.2°Brix); (b) strawberry juice (7.2°Brix). (Data from Aguiló-Aguayo, I., Soliva-Fortuny, R., and Martín-Belloso, O., *International Journal of Food Science and Technology*, 44, 2268–2277, 2009.)

result in a small reduction in particle sedimentation and serum separation, and an increase in its consistency, which improves its sensory acceptance, thereby reducing the need for the addition of hydrocolloids.

On the other hand, cashew apple juice shows a reduction in consistency due to the HPH process (Figure 6.43, Leite et al., 2013), which is similar behavior to pineapple pulp (Silva et al., 2010). This reduction is explained by the differences in the juice's tissues, cell composition, and shape. When the cashew apple juice is processed by HPH, the consequent cell disruption results in particles with a less rough shape and a considerable amount of very small particles, whose resistance to flow is smaller than the original product (Leite et al., 2013).

Additionally, Figures 6.44 through 6.46 show the reduction in the consistency of polysaccharides due to HPH, ultrasound, and irradiation processing, mainly related

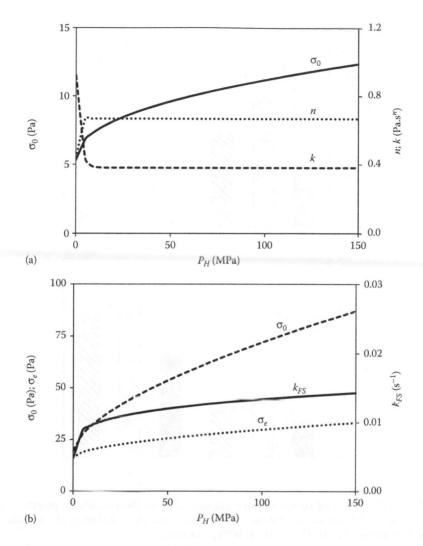

FIGURE 6.41 Effect of homogenization pressure (P_H) on the rheology of tomato juice (4.5°Brix): (a) steady-state shear properties (Herschel–Bulkley model); (b) time-dependent flow (Figoni–Shoemaker model). (From Augusto, P.E.D., Ibarz, A., and Cristianini, M., *Journal of Food Engineering*, 111(4), 570–579, 2012c. With permission.)

to a reduction in their molecular weight (Harte and Venegas, 2010). The results for polysaccharides are important not only considering their use as hydrocolloids in fruit juices, but also as their behaviour is similar to the behavior expected and observed for the juice serum (Augusto et al., 2012b). Moreover, the results highlight the potential for using rheological procedures to evaluate the changes in the molecular weight of polysaccharides, as their intrinsic viscosity ([η]) depends only on the dimensions of their chains (Rao, 1999).

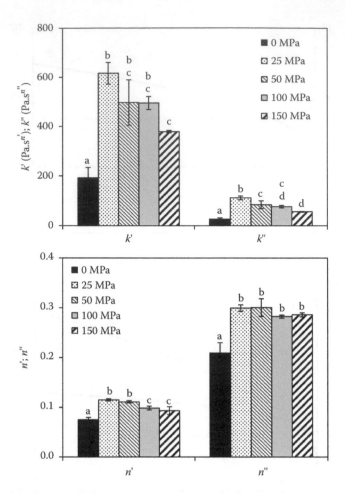

FIGURE 6.42 Effect of homogenization pressure (P_H) on the viscoelastic properties of tomato juice (4.5°Brix). (From Augusto, P.E.D., Ibarz, A., and Cristianini, M., *Journal of Food Engineering*, 114(1), 57–63, 2013a. With permission.)

6.5 CONCLUSIONS

Fruit juices and derivatives are complex products, whose rheological properties are important to guarantee process and product optimization. Fruit products show a complex rheology, described by non-Newtonian behavior, with time-dependent, shear-thinning, and viscoelastic properties. Therefore, the effect of the composition and processing conditions on those properties must be suitably evaluated and known to guarantee high-quality products.

Moreover, each vegetal product shows a different behavior in relation to its processing, which highlights the need to evaluate each fruit product independently, and that it is not possible to predict a general behavior. Therefore, there is still a need

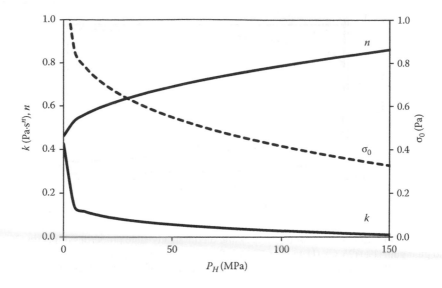

FIGURE 6.43 Effect of homogenization pressure (P_H) on the steady-state shear properties of cashew apple juice (10°Brix) (Herschel–Bulkley model). (Data from Leite, T.S., Augusto, P.E.D., and Cristianini, M., Effect of high pressure homogenization on microstructure of cashew apple juice. In: *Proceedings of the International Nonthermal Food Processing Workshop: Research and Innovation towards Competitiveness*, 2013.)

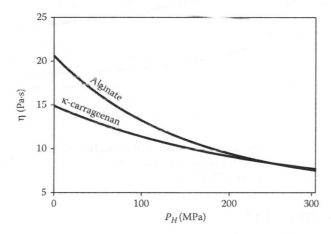

FIGURE 6.44 Effect of homogenization pressure (P_H) on the viscosity of alginate (0.3%) and κ-carrageenan (0.2%) (25°C; data from Harte, F. and Venegas, R., *Journal of Texture Studies*, 41, 49–61, 2010).

to better understand the effect of product composition and process conditions on the rheological properties of food products, with integrated studies correlating the steady-state shear, the time-dependent flow, and the viscoelastic properties with the structure and functions of the product. In fact, rheology has been shown to be an interesting tool to conduct those studies.

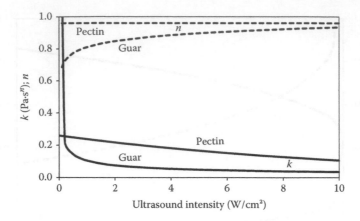

FIGURE 6.45 Effect of ultrasound processing on the steady-state properties of pectin (2%) and guar gum (1%) (25°C). (Data from Tiwari, B.K., Muthukumarappan, K., O'Donnell, C.P., and Cullen, P.J., *International Journal of Food Properties*, 13(2), 223–233, 2010).

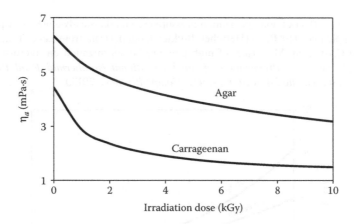

FIGURE 6.46 Effect of irradiation processing on the steady-state properties of agar (1%, 60°C) and carrageenan (1%) (50°C). (Data from Aliste, A.J., Vieira, F.F., and Mastro, N.L.D., *Radiation Physics and Chemistry,* 57, 305–308, 2000.)

6.6 NOMENCLATURE

$\alpha, \beta, \lambda, \psi$	general constant values used in functions that describe rheological parameters (–)
γ	strain (–)
$\dot{\gamma}$	shear rate (Equation 6.2) (s^{-1})
δ	phase angle (–)
$\tan \delta$	loss tangent (Equation 6.20) (–)
ϕ	particle volume fraction (–)
ϕ_m	maximum packing fraction of solids (–)

η	viscosity (Equation 6.3) (Pa·s)
η_a	apparent viscosity (Equation 6.4) (Pa·s)
η_p	plastic viscosity in the Bingham model (Equation 6.7) (Pa·s)
η_r	relative viscosity (Equation 6.38) (Pa·s)
η_0	initial viscosity in the Falguera–Ibarz model (Equation 6.9) (Pa·s)
η_∞	equilibrium viscosity in the Falguera–Ibarz model (Equation 6.9) (Pa·s)
η^*	complex viscosity (Equation 6.22) (Pa·s)
$[\eta]$	intrinsic viscosity (Pa·s)
σ	shear stress (Equation 6.1) (Pa)
σ_0	yield stress, HB and Bingham models (Equations 6.7 and 6.8) (Pa)
σ_0	initial stress in the Figoni–Shoemaker model (Equation 6.10) (Pa)
σ_e	equilibrium stress in the Figoni–Shoemaker and Hahn–Ree–Eyring models (Equations 6.10 and 6.12) (Pa)
ω	oscillatory frequency (Hz)
A	a general rheological variable (f(variable))
A_C	preexponential parameter related to the effect of concentration (Equation 6.33) (f(variable))
A_{HRE}	structural parameter in the Hahn–Ree–Eyring model (Equation 6.12) (Pa)
A_T	Arrhenius's preexponential parameter model (Equation 6.32) (f(variable))
A_{TC}	preexponential parameter related to the effect of temperature and concentration (Equation 6.34) (f(variable))
A_W	structural parameter in the Weltman model (Equation 6.11) (Pa)
B	factor related to the effect of concentration (Equation 6.33) (C^{-1})
B_{HRE}	kinetic parameter in the Hahn–Ree–Eyring model (Equation 6.12) (Pa·s^{-1})
B_W	kinetic parameter in the Weltman model (Equation 6.11) (Pa·s^{-1})
C	product concentration (°Brix, %, –)
Ea	activation energy in Arrhenius's model (Equation 6.32) (J·mol^{-1})
G	elastic modulus (Equation 6.13) (Pa)
G_0	instantaneous elastic modulus, associated with the Maxwell spring (Equation 6.31) (Pa)
G_1	retarded elastic modulus, associated with the Kelvin–Voigt spring (Equation 6.31) (Pa)
G'	storage modulus (Equation 6.18) (Pa)
G''	loss modulus (Equation 6.19) (Pa)
G^*	complex modulus (Equation 6.21) (Pa)
J	compliance (Equation 6.28) (Pa^{-1})
J_∞	residual compliance corresponding to the permanent deformation of the Maxwell dashpot (Equation 6.31) (Pa^{-1})

J_{KV} recovery compliance due to the Kelvin–Voigt element (Equation 6.31) (Pa^{-1})

k consistency coefficient, HB and Ostwald–de Waele models (Equations 6.5 and 6.8) ($Pa \cdot s^n$)

k', k'' consistency coefficient in power law model of viscoelastic properties (Equations 6.23 and 6.24) ($Pa \cdot s^{n'}$, $Pa \cdot s^{n''}$)

k_B Boltzmann constant ($= 1.38 \cdot 10^{-23}$ J K^{-1})

k_{FS} kinetic parameter in the Figoni–Shoemaker model (Equation 6.10) (s^{-1})

k_{FI} viscosity decrease parameter in the Falguera–Ibarz model (Equation 6.9) (–)

n flow behavior index, HB and Ostwald–de Waele models (Equations 6.5 and 6.8) (–)

n', n'' behavior index in power law model of viscoelastic properties (Equations 6.23 and 6.24) (–)

Pe Peclet number (Equation 6.6) (–)

R constant of the ideal gases ($= 8.314$ Pa m^3 mol^{-1} K^{-1})

$\bar{r}_{particle}$ mean suspended particle radius (m)

t time (s)

T absolute temperature (K)

x mass fraction (–)

REFERENCES

Aguiló-Aguayo, I., Soliva-Fortuny, R., Martín-Belloso, O. (2009). Changes in viscosity and pectolytic enzymes of tomato and strawberry juices processed by high-intensity pulsed electric fields. *International Journal of Food Science and Technology*, 44, 2268–2277.

Ahmed, J., Ramaswamy, H. S. (2006). Viscoelastic and thermal characteristics of vegetable puree-based baby foods. *Journal of Food Process Engineering*, 29, 219–233.

Ahmed, J., Ramaswamy, H. S. (2007). Dynamic and steady shear rheology of fruit puree based baby foods. *Journal of Food Science and Technology*, 44(6), 579–585.

Aliste, A. J., Vieira, F. F., Mastro, N. L. D. (2000). Radiation effects on agar, alginates and carrageenan to be used as food additives. *Radiation Physics and Chemistry*, 57, 305–308.

Altan, A., Kus, S., Kaya, A. (2005). Rheological behaviour and time dependent characterization of gilaboru juice (*Viburnum opulus* L.). *Food Science and Technology International*, 11(2), 129–137.

Alvarez, M. D., Fernández, C., Canet, W. (2004). Rheological behavior of fresh and frozen potato puree in steady and dynamic shear at different temperatures. *European Food Research Technology*, 218, 544–553.

Augusto, P. E. D., Falguera, V., Cristianini, M., Ibarz, A. (2011a). Influence of fibre addition on the rheological properties of peach juice. *International Journal of Food Science and Technology*, 46, 1086–1092.

Augusto, P. E. D., Cristianini, M., Ibarz, A. (2011b). Using the Mitschka-Briggs-Steffe method for evaluation of cactus pear concentrated pulps rheological behavior. *International Journal of Food Engineering*, 7, 14.

Augusto, P. E. D., Cristianini, M., Ibarz, A. (2012a). Effect of temperature on dynamic and steady-state shear rheological properties of siriguela (*Spondias purpurea* L.) pulp. *Journal of Food Engineering*, 108(2), 283–289.

Augusto, P. E. D., Ibarz, A., Cristianini, M. (2012b). Effect of high pressure homogenization (HPH) on the rheological properties a fruit juice serum model. *Journal of Food Engineering*, 111(2), 474–477.

Augusto, P. E. D., Ibarz, A., Cristianini, M. (2012c). Effect of high pressure homogenization (HPH) on the rheological properties of tomato juice: Time-dependent and steady-state shear. *Journal of Food Engineering*, 111(4), 570–579.

Augusto, P. E. D., Falguera, V., Cristianini, M., Ibarz, A. (2012d). Rheological behavior of tomato juice: Steady-state shear and time-dependent modeling. *Food and Bioprocess Technology*, 5(5), 1715–1723.

Augusto, P. E. D., Ibarz, A., Cristianini, M. (2013a). Effect of high pressure homogenization (HPH) on the rheological properties of tomato juice: Viscoelastic properties and the Cox–Merz rule. *Journal of Food Engineering*, 114(1), 57–63.

Augusto, P. E. D., Ibarz, A., Cristianini, M. (2013b). Effect of high pressure homogenization (HPH) on the rheological properties of tomato juice: Creep and recovery behaviour. *Food Research International*, 54, 169–176.

Augusto, P. E. D., Tribst, A. A., Cristianini, M. (2013c). Chapter 405: Thermal processes, commercial sterility (retort). In: Batt, C., Tortorello, M. L. (Eds.). *Encyclopedia of Food Microbiology*, 2nd edn. Elsevier (*in press*).

Bayod, E., Månsson, P., Innings, F., Bergenståhl, B., Tornberg, E. (2007). Low shear rheology of concentrated tomato products. Effect of particle size and time. *Food Biophysics*, 2, 146–157.

Canet, W., Alvarez, M. D., Fernández, C., Luna, P. (2005). Comparisons of methods for measuring yield stresses in potato puree: Effect of temperature and freezing. *Journal of Food Engineering*, 68, 143–153.

Cepeda, E., Villarán, M. C., Ibarz, A. (1999). Rheological properties of cloudy and clarified juice of *Malus floribunda* as a function of concentration and temperature. *Journal of Texture Studies*, 30, 481–491.

Córdoba, A., Camacho, M. M., Martínez-Navarrete, N. (2012). Rheological behaviour of an insoluble lemon fibre as affected by stirring, temperature, time and storage. *Food and Bioprocess Technology*, 5, 1083–1092.

Da Silva, J. A. L., Rao, M. A. (1992). Viscoelastic properties of food hydrocolloid dispersions. In: Rao, M. A., Steffe, J. F. (Eds.). *Viscoelastic Properties of Foods*, pp. 285–315. London: Elsevier Science.

Dogan, H., Kokini, J. L. (2007). Rheological properties of foods. In: Heldman, D. R., Lund, D. B. (Eds.). *Handbook of Food Engineering*, 2nd edn, pp. 1–124. Boca Raton, FL: Taylor & Francis.

Dutta, D., Dutta, A., Raychaudhuri, U., Chakraborty, R. (2006). Rheological characteristics and thermal degradation kinetics of beta-carotene in pumpkin puree. *Journal of Food Engineering*, 76, 538–546.

Falguera, V., Ibarz, A. (2010). A new model to describe flow behaviour of concentrated orange juice. *Food Biophysics*, 5, 114–119.

Falguera, V., Vélez-Ruiz, J. F., Alins, V., Ibarz, A. (2010). Rheological behaviour of concentrated mandarin juice at low temperatures. *International Journal of Food Science and Technology*, 45, 2194–2200.

Figoni, P. I., Shoemaker, C. F. (1983). Characterization of time dependent flow properties of mayonnaise under steady shear. *Journal of Texture Studies*, 14, 431–442.

Fischer, P., Pollard, M., Erni, P., Marti, I., Padar, S. (2009). Rheological approaches to food systems. *Comptes Rendus Physique*, 10, 740–750.

Genovese, D. B., Rao, M. A. (2005). Components of vane yield stress of structured food dispersions. *Journal of Food Science*, 70(8), E498–E504.

Genovese, D. B., Lozano, J. E., Rao, M. A. (2007). The rheology of colloidal and noncolloidal food dispersions. *Journal of Food Science*, 72(2), R11–R20.

Giner, J., Ibarz, A., Garza, S., Xhian-Quan, S. (1996). Rheology of clarified cherry juices. *Journal of Food Engineering*, 30, 147–154.

Goksel, M., Dogan, M., Toker, O. S., Ozgen, S., Sarioglu, K., Oral, R. A. (2013). The effect of starch concentration and temperature on grape molasses: Rheological and textural properties. *Food and Bioprocess Technology*, 6, 259–271.

Gunasekaran, S., Ak, M. M. (2000). Dynamic oscillatory shear testing of foods—Selected applications. *Trends in Food Science and Technology*, 11, 115–127.

Hahn, S. J., Ree, T., Eyring, H. (1959). Flow mechanism of thixotropic substances. *Industrial and Engineering Chemistry*, 51, 856–857.

Harte, F., Venegas, R. (2010). A model for viscosity reduction in polysaccharides subjected to high-pressure homogenization. *Journal of Texture Studies*, 41, 49–61.

Ibarz, A., Pagán, J., Miguelsanz, R. (1992). Rheology of clarified fruit juices. II: Blackcurrant juices. *Journal of Food Engineering*, 15(1), 63–73.

Ibarz, A., Barbosa-Cánovas, G. V. (2003). *Unit Operations in Food Engineering*. Boca Raton, FL: CRC Press.

Ibarz, R., Falguera, V., Garvín, A., Garza, S., Pagan, J., Ibarz, A. (2009). Flow behavior of clarified orange juice at low temperatures. *Journal of Texture Studies*, 40, 445–456.

Ibrahim, G. E., Hassan, M. I., Abd-Elrashid, A. M., El-Massry, K. F., Eh-Ghorab, A. E., Manal, M. R., Osman, F. (2011). Effect of clouding agents on the quality of apple juice during storage. *Food Hydrocolloids*, 25, 91–97.

Koocheki, A., Taherian, A. R., Bostan, A. (2013). Studies on the steady shear flow behavior and functional properties of *Lepidium perfoliatum* seed gum. *Food Research International* 50, 446–456.

Kubo, M. T. K., Augusto, P. E. D., Cristianini, M. (2013). Effect of high pressure homogenization (HPH) on the physical stability of tomato juice. *Food Research International*, 51, 170–179.

Leite, T. S., Augusto, P. E. D., Cristianini, M. (2013). Effect of high pressure homogenization on microstructure of cashew apple juice. In: *Proceedings of the International Nonthermal Food Processing Workshop: Research and Innovation Towards Competitiveness*, Florianópolis, 2013.

Massa, A., González, C., Maestro, A., Labanda, J., Ibarz, A. (2010). Rheological characterization of peach purees. *Journal of Texture Studies*, 41, 532–548.

Metzner, A. B. (1985). Rheology of suspensions in polymeric liquids. *Journal of Rheology*, 29(6), 739–775.

Noomhorm, A., Tansakul, A. (1992). Effect of pulper-finisher operation on quality of tomato juice and tomato puree. *Journal of Food Process Engineering*, 15(4), 229–239.

Ramos, A. M., Ibarz, A. (1998). Thixotropy of orange concentrate and quince puree. *Journal of Texture Studies*, 29, 313–324.

Rao, M. A. (1999). *Rheology of Fluid and Semisolid Foods: Principles and Applications*. Gaithersburg, MD: Aspen.

Rao, M. A. (2005). Rheological properties of fluid foods. In: Rao, M. A., Rizvi, S. S. H., Datta, A. K. (Eds). *Engineering Properties of Foods*, 3rd edn, pp. 41–100. Boca Raton, FL: CRC Press.

Rao, M. A., Cooley, H. J., Liao, H. J. (1999). High temperature rheology of tomato puree and starch dispersion with a direct-drive viscometer. *Journal of Food Process Engineering*, 22, 29–40.

Rao, M. A., Cooley, H. J., Vitali, A. A. (1984). Flow properties of concentrated juices at low-temperatures. *Food Technology*, 38(3), 113–119.

Ros-Polski, V. (2011). Development of a pressurized capillary rheometer and optimization of thermal treatment of fluids at high temperatures. PhD thesis, University of Campinas.

Sato, A. C. K., Cunha, R. L. (2009). Effect of particle size on rheological properties of jaboticaba pulp. *Journal of Food Engineering*, 91, 566–570.

Servais, C., Jones, R., Roberts, I. (2002). The influence of particle size distribution on the processing of foods. *Journal of Food Engineering*, 51, 201–208.

Shamsudin, R., Daud, W. R. W., Takrif, M. S., Hassan, O., Ilicali, C. (2009). Rheological properties of Josapine pineapple juice at different stages of maturity. *International Journal of Food Science and Technology*, 44, 757–762.

Shamsudin, R., Ling, C. S., Adzahan, N. M., Wan, W. R. (2013). Rheological properties of ultraviolet-irradiated and thermally pasteurized Yankee pineapple juice. *Journal of Food Engineering*, 116, 548–553.

Sharoba, A., Ramadan, M. F. (2011). Rheological behavior and physicochemical characteristics of goldenberry (*Physalis peruviana*) juice as affected by enzymatic treatment. *Journal of Food Processing and Preservation*, 35, 201–219.

Silva, V. M., Sato, A. C. K., Barbosa, G., Dacanal, G., Ciro-Velásquez, H. J., Cunha, R. L. (2010). The effect of homogenisation on the stability of pineapple pulp. *International Journal of Food Science and Technology*, 45, 2127–2133.

Steffe, J. F. (1996). *Rheological Methods in Food Process Engineering*, 2nd edn. East Lansing, MI: Freeman Press.

Sun, A., Gunasekaran, S. (2009). Yield stress in foods: Measurements and applications. *International Journal of Food Properties*, 12, 70–101.

Tabilo-Munizaga, G., Barbosa-Cánovas, G. V. (2005). Rheology for the food industry. *Journal of Food Engineering*, 67, 147–156.

Takada, N., Nelson, P. E. (1983). Pectin–protein interaction in tomato products. *Journal of Food Science*, 48(5), 1408–1411.

Tanglertpaibul, T., Rao, M. A. (1987). Rheological properties of tomato concentrates as affected by particle size and methods of concentration. *Journal of Food Science*, 52(1), 141–145.

Tiwari, B. K., Muthukumarappan, K., O'Donnell, C. P., Cullen, P. J. (2010). Rheological properties of sonicated guar, xanthan and pectin dispersions. *International Journal of Food Properties*, 13(2), 223–233.

Tonon, R. V., Alexandre, D., Hubinger, M. D., Cunha, R. L. (2009). Steady and dynamic shear rheological properties of açai pulp (*Euterpe oleraceae* Mart.) *Journal of Food Engineering*, 92, 425–431.

Tsai, S. C., Zammouri, K. (1988). Role of interparticular van der Waals force in rheology of concentrated suspensions. *Journal of Rheology*, 32(7), 737–750.

Vitali, A. A., Rao, M. A. (1982). Flow behavior of guava puree as a function of temperature and concentration. *Journal of Texture Studies*, 13(3), 275–289.

Vitali, A. A., Rao, M. A. (1984). Flow properties of low-pulp concentrated orange juice— Serum viscosity and effect of pulp content. *Journal of Food Science*, 49(3), 876–881.

Wei, Y. P., Wang, C. S., Wu, J. S. B. (2001). Flow properties of fruit fillings. *Food Research International*, 34, 377–381.

Weltman, R. N. (1943). Breakdown of thixotropic structure as function of time. *Journal of Applied Physics*, 14, 343–350.

Yoo, B., Rao, M. A. (1994). Effect of unimodal particle size and pulp content on rheological properties of tomato puree. *Journal of Texture Studies*, 25(4), 421–436.

7 Assessing Juice Quality
Analysis of Organoleptic Properties of Fruit Juices

Gemma Echeverría and María Luisa López

CONTENTS

7.1 Introduction 137
7.2 Sensory Attributes of Fruit Juice 138
7.3 How to Measure Fruit Juice Quality Using Sensory Evaluation? 139
7.4 Advantages and Disadvantages of Sensory Analysis to Measure
    Fruit Juice Quality 141
7.5 Applications 142
    7.5.1 New Product Development 143
    7.5.2 Marketing and Consumer Characteristics 143
    7.5.3 Comparison of Sensory and Instrumental Measurements 144
    7.5.4 Assessing Product Quality 145
          7.5.4.1 Effect of Processing Conditions: Temperature 145
          7.5.4.2 Effect of Product Properties: Composition,
                   Ingredients, and Concentration 146
          7.5.4.3 Effect of Unit Operations and Processing 146
7.6 Conclusions 147
References 147

7.1 INTRODUCTION

Fruit juice is known as a healthy food product, and is currently consumed by a large percentage of the global consumer population (Verbeke 2005). Fruits are healthy foods because they are rich in antioxidants, vitamins, dietary fiber, and minerals. In addition, fruits do not contain any dairy allergens such as casein and lactose (Luckow and Delahunty 2004). It has also been suggested that fruit juice serves as a good medium for probiotics (Tuorila and Cardello 2002). All these characteristics of fruit juice are very important in the purchasing decisions of consumers. However, another significant factor affecting consumer satisfaction, and consequently influencing the purchasing decision, is the quality of the product. Quality is a key product component, and it can be determined using objective or subjective measurements. Objective evaluation involves the use of laboratory instruments with no involvement of the senses. Subjective evaluation is done by either trained or untrained human observers (OSU 1998). Food industries often utilize sensory evaluation techniques to test products. The quality of juice is often assessed in terms of three main sensory properties: appearance, flavor, and texture. The visual perception of color is the main appearance attribute in fruit juices and results from the activation of the retina by electromagnetic waves in the visible spectrum. Flavor characteristics include taste and odor. Taste sensations are produced as substances dissolved in the saliva interact with the taste buds in the papillae on the tongue (Weaver and Daniel 2003) and odor sensations are created by those substances that are volatile enough to enter the air in the sensory region and are partially soluble in the mucus that covers receptors (Masson and Nottingham 2002). The texture attributes of juices comprise all these traits, influencing mouthfeel, and the most important texture attribute is viscosity. These three attribute categories are expressed as a continuum and not as discrete properties.

7.2   SENSORY ATTRIBUTES OF FRUIT JUICE

The sensory evaluation of fruit juices is important to many industries that sell consumer goods and food products, because the human senses integrate their input, so that changes in one sense can be perceived as changes in another. For example, a change in a product's odor can sometimes be perceived as a change in taste. In order to successfully sell the product, consumer appeal and target consumer populations should be considered (Moskowitz 1988). According to Harker et al. (2003), to bear in mind consumer requirements in the development of new products is as important for the fresh fruit sector as it is for manufactured foods.

Appearance is an important aspect, as it is the first subjective evaluation made of juice quality. The product has to pass visual assessment before the consumer can or will consider other parameters such as flavor and texture. As has been mentioned above, color is the most important appearance attribute in fruit juices.

Factors that should be considered in evaluating product appearance include:

- *Use of standard conditions*: light source (type, intensity, and color), background, and style of presentation (unless tested)
- *Selection of appearance attribute(s) for inclusion on score sheet*: should be masked to eliminate unwanted interactions when assessing parameters involving other senses; color charts/standards aid in rating

In relation to smell, it is relevant to point out that odor is the major component of a food flavor, and the human nose is much more sensitive than analytical instruments. This higher sensitivity of the nose justifies the use of sensory measurements during the evaluation of fruit juice quality. In addition, fruit juices contain numerous compounds of varying volatility that may make analytical interpretation difficult (e.g., strong peaks may produce a weak odor whereas weak peaks may produce a strong odor), while human smell perceives a mixture with absolute perfection.

Strictly speaking, taste involves only those sensations mediated by the gustatory nerve fibers, and these sensations have five basic qualities: sweet, sour, bitter, salty, and umami. The first three are the ones most commonly found in fruit juices.

A taste response requires an aqueous solution of the substance (stimulus) to contact the taste buds. Therefore, saliva secretions are important in terms of ensuring contact between the product and the taste buds. Saliva production is generally stimulated by chewing, as well as the appearance and odor of the food. The taste receptors are the taste buds and these are mounted on papillae (folds in the skin of the tongue). The area of greatest response is the top of the tongue. Other areas in the mouth and throat where taste buds are situated include the palate, pharynx, larynx, tonsils, epiglottis, lips, cheeks, the underside of the tongue, and the floor of the mouth (Meilgaard et al. 2007). Having described the five basic tastes, it is obvious that foods, and in particular fruit juices, are a very complex system that contains many different taste compounds and therefore many different tastes. The fact that there are only five basic tastes, and yet we are able to detect hundreds of different taste sensations, is due to a series of complex taste interactions that can range from simple two-way interactions to complex five-way interactions (Masson and Nottingham 2002).

Texture attributes in liquids, as in the case of fruit juices, mainly comprise viscosity. Instrumental methods only measure one aspect of "texture" and again cannot relate the complex interactions that produce the perception of food texture.

7.3 HOW TO MEASURE FRUIT JUICE QUALITY USING SENSORY EVALUATION?

There are two basic categories of sensory methods: analytical and affective (Figure 7.1). They are separate types of methods because they answer different questions.

The techniques that measure the product sensation are considered objective measurements and are either discriminative (difference tests) or descriptive. The former techniques answer the question: Have the differences between products been perceived and at what confidence level? The latter method identifies specific types of differences and their magnitudes (Stone and Sidel 2004).

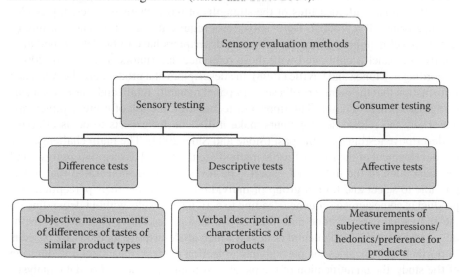

FIGURE 7.1 Sensory evaluation methods, tests, and applications.

In the fruit juice industry, discriminative techniques are commonly used to test for ingredient substitutions when the objective is to maintain product similarity (Civille and Oftedal 2012). Discrimination methods include paired comparison, duo-trio, triangle, and dual standard, to name the most frequently used methods. Each offers advantages and disadvantages, but none of them is more sensitive than the others. The choice of method is determined by the objective and the type of product. Attribute difference tests usually determine in what sense a certain attribute differs between samples. Overall difference tests determine the sensory difference that may exist between samples (Meilgaard et al. 2007). The sensory test measures whether any differences detected are statistically significant by analyzing the sensory data. After statistical analysis, the researchers can make a meaningful interpretation from the results of the data (Meilgaard et al. 2007). Difference tests are often used for difference evaluations in quality control at various stages of product development or modification, or to screen experiments prior to consumer testing.

Descriptive analysis is another objective sensory technique, and requires a highly trained panel. Descriptive methods document the qualitative and quantitative sensory aspects of a product. The qualitative aspects of fruit juices include specific appearance, aroma, flavor, and texture characteristics. The quantitative aspect is the intensity of each of the attributes. Descriptive analysis methods include: Flavor Profile®, Texture Profile®, Spectrum Analysis®, and Quantitative Descriptive Analysis (QDA®). These methods provide product descriptions with numerical measures of strength. Whichever method is chosen, the sensory staff must understand the process sufficiently to reach an informed decision. There are two basic issues to consider: The first is whether the subjects develop a language to describe the products or the sensory staff train the subjects to respond to specific attributes; the second is how the responses are analyzed. A detailed discussion of this topic can be found in Stone and Sidel (2004). Descriptive analysis is probably the most powerful and useful of all the sensory methods. It identifies all of a product's perceived characteristics along with measures of the strengths of those characteristics. It provides a "fingerprint" of a product. Descriptive tests require the selection and training of tasting panel members. Next, the reference descriptors have to be determined and, finally, the panel is calibrated with those reference descriptors (Pérez et al. 2007). According to Muñoz and Civille (1998), the descriptors of a product are the reference information that the members of a sensory panel mentally retain and share when carrying out tasting exercises. The impact of technology, the use of more complex raw materials, and related developments make it difficult for experts to be as effective in descriptive testing as in the past (Stone and Sidel 2004). The main challenges for the development of the Flavor Profile method are the formal descriptive analysis and the separation of the individual expert. The investigators demonstrated that it was possible to select and train a group of individuals to describe their perception of a product in some agreed sequence, leading to actionable results without depending on the individual expert (Stone and Sidel 2004). Before describing specific test methods, a review of the fundamental issues on which all descriptive methods are based is important. This includes the participants' selection process, the extent and duration of the study, the quantification of the panel, and finally the method of data analysis. Sensory evaluation must have tools with which to work, including the methods used to evaluate the products, such as difference tests and acceptance/preference tests (Stone and Sidel 2004). While conducting sensory evaluation, the researcher should be familiar with all the different sensory methods to be used in order to apply them properly. Understanding alternative test methods also reduces unwarranted reliance on a single method to test options and solve problems. The selected panelists must be qualified to participate in the training. Failure to use appropriately qualified panelists has a significant impact on the credibility of the study. There must be a formal program for participants' selection, so as to improve the level of sensitivity, to match the panel with a specific sensory problem, and to increase confidence in the conclusions derived from the test results (Stone and Sidel 2004). The individuals selected should have normal acuity and perception, above-average interest in odor and flavor work, and the ability to work cooperatively with others in a group setting. These personal qualities are determined by test scores and through a personal interview (Moskowitz 1988). Once individuals have indicated a willingness to participate, they are required to take part in a series of screening tests to determine their level of skill. A threshold test is designed to determine the minimum concentration at which a stimulus can be detected as different from a blank (detection threshold) or can be recognized as having a typical taste (Moskowitz 1988).

The second branch of sensory evaluation focuses on the consumer response. These techniques measure the subjective personal reactions of consumers, such as acceptance (liking) or preference. The tests used to measure these subjective reactions are called affective tests (Meilgaard et al. 2007). How consumers perceive product attributes is a critical aspect in the food choice process (Kupiec and Revell 2001). Several studies have been conducted to examine how consumers evaluate different product attributes in numerous food products. Health, nutrition, taste, price, and convenience are some of the criteria that consumers use to determine which product is more attractive (Bech-Larsen et al. 2001). Consumers face many tradeoffs in their food choices, for example, between nutrition and price, or nutrition and convenience (Blaylock et al. 1999). There are two main types of affective methods: the paired preference and the nine-point hedonic scale. From a sensory perspective, the nine-point hedonic scale is more useful because it provides a measure of liking for each product, the magnitude of the difference in liking among the products, and enables the use of parametric statistics, such as the analysis of variance, to identify significant product differences. Overall, it is a more efficient methodology, enabling one to test multiple products as opposed to multiple paired comparisons. However, if one wants to know which of two products is preferred, then the paired comparison is more appropriate. Method selection should be determined primarily by the testing objectives. Other factors that impact choice are the time line, the availability of qualified subjects, and, of course, the availability of the product (Stone and Sidel 2004).

7.4 ADVANTAGES AND DISADVANTAGES OF SENSORY ANALYSIS TO MEASURE FRUIT JUICE QUALITY

Sensory analysis is the measurement of consumer responses to sensory stimuli. It is used in grading, consumer preferences, quality assurance, shelf-life testing, product development, and research. The advantages and disadvantages of employing sensory analysis depend, of course, on the type of sensory method used. In general, some significant advantages are listed below:

- The method gives real answers regarding consumer quality.
- Objective methods are more reliable, accurate, and reproducible. However, they must be correlated to sensory evaluation to indicate a consumer response.
- Sensory panels help manufacturers, scientists, food technologists, and so on to gain a clear perception of what ordinary consumers may experience.
- Sensory panel testing can be much more rapid than most nonsensory methods.
- Sensory panelists use more than one sense, making them more flexible subjects.
- Sensory panelists can be very sensitive and good at detecting minute differences in product characteristics.
- It is acceptable to write sensory panels into specifications for quality.
- Laboratory facilities are not required to conduct the descriptive analysis of a product. This makes sensory panels a feasible proposition to study products.

In contrast, some disadvantages are:

- The process is time-consuming.
- Sensory panelists may become fatigued with the entire process of testing and assessing descriptive data.
- Assessors may be subject to biases, for example, due to loss of interest or distractions.
- To ensure precision in the analysis and interpretation of the descriptive data, several assessors may be required, making it an expensive proposition.
- The entire process of recruiting and training sensory panelists can be a time-consuming and costly process.
- It may not be easy to replace assessors quickly, as incoming assessors will require intensive training to develop the requisite expertise for the job.
- The sensory panel method may be more expensive than some nonsensory methods.
- The panelists may not be good at quantifying perceptions.
- The interpretation of results may be problematic and open to dispute.

7.5 APPLICATIONS

There are multiple applications of sensory evaluation in the fruit juice industry: for example, to study the development of new products or improve existing ones, to select new raw materials, to assess or change the process to elaborate fruit juices in order to achieve better juice quality or reduce the cost of production, to revise marketing and discover more about consumer preferences, and to obtain a correlation between objective or analytical measurements and subjective or consumer preferences. Among these, the most relevant applications have been clustered as shown below:

- Research and development (long-term studies)
- Specifications for quality assurance and quality control purposes
- Tracking sensory changes over time

- Long-term changes for shelf-life/packaging studies
- Short-term intensity measurement of specific attributes

7.5.1 NEW PRODUCT DEVELOPMENT

Developing products that are successful is a difficult and time-consuming process. The published evidence shows that the success rate is very low so there is always a search for ways to increase it. This low rate of success has been attributed to many factors, some on their own, but most often reflecting a combination of problems. Competition is intense, time lines are short, strategies change, targets move, raw materials are unavailable, and so on (Stone and Sidel 2007).

The development of new products requires an in-depth analysis of two factors. The first is to identify consumer responses to this new product in advance and the second is to know its sensory profile, as described by a trained panel, in order to anticipate consumer acceptance. In relation to consumer responses, Tuorila and Cardello (2002) conducted an experiment with juices containing functional ingredients, in which they determined the following: To what extent are consumers willing to accept an inferior taste to achieve a beneficial health effect? Does the acceptance of an inferior taste depend on the type of health benefit expected to be achieved? And does the acceptance depend on the required frequency and overall duration of consumption? The results revealed that the consumption of a functional juice will be inversely related to the severity of off-flavor and to the required frequency and duration of consumption. Kozlowska et al. (2003) also evaluated the effect of various test locations and contexts on hedonic responses to experimental apple juices with different sucrose levels, and investigated the predictive value of the results on juice consumption at home by the elderly in comparison with young subjects. The results obtained confirmed a shift toward higher sucrose levels in the elderly compared with young adults, and provided additional evidence that, with an increase in the volume ingested and repeated exposure, the preferred sucrose concentration decreases, regardless of the age of the consumers. Moreover, they found that a correlation between hedonic judgments and intake was lower in the elderly than in young subjects.

Concerning the sensory profile of new products, Carbonell et al. (2007) developed a list of descriptors to evaluate fresh and processed mandarin juices via the conventional sensory profile method and selected a group of assessors for future research in this field. There is a limited amount of available literature relating to mandarin juices, and that which does exist is focused on their composition (Moshonas and Shaw 1997; Trifiro et al. 1999), on detecting additions of mandarin juice to orange juice (Knight 2000), or on comparing the effects of heat treatment conditions on the acceptability of chilled juices (Sentandreu et al. 2005); but little is known about the suitability of the different varieties of mandarins for juice production. Hence, the main aim of the work carried out by Carbonell et al. (2007) was to use this group of trained assessors and the descriptor list developed to evaluate such suitability.

7.5.2 MARKETING AND CONSUMER CHARACTERISTICS

Consumer expectations and their interests when buying food are important factors that need to be understood to improve the food industry, because a continuous change has been noticed in eating habits and the search for products that are healthier, despite the lifestyles of the twenty-first century (Gadioli et al. 2013). In addition, consumer characteristics, including familiarity, buying habits, and demographics, can influence purchasing choices. Conceivably, consumers can gain utility from the potential health-promoting aspects of products, as well as their sensory quality (Ares et al. 2008, 2010; Carrillo et al. 2011).

A good strategy of marketing involves knowing consumers' opinions. Preference mapping techniques, combining the use of consumer and sensory data to identify the attributes that drive consumer preferences, are used to optimize products (Greenhoff and MacFie 1999).

Expected sensory characteristics can affect purchase decision making (Deliza and MacFie 1996; Garber et al. 2003; Hutchings 2003). The sensory attraction of a food product and the visual appearance of its packaging are powerful influences on consumer acceptability (Tuorila and Pangborn 1988; Cardello 1994). Packaging attributes can persuade consumers to purchase the product, and sensory attributes will confirm if they like it. This process may be determined if the buyer repeats the purchase (Munrray and Delahunty 2000).

Other authors such as Lawless et al. (2013) carried out consumer-driven approaches to balance the nutraceutical and sensory qualities of products and to optimize consumer utility. Black cherry, Concord grape, and pomegranate juice blends are prime candidates for the nutraceutical juice market because of their inherent health-oriented characteristics and portable convenience. Merely applying instrumental measures of nutraceutical levels to optimization models does not incorporate how consumers value those attributes; thus, an optimization that applied consumer value to antioxidants in juice products was used, the principle of which could aid in the future development of nutraceutical beverages. Bett-Garber and Lea (2013) worked with blueberry juices and developed a lexicon to describe these juices. This lexicon provides a means to evaluate blueberry juice flavor, whether freshly pressed or processed. These descriptors facilitated the monitoring of the changes in flavor during processing and storage, and assisted processors to determine the impact of processing methods on the quality of product flavor. They were also useful to evaluate how cultivation and production practices affected juice flavor. Lawless et al. (2012a) assessed consumers' willingness to pay for nutraceuticals through nonhypothetical experimental auctions. Nonhypothetical value elicitation methods use real money and products to advantageously eliminate hypothetical bias. Experimental auctions allow product attributes such as nutraceutical status to be assessed along with sensory characteristics; hence, auctions can more easily capture all aspects of a product that contribute to consumer preferences. Understanding how consumers value all attributes can provide crucial information about the sustainability of a product in the marketplace.

7.5.3 COMPARISON OF SENSORY AND INSTRUMENTAL MEASUREMENTS

As has been mentioned, descriptive analysis provides a sensory profile of a product. When that information is combined with its physicochemical measurements and consumer preferences, it becomes an integral part of a company's product market strategy. It is especially useful to know what product attributes best fit the physicochemical measurements and have more influence on consumer preferences. Concomitantly, we can identify which formulations, operations, and processes optimize them.

Ravi et al. (2010) studied the influence of the addition of white pumpkin juice to orange juice, considering different variations and analyzing the physicochemical, nutritional, and sensory properties of this new blend. The results showed that the blend of orange and white pumpkin juice enhanced the nutritional quality without affecting the taste and flavor of the juice.

Citrus juices are well known as complex mixtures of aromatic volatiles and non-volatile components. Although aromatic volatiles are generally present at trace levels, they are essential to characterize the aroma of citrus juices. Cheong et al. (2012) revealed a strong correlation in grapefruit juices between their chemical components and some flavor attributes.

7.5.4 ASSESSING PRODUCT QUALITY

During product development, sensory properties are heavily emphasized as important factors in the final product (Lawless et al. 2012b). To optimize products, important factors affecting such variables must be correctly identified. Additionally, more than one optimal point may be present (Gacula 1993). Optimization techniques can help to develop ideal products and to promote an understanding of the sensory characteristics that consumers value (Lattey et al. 2007).

7.5.4.1 Effect of Processing Conditions: Temperature

Fresh fruit juices are highly susceptible to spoilage, since fluid components (enzymes, organic acids, carbohydrates, etc.) are in contact with air and microorganisms from the environment during handling (Mosqueta-Melgar et al. 2012). Thus, if juices are not rapidly heated, microbial, enzymatic, chemical, and physical deterioration quickly takes place and a shorter shelf life is observed (Bates et al. 2001). Although thermal treatment may avoid spoiling of juices, significant damage to the organoleptic, nutritional, and physicochemical properties of fluid foods may occur (Yeom et al. 2000; Espachs-Barroso et al. 2003; Elez-Martínez et al. 2006). For this reason, it is of vital importance to assess, with sensory analysis, the effect that temperature produces on the organoleptic quality of fruit juices. Several authors have discovered that the heating process influences the constituents of volatile fractions and this is mainly related to the production of off-flavors in mandarin juices (Pérez-López and Carbonell-Barrachina 2006; Pérez-López et al. 2006, 2007). Heating reduces levels of aroma impact compounds such as ethyl butanoate, linalool, neral, and geranial, and creates off-flavors such as 4-vinylguaiacol, p-cymene, α-terpineol, furaneol, and carvone in processed orange juice. When these compounds causing off-flavors were added to fresh juice, they produced the characteristic odor of aged or heat-abused juice (Ruiz Perez-Cacho and Rouseff 2008). A study of the heat-treatment conditions of chilled mandarin and orange juices (Sentandreu et al. 2005) concluded that pasteurization at 85°C for 10 s satisfactorily inactivates clarifying enzymes with minimal loss of acceptability. On the other hand, juices treated under these heat conditions presented the same acceptability as those stabilized by pulsed electric fields (Sentandreu et al. 2006). Leizerson and Shimoni (2005) examined the influence of ohmic heating on the sensory quality of orange juice. The assessors could not differentiate between fresh and ohmic-heated juice. Thus, ohmic heating produced a juice that retained most of the sensory attributes of the initial juice and still reduced microbial and enzymatic activity to required levels. The lower initial heat load during pulsed electric field treatment might induce fewer chemical reactions, resulting in greater retention of the initial flavor compounds.

7.5.4.2   Effect of Product Properties: Composition, Ingredients, and Concentration

The application of sensory evaluation in the development of fortified fruit juices is commonly used in the industry. Often, the ingredient that is being fortified imparts a distinct flavor or texture change. Sensory testing can aid in knowing how this new ingredient is perceived by consumers and allows a reduction of the possible off-flavors generated (Civille and Oftedal 2012). We can also observe the utility of a sensory analysis in the manufacturing and consumption of pomegranate and pomegranate-based products, which have increased. Many products use pomegranate as a main flavor component or as an addition to other flavors in juices. The research, using trained sensory panels, provides sensory terms that can be used to describe the flavor characteristics of pomegranate juices. This information is useful to product developers, researchers, and technologists in understanding the characteristics of pomegranate flavor and using those attributes to create new products, adapt other products, and study quality control and shelf-life issues (Koppel and Chambers 2010).

7.5.4.3   Effect of Unit Operations and Processing

The sensory aspects of fruit juices are greatly impaired by storage conditions. Color, for instance, is an aspect of great importance, as it impacts consumers' perception of quality. Gollucke et al. (2008) demonstrated that the proper storage of grape juice is capable of preserving its sensory characteristics. Moreover, cultivar differences of the same fruit species affect the sensory stability of juices. In practical terms, the use of blends may be useful for commercial grape juice producers to obtain an optimal product that combines high-quality taste and stability.

In general, good sensory qualities of juice, especially apple juice, are considered by consumers to be more important than price (Harker et al. 2002). For the best sensory qualities of apple juice, many researchers have paid attention to the changes in quality and the methods of preventing losses in quality of the product during processing (Özoğlu and Bayindirli 2002). Using sensory evaluation, Komthong et al. (2006) investigated the changes in the odors of apple juice during enzymatic browning after squeezing the fruit at different time points. A trained panel detected that fresh, fruity, and apple-like odors temporarily increased in the first 2 h of browning, and gradually decreased thereafter. Mechanically squeezed orange juice contains higher concentration levels of limonene than fresh hand-extracted juice, as it is also present in the peel oil (Moshonas and Shaw 1994). Moreover, many reports have mentioned that the high concentration of this terpene is associated with off-odors or a negative sensory mouthfeel commonly referred to as peel burn (Ruiz Perez-Cacho and Rouseff, 2008).

The commercial processes of concentrating fruit juice usually involve the removal of water at high temperature in a slight vacuum for short time periods, followed by the recovery and concentration of volatile aromas and their addition back into the concentrated product. These juices are designated as reconstituted from concentrate (RFC). In a study of orange juices using a sensory survey, some canned RFC juices were not perceived as orange juice. These juices were described by a trained panel as tropical fruit/grapefruit, heated/caramel, and moldy, whereas fresh, hand-squeezed orange juices completely lacked these sensory descriptors. The atypical aroma was attributed to the strong contribution of sulfur volatiles such as methanethiol, 1-*p*-menthene-8-thiol, 2-methyl-3-furanthiol, and dimethyl trisulfide contained in RFC juices (Ruiz Perez-Cacho et al., 2007).

7.6 CONCLUSIONS

Sensory evaluation has two main branches of application. The first concerns consumer understanding, which is focused on measuring the perception of product attributes as filtered through the consumers' screen of expectations. The second includes all the techniques that measure product sensation. These techniques are considered objective measurements and are either discriminative or descriptive. Consumer evaluation can provide valuable information to fruit juice producers and marketers about consumer preferences, while objective sensory analysis may deliver valuable information to the product development process.

REFERENCES

Ares, G., Gimenez, A., and Deliza, R. (2010). Influence of three non-sensory factors on consumer choice of functional yogurts over regular ones. *Food Quality and Preference* 21: 361–367.

Ares, G., Gimenez, A., and Gambaro, A. (2008). Uruguayan consumers' perception of functional foods. *Journal of Sensory Studies* 23: 614–630.

Bates, R.P., Morris, J.R., and Crandall, P.G. (2001). *Principles and Practices of Small- and Medium-Scale Fruit Juice Processing*. Rome: FAO.

Bech-Larsen, T., Grunert, K.G., and Poulsen, J.B. (2001). The acceptance of functional foods in Denmark, Finland, and the United States. MAPP Working Paper No. 73. Aarhus, Denmark: MAPP.

Bett-Garber, K.L. and Lea, J.M. (2013). Development of flavor lexicon for freshly pressed and processed blueberry juice. *Journal of Sensory Studies* 28: 161–170.

Blaylock, J., Smallwood, D., Kassel, K., Variyam, J., and Aldrich, L. (1999). Economics, food choices, and nutrition. *Food Policy* 24: 269–286.

Carbonell, L., Izquierdo, L., and Carbonell, I. (2007). Sensory analysis of Spanish mandarin juices. Selection of attributes and panel performance. *Food Quality and Preference* 18: 329–341.

Cardello, A.V. (1994). Consumer expectations and their role in food acceptance. In MacFie, H.J.H. and Thompson, D.M.H. (eds), *Measurement of Food Preferences*, pp. 253–297. London: Blackie Academic Press.

Carrillo, E., Varela, P., Salvador, A., and Fiszman, S. (2011). Main factors underlying consumers' food choice: A first step for the understanding of attitudes toward "healthy eating". *Journal of Sensory Studies* 26: 85–95.

Cheong, M.W., Liu, S.Q., Zhou, W., Curran, P., and Yu, B. (2012). Chemical composition and sensory profile of pomelo (*Citrus grandis* (L.) Osbeck) juice. *Food Chemistry* 135: 2505–2513.

Civille, G.V. and Oftedal, K.N. (2012). Sensory evaluation techniques—Make "good for you" taste "good". *Physiology and Behavior* 107: 598–605.

Deliza, R. and MacFie, H.J.H. (1996). The generation of sensory expectation by external cues and its effect on sensory perception and hedonic ratings: A review. *Journal of Sensory Studies* 11: 103–128.

Elez-Martínez, P., Soliva-Fortuny, R., and Martín-Belloso, O. (2006). Comparative study on shelf life of orange juice processed by high-intensity pulsed electric fields or heat treatment. *European Food Research and Technology* 222: 321–329.

Espachs-Barroso, A., Barbosa-Cánovas, G.V., and Martín-Belloso, O. (2003). Microbial and enzymatic changes in fruit juice induced by high-intensity pulsed electric fields. *Food Reviews International* 19: 253–273.

Gacula, M.C. (1993). *Design and Analysis of Sensory Optimization*. Trumbull, CT: Food and Nutrition Press.

Gadioli, I.L., Pineli, L.L., Rodriges, J.S., Campos, A.B., Gerolim, I., and Chiarello, M. (2013). Evaluation of packing attributes of orange juice on consumers' intention to purchase by conjoint analysis and consumer attitudes expectation. *Journal of Sensory Studies* 28: 57–65.

Garber Jr., L., Hyatt, E.M., and Starr Jr., R.G. (2003). Measuring consumer response to food products. *Food Quality and Preference* 14: 3–15.

Gollucke, A.P.B., Souza, J.C., and Tavares, D.Q. (2008). Sensory stability of concord and Isabel concentrated grape juices during storage. *Journal of Sensory Studies* 23: 340–353.

Greenhoff, K. and MacFie, H.J.H. (1999). Preference mapping in practice. In MacFie, H.J.H. and Thomson, D.M.H. (eds), *Measurement of Food Preferences*, pp. 137–165. Gaithersburg, MD: Aspen.

Harker, F.R., Gunson, F.A., and Jaeger, S.R. (2003). The case for fruit quality: An interpretative review of consumer attitudes, and preferences for apples. *Postharvest Biology and Technology* 28: 333–347.

Harker, F.R., Marsh, K.B., Young, H., Murray, S.H., Gunson, F.A., and Walker, S.B. (2002). Sensory interpretation of instrumental measurements 2: Sweet and acid taste of apple juice. *Postharvest Biology and Technology* 24: 241–250.

Hutchings, J.B. (2003). *Expectations and the Food Industry: The Impact of Color and Appearance*. New York: Kluwer Academic/Plenum.

Knight, A. (2000). Development and validation of a PCR-based heteroduplex assay for the quantitative detection of mandarin juice in processed orange juices. *Agro Food Industry Hi-Tech* 11(2): 7–8.

Komthong, P., Katoh, T., Igura, N., and Shimoda, M. (2006). Changes in the odours of apple juice during enzymatic browning. *Food Quality and Preference* 17: 497–504.

Koppel, K. and Chambers, E. (2010). Development and application of a lexicon to describe the flavor of pomegranate juice. *Journal of Sensory Studies* 25: 819–837.

Kozlowska, K., Jeruszka, M., Matuszewska, I., Roszkowski, W., Barylko-Pikielna, N., and Brzozowska, A. (2003). Hedonic tests in different locations as predictors of apple juice consumption at home in elderly and young subjects. *Food Quality and Preference* 14: 653–661.

Kupiec, B. and Revell, B. (2001). Measuring consumer quality judgments. *British Food Journal* 103: 7–22.

Lattey, K.A., Bramley, B.R., Francis, I.L., Herderich, M.J., and Pretorius, S. (2007). Wine quality and consumer preferences: Understanding consumer needs. *Wine Industry Journal* 22: 31–39.

Lawless, L.J.R., Nayga, R.M., Akaichi, F., Meullenet, J.F., Threfall, R.T., and Howard, L.R. (2012a). Willingness-to-pay for nutraceutical-rich juice blend. *Journal of Sensory Studies* 27: 375–383.

Lawless, L.J.R., Threfall, R.T., Meullenet, J.F., and Howard, L.R. (2012b). Consumer-based optimization of blackberry, blueberry and concord juice blends. *Journal of Sensory Studies* 27: 439–450.

Lawless, L.J.R., Threfall, R.T., Meullenet, J.F., and Howard, L.R. (2013). Applying a mixture design for consumer optimization of black cherry, concord grape and pomegranate juice blends. *Journal of Sensory Studies* 28: 102–112.

Leizerson, S. and Shimoni, E. (2005) Stability and sensory shelf life of orange juice pasteurized by continuous ohmic heating. *Journal of Agricultural and Food Chemistry* 53(10): 4012–4018.

Luckow, T. and Delahunty, C. (2004). Which juice is "healthier"? A consumer study of probiotic non-dairy juice drinks. *Food Quality and Preference* 15: 751–759.

Mason, R.M. and Nottingham, S.L. (2002). Sensory evaluation manual. Alimentos Food Available at: http://es.scribd.com/doc/8940001/Sensory-Evaluation-Manual-.

Meilgaard, M.C., Civille, G.V., and Carr, B.T. (2007). *Sensory Evaluation Techniques*, 4th edn. Boca Raton, FL: CRC Press.

Moshonas, M.G. and Shaw, P.E. (1994). Quantitative determination of 46 volatile constituents in fresh, unpasteurized orange juices using dynamic headspace gas chromatography. *Journal of Agricultural and Food Chemistry* 42(7): 1525–1528.

Moshonas, M.G. and Shaw, P.E. (1997). Quantitation of volatile constituents in mandarin juices and its use for comparison with orange juices by multivariate analysis. *Journal of Agricultural and Food Chemistry* 45(10): 3968–3972.

Moskowitz, H. (1988). *Applied Sensory Analysis of Foods*, vol. I. Boca Raton, FL: CRC Press.

Mosqueta-Melgar, J., Raybaudi-Massilia, R.M., and Martín-Belloso, O. (2012). Microbiological shelf life and sensory evaluation of fruit juices treated by high-intensity pulsed electric fields and antimicrobials. *Food and Bioproducts Processing* 90: 205–214.

Muñoz, A.M. and Civille, G.V. (1998). Universal, product and attribute scaling and the development of common lexicons in descriptive analysis. *Journal of Sensory Studies* 13: 57–75.

Munrray, J.M. and Delahunty, C.M. (2000). Mapping consumer preference for sensory and packaging attributes of cheddar cheese. *Food Quality and Preference* 5: 419–435.

Oregon State University. (1998). Moore family center for whole grain foods, nutrition and preventive health. College of Public Health and Human Sciences, Oregon State University. Available at: http://food.oregonstate.edu/sensory/dena.html.

Özoğlu, H. and Bayindirli, A. (2002). Inhibition of enzymatic browning in cloudy apple juice with selected antibrowning agents. *Food Control* 13: 213–221.

Pérez, J., Toledano, M.A., and Lafuente, V. (2007). Descriptive sensory analysis in different classes of orange juice by a robust free-choice profile method. *Analytica Chimica Acta* 595: 238–247.

Pérez-López, A.J. and Carbonell-Barrachina, A.A. (2006). Volatile odour components and sensory quality of fresh and processed mandarin juices. *Journal of the Science of Food and Agriculture* 86: 2404–2411.

Pérez-López, A.J., López-Nicolás, J.M., and Carbonell-Barrachina, A.A. (2007). Effects of organic farming on minerals contents and aroma composition of Clemenules mandarin juice. *European Food Research and Technology* 225: 255–260.

Pérez-López, A.J., Saura, D., Lorente, J., and Carbonell-Barrachina, A.A. (2006). Limonene, linalool, α-terpineol, and terpinen-4-ol as quality control parameters in mandarin juice processing. *European Food Research and Technology* 222: 281–285.

Ravi, U., Menon, L., Aruna, M., and Jananni, B.K. (2010). Development of orange-white pumpkin crush and analysis of its physicochemical, nutritional and sensory properties. *American-Eurasian Journal of Agricultural and Environmental Sciences* 8: 44–49.

Ruiz Perez-Cacho, P., Mahattanatawee, K., Smoot, J.M., and Rouseff, R. (2007). Identification of sulfur volatiles in canned orange juices lacking orange flavor. *Journal of Agricultural and Food Chemistry* 55(14): 5761–5767.

Ruiz Perez-Cacho, P. and Rouseff, R. (2008). Processing and storage effects on orange juice aroma: A review. *Journal of Agricultural and Food Chemistry* 56: 9785–9796.

Sentandreu, E., Carbonell, L., Carbonell, J.V., and Izquierdo, L. (2005). Effects of heat treatment conditions on fresh taste and on pectinmethylesterase activity of chilled mandarin and orange juices. *Food Science and Technology International* 11: 217–222.

Sentandreu, E., Carbonell, L., Rodrigo, D., and Carbonell, J.V. (2006). Pulse electric-fields versus thermal treatment: Equivalent processes to obtain equally acceptable citrus juices. *Journal of Food Protection* 69: 2016–2018.

Stone, H. and Sidel, J.L. (2004). *Sensory Evaluation Practices*, 3rd edn. New York: Academic Press/Elsevier.

Stone, H. and Sidel, J.L. (2007). Sensory research and consumer-led food product development. In MacFie, H.J.H. (ed.), *Consumer-Led Food Product Development*. Cambridge, UK: Woodhead.

Trifiro, A., Saccani, G., Bazzarini, R., Zoni, C., Zanotti, A., and Gherardi, S. (1999). Composition of mandarin and clementine juices of Italian production. *Industria Conserve* 74(2): 125–132.

Tuorila, H. and Cardello, A.V. (2002). Consumer responses to an off-flavor in juice in the presence of specific health claims. *Food Quality and Preference* 13: 561–569.

Tuorila, H. and Pangborn, R.M. (1988). Prediction of reported consumption of selected fat-containing foods. *Appetite* 11: 341–352.

Verbeke, W. (2005). Consumer acceptance of functional foods: Socio-demographic cognitive and attitudinal determinants. *Food Quality and Preference* 16(1): 45–57.

Weaver, M.C. and Daniel, R.J. (2003). *The Food Chemistry Laboratory: A Manual for Experimental Foods, Dietetics, and Food Scientists*, 2nd edn. Boca Raton, FL: CRC Press.

Yeom, H.W., Streaker, C.B., Zhang, Q.H., and Min, D.B. (2000). Effects of pulsed electric fields on the quality of orange juice and comparison with heat pasteurization. *Journal of Agricultural and Food Chemistry* 48: 4597–4605.

8 Utilization of Enzymes in Fruit Juice Production

Jordi Pagán

CONTENTS

8.1 Cell Wall Structure and Polysaccharide Components in Fruits 151
    8.1.1 Cell Wall Structure 151
    8.1.2 Pectin 152
    8.1.3 Cellulose and Hemicelluloses 153
    8.1.4 Starch 154
8.2 Enzymes Used in Fruit Processing 155
    8.2.1 Fruit Juice Problems Caused by Polysaccharides 155
    8.2.2 Industrial Enzyme Preparations 155
    8.2.3 Pectinases 158
    8.2.4 Cellulases and Hemicellulases 161
    8.2.5 Other Enzymes in Enzymatic Mixtures for Juice Treatment 161
    8.2.6 Enzymatic Activity Determination for Enzymatic Mixtures
        for Juice Treatment 162
    8.2.7 Methods of Immobilized Pectinolytic Enzymes in Fruit Processing 164
        8.2.7.1 Application of Native and Immobilized Pectinases
            in Ultrafiltration of Apple Juice 165
        8.2.7.2 Immobilized Pectinases in Mash Treatment and
            in Apple Juice Clarification 166
References 166

8.1 CELL WALL STRUCTURE AND POLYSACCHARIDE COMPONENTS IN FRUITS

8.1.1 CELL WALL STRUCTURE

Plant cells walls are complex in nature and are composed mostly of polysaccharides. The distribution of the components of a plant cell was proposed for the first time by Northcote (in 1958) and was confirmed by microscopy and electron micrography (Albersheim et al., 1960). This distribution includes a middle lamella, a primary wall, and a secondary wall. In the past three decades, the view of cell wall structure has been revised several times as new information about wall components, polymer structures, and interpolymer associations has become available (Ariel et al., 2007). The middle lamella forms one amorphous intercellular layer between the primary walls of adjacent cells and is considered the first material deposited by the cytoplasm. It is a cellulose-free zone and is composed of pectic polymers in its free form and calcium salts. The primary wall is the structure that expands to accommodate cell growth. It is composed of three polymer networks in a mesh-like structure: the pectins, cellulose–xyloglucan framework, and structural glycoproteins (Cosgrove, 1997). Moreover, phenolic esters ionically and covalently bind minerals, and enzymes complete the structure of the wall. Pectin is formed with three components: homogalacturonan (HG), rhamnogalacturonan-I (RGI), and rhamno-galacturonan-II (RGII) (Zhan et al., 1998). Except for RGII, these galacturonans do not show a stable definite structure (O'Neill et al., 2004). Typically, the components of the pectin backbone are HG and the core of RGI, the latter being branched with neutral sugar side chains (some combination of arabinan and arabinogalactan I and II) (Coenen et al., 2007). Another model proposes RGI is the main pectin backbone and HG and RGII form the side chains (Vincken et al., 2003). These models are typically representations of the wall structural components, which collectively provide a static view of the overall architecture. One interesting aspect of these models is that they generally incorporate the results of research conducted on many divergent aspects of wall structure and composition. Different models have been proposed in the past (Talbott and Ray, 1992). However, while fundamental components are common to all these models, there is less agreement in terms of the bonding interactions and their distributions within the wall (Ariel et al., 2007). The most frequently cited models were presented by Carpita and Gibeaut (1993) and describe the cell wall as composed of two polysaccharide networks. One comprises cellulose micro-fibrils cross-linked by hemicelluloses (most often xyloglucans or xylans); a simple analogy of this network is that of the steel and wire grids in a reinforced concrete slab. The other network, the pectin polysaccharides, would be the concrete (Ariel et al., 2007). Turgor in the cell plant is produced by the water entrapped by different polysaccharides. Pressure is produced by a solution against the semiperme-able membrane enclosing the cell due to osmotic pressure differences between the inside and outside of the cell. Cell turgor has a major function in determining tissue strength and changes in turgor are an integral part of fruit softening (Harker et al., 1997). A positive relationship between cell turgor and tissue puncture firmness was observed in cultivars with different softening rates (Tong et al., 1999). Fruit treated with a solution of calcium chloride had higher turgor and lower internal air space and was firmer than nontreated fruit after storage (Saftner et al., 1998). When turgor was modified by soaking the tissue in several solutions of mannitol, the fruit tissue failed by cell rupture at high turgor and by cell debonding at low turgor, and failure force under compression was reduced as turgor decreased (Lin and Pitt, 1986).

The most important cell wall polysaccharides in fruits are discussed in the following subsections.

8.1.2 PECTIN

Pectin is a polysaccharide with two fundamental constituents: polygalacturonic acid (PGA), which is made of helical homopolymers of (1-4)-α-galactosyluronic acid (GalA), and RGI, which is made of contorted rod-like heteropolymers of repeating (1-2)-α-rhamnosyl-(1-4)α-GalA disaccharide units (Lau et al., 1987). The rhamnosyl units may also interrupt long runs of PGA (Jarvis, 1984). An unusual RGII has the richest diversity of sugars and linkage structures known (Darvill et al., 1978). The molecule is too scarce to be a major structural polymer, but the complex form led the authors to suggest that it is a signal molecule (Carpita and Gibeaut, 1993). The PGAs contain up to about 200 GalA units and are about 100 nm long. The best-documented RGs are isolated from the cell walls by enzymic digestion with PGAse (Lau et al., 1987), but the length of RGI is unknown because there may be stretches of PGA on their ends. The helical chains of PGAs can condense by cross-linking with Ca^{2+} to form "junction zones" (Rees, 1977), linking two antiparallel chains (Jarvis, 1984). Just how many contiguous unesterified GalA residues are needed to form stable junction zones and the extent to which several chains can stack to form the multiple "eggbox" structures are not known *in vivo* or *in vitro*. At low Ca^{2+} concentrations, two chains are thought to form a stable junction with maximum strength at about 14 GalA units (Jarvis, 1984). If sufficient Ca^{2+} is present, some interrupting esterified GalA can be tolerated in the stable junction zone. With excess Ca^{2+} available, four-chain or higher-order stacking of PGA chains is possible (Jarvis, 1984). Stretches of PGA at the ends or within RG could link these two types of polymers, but the rhamnosyl units of RGI and their side chains interrupt the Ca^{2+} junctions. In addition to the Ca^{2+}-binding junction zones, pectins in some species may be cross-linked to other pectins and noncellulosic polysaccharides by ester linkages with dihydroxycinnamic acids such as diferulic acid (Fry, 1986). The pectin contents in several fruits are shown in Table 8.1.

8.1.3 CELLULOSE AND HEMICELLULOSES

Cellulose is the main structural fiber in the plant kingdom. It is a long-chain polysaccharide made up of 7,000–15,000 glucose monomer units, which are alternately rotated at 180° (Gibson, 2012). Cellulose molecules align to form microfibrils,

---

TABLE 8.1
Comparison of Fresh-Weight Pectin Content Values (%) as Calcium Pectate in Fruits

Product	Range	Average
Apples	0.71–0.84	0.78
Apricots	0.71–1.32	1.02
Blackberries	0.68–1.19	0.94
Cherries	0.24–0.54	0.39
Grapefruit	3.30–4.50	3.90
Lemons	2.80–2.99	2.90
Oranges	2.34–2.38	2.36
Raspberries	0.97	0.97

Source: Baker, R.A., *Journal of Food Science Institute of Food Technologists* 62, 225, 1997. With permission.

---

with a diameter of about 3–4 nm (Hori et al., 2002). The microfibrils have both crystalline and noncrystalline regions that merge together (Fernandes et al., 2011). The cellulose microfibrils themselves are aligned and bound together into fibril aggregates (or macrofibrils), roughly 10–25 nm in diameter, by a matrix of hemicellulose and either pectin or lignin (Donaldson, 2007). Hemicelluloses are plant cell wall polysaccharides that are not solubilized by water but are solubilized by aqueous alkali. Other hemicellulosic polysaccharides include xylan, glucuronoxylan, arabinoxylan, mannan, glucomannan, and galactoglucomannan. Hemicelluloses are also defined chemically as plant cell wall polysaccharides that have a backbone of 1,4-linked β-D-pyranosyl residues in which O-4 is in the equatorial orientation. The structural similarity between the hemicelluloses and cellulose most likely results in a conformational homology that can lead to a strong noncovalent association of hemicellulose with cellulose microfibrils. Xyloglucan is the quantitatively predominant hemicellulosic polysaccharide in the primary walls of dicotyledons. Xyloglucan may account for up to 20% of the dry weight of the primary wall. Xyloglucan has a backbone composed of 1,4-linked β-D-Glc$p$ residues. Up to 75% of these residues are substituted at O6 with mono-, di-, or triglycosyl side chains. Glycoproteins, a minor constituent of the cell wall, are also thought to be involved in the cross-linking. Xylans are heterogeneous polymers of the secondary wall and are the main component of hemicelluloses deposited during differentiation of the xylem (Bolwell, 1993). They broadly consist of 1,4-linked β-D-xyl$p$ residues, substituted with 4-O-methyl-D-glucuronic acid, arabinose, and acetate. There are at least six types of linkages involved in their biosynthesis. In dicotyledons, the 4-O-methylglucuronic acid side chain is the main substituent attached to C-2 positions. The acetyl content varies between 10% and 70% (Biely et al., 1985).

The mannans are a set of heterogeneous glycans widespread among green algae and terrestrial plants. Structurally, these polysaccharides contain β(1→4)-linked residues of either mannose (Man) or a combination of glucose (Glc) and Man. This backbone may also be substituted with α(1→6)-linked galactose (Gal) short side chains. Several types of mannans have been characterized: (i) pure mannans that contain >95% Man and that can adopt paracrystalline structures; (ii) galactomannans that contain >5% Gal; (iii) glucomannans with Glc and Man residues in the backbone; and (iv) (Gal–Glc)-mannans (Scheller and Ulvskov, 2010). Dried pears, for example, are mainly composed of cellulose (33%), pectins (32%), glucuronoxylans (30%), xyloglucans (3%), and mannans (1%) (Alasalvar and Shahidi, 2013).

8.1.4 STARCH

Starch is a polysaccharide that comprises two types of molecules: amylose (normally 20%–30%) and amylopectin (normally 70%–80%). Both consist of polymers of α-D-glucose units. In amylose these are linked (1α→4)-, with the ring oxygen atoms all on the same side, whereas in amylopectin about one residue in every twenty or so is also linked (1α→6)-, forming branch points. The relative proportions of amylose to amylopectin and (1α→6)- branch points both depend on the source of the starch. Although it is a very minority polysaccharide in fruits, starch is also included in the analytical determinations in fruit juices.

8.2 ENZYMES USED IN FRUIT PROCESSING

8.2.1 FRUIT JUICE PROBLEMS CAUSED BY POLYSACCHARIDES

Fruit juices contain colloids that can lead to problems during the filtration process. These colloids can be part of the fruit itself during fruit ripening (Barros et al., 2004). Pectins, celluloses, and hemicelluloses are gel-forming agents present in fruit juices; their fiber-like structures impede the clarification process by significantly reducing flux and yield (Srimanta et al., 2008). Pectins can cause problems in the food industry by giving rise to turbidity and viscosity during the extraction, filtration, and clarification of fruit juices (Fernández-González et al., 2005). In fact, the presence of pectic substances in fruit juices causes a considerable increase in their viscosity, thereby impeding filtration and subsequent concentration processes (Biscaro and Cano, 2010). The starch present in the fruit juices can also lead to difficulties during clarification and can give rise to a secondary haze in juices and therefore should not be present in clarified juices (Carrin et al., 2004). Polysaccharides like pectin and hemicellulose can form flocks with proteins present in the juices. These problems can be solved with the addition of industrial enzyme preparations.

8.2.2 INDUSTRIAL ENZYME PREPARATIONS

Industrial enzyme preparations are macerating enzyme complexes containing mainly pectinases, cellulases, and hemicellulases that are used for extraction and clarification of fruit and vegetable juices to increase the yield of juices and to remove clogging from filters. The reported improvements in juice flux by means of maceration and depectination are summarized in Table 8.2 (Echavarría et al., 2011c). Most enzyme components of the enzyme preparations are obtained from filamentous fungi, especially *Aspergillus niger*, or other microorganisms by submerged culture fermentation (Figure 8.1) or solid substrate fermentation. In many cases, its strains have been genetically transformed in order to increase the yield of enzyme protein. Figure 8.2 shows the steps to apply enzyme treatment in the industrial fruit juice extraction process. The use of macerating enzymes increases both yield and process performance without additional capital investment (Kuhad et al., 2011). The authors also report that these enzyme mixtures are used for improved mash treatment, improving the yield of extracted juice. The macerating enzymes are used to improve cloud stability and texture and decrease viscosity of the nectars and purees from different tropical fruits such as mango, peach, papaya, plum, apricot, and pear (Bhat, 2000). Texture, flavor, and aroma properties of fruits and vegetables can be improved by reducing excessive bitterness of citrus fruits by infusion of enzymes such as pectinases and β-glucosidases (Rai et al., 2007). The use of macerating enzymes not only improves the cloud stability and texture of nectars and purees, but also rapidly decreases their viscosity (Grassin and Fauquembergue, 1996). Thus, the macerating enzymes play a key role in food biotechnology and their demand will likely increase for extraction of juice from a wide range of fruits and vegetables (Dourado et al., 2002). Furthermore, infusion of pectinases and β-glucosidases has also been shown to alter the texture, flavor, and other sensory properties such as aroma and volatile characteristics of fruits and vegetables (Karmakar and Ray, 2011). The widespread and more efficient use of microbial enzymes in the preparation of wines

TABLE 8.2
Effect of Enzymatic Pretreatment of Fruit Juices on Filtration

Pretreatment	Comments	References
Maceration	Black currant juice treated with prepress maceration with 10 different pectinolytic enzymes (Pectinex BE®, Novozymes) consistently resulted in the best responses regarding anthocyanin yields, phenols, and low juice turbidity. The cloudiness of citrus juices, purees, and nectars was stabilized.	Landbo and Meyer (2004)
Depectinization	Cherry juice was treated with Pectinex Smash® (Novozymes), a protease preparation derived from *Aspergillus* spp. The protease treatment resulted in a significant reduction in immediate turbidity. Protease addition may be a workable alternative measure for decreasing immediate turbidity levels.	Pinelo et al. (2010)
Depectinization	The influence of enzymatic treatment using enzyme concentrations of 20, 100, and 300 mg/L, a time of 90 min, and a temperature of 40°C for depectinization was studied in cherry juice and pineapple (*Ananas comosus*) juice. A lower permeate flow rate was found for the polysulfone hollow-fiber membrane. Due to the increase in permeate flow rate is economically advantageous to ultrafilter depectinized juice treated with an enzyme concentration of 20 mg/L.	Barros et al. (2004)
Depectinization	Peach juice was clarified using the enzymatic hydrolysis Pectinex AFP® L3 (Novozymes) to reduce the viscosity of the juice and its pulp content, and consequently to increase juice extraction. Physical and chemical analyses showed that enzymatic treatment is effective for reducing peach pulp viscosity, pulp content, and turbidity and does not influence other juice parameters such as pH, total acidity, vitamin C, and soluble solids. Hydrolysis at 25°C for 60 min yielded the best results for the reduction in pulp (48%) and viscosity (68%).	Santón et al. (2008)
Depectinization	To prevent fouling the membrane, black currant juice was depectinized with Panzym Super E® (Novozymes) liquid enzyme preparation. The UF was carried out at a transmembrane pressure of 2 bars and an operating temperature of 25°C. The effect of processing on the valuable anthocyanin and flavonol content of the juices was examined. The results indicate that enzymatic treatment increases the valuable compound content of the juice.	Pap et al. (2012)

TABLE 8.2   (Continued)
Effect of Enzymatic Pretreatment of Fruit Juices on Filtration

Pretreatment	Comments	References
Enzyme immobilization	The catalytic behavior of a mixture of pectic enzymes in a pectin aqueous solution covalently immobilized on different supports was analyzed. No differences were observed at low circulation rates, while at higher recirculation rates, the time required to obtain complete pectin hydrolysis in the fluidized reactor was found to be 0.25 times shorter than in the packed bed reactor: 131 min for the packed reactors and 41 min for the fluidized reactors.	Diano et al. (2008)
Coimmobilization	The process was applied in the clarification of apple juice and the potential of coimmobilized pectinase amylase by physical adsorption on a UF hollow-fiber membrane was studied. The concentration of reaction products increased by up to 50% with the pectin concentration, and the starch content changed from 3.85 to 5.00 mg/mL. The reference permeate flux was improved when starch was added to the substrate, regardless of its concentration.	Carrin et al. (2004)
Previous enzymatic recirculation	Apple juice and model solution containing pectins were assessed through tubular membranes of 100 and 300 kDa (one and three channels). In order to obtain a higher permeate flow, the fluids were pretreated with pectinolytic enzymes recirculating through a tubular membrane at different concentrations and treatment times. Depectinization increased the permeate flow for the model solution and apple juice by 67.52% and 53.11% when the pectinolytic enzyme preparation recirculated across the tubular membrane.	Echavarría et al. (2011a)

Source: Adapted from Echavarría, A.P., Torras, C., Pagán, J., and Ibarz, A., *Food Engineering Reviews*, 3, 136–158, 2011. With permission.

and fruit juices started in the 1960s. The best performance achieved in the manufacture of fruit juices is obtained by adding enzymes in the phase immediately after the pulp has been mashed and heated. This pulp is first stirred in a holding tank for an appropriate time so that polyphenols are oxidized, otherwise they could inhibit the activity of the hydrolase enzymes added. To get the best results, the conditions of dose, temperature, application time, and pH have to be those in which the enzymatic mixture reaches its maximum activity. These have to be known previously using the data provided by

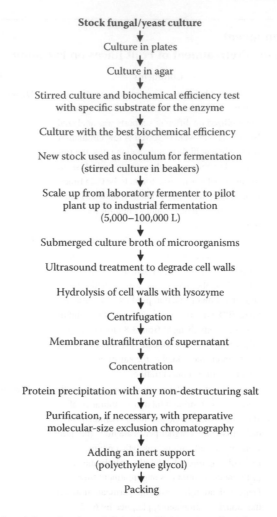

Stock fungal/yeast culture
↓
Culture in plates
↓
Culture in agar
↓
Stirred culture and biochemical efficiency test
with specific substrate for the enzyme
↓
Culture with the best biochemical efficiency
↓
New stock used as inoculum for fermentation
(stirred culture in beakers)
↓
Scale up from laboratory fermenter to pilot
plant up to industrial fermentation
(5,000–100,000 L)
↓
Submerged culture broth of microorganisms
↓
Ultrasound treatment to degrade cell walls
↓
Hydrolysis of cell walls with lysozyme
↓
Centrifugation
↓
Membrane ultrafiltration of supernatant
↓
Concentration
↓
Protein precipitation with any non-destructuring salt
↓
Purification, if necessary, with preparative
molecular-size exclusion chromatography
↓
Adding an inert support
(polyethylene glycol)
↓
Packing

FIGURE 8.1   Industrial production of the microbial enzyme flowchart.

the manufacturer; however, it may be necessary to carry out a study of the optimization of the process variables such as temperature, pH, time, and enzyme concentration in the laboratory or pilot plant. (Aehle, 2007) describes the effect of enzymatic treatment in fruit juice clarification Table 8.3.

8.2.3 PECTINASES

Pectinases are today one of the leading enzymes used in the commercial fruit juice processing sector (Kashyap et al., 2001). These enzymes catalyze the degradation of pectin molecules. According to the catalyzed reactions, three types of pectic enzymes are known: de-esterifying enzymes (pectinesterases), depolymerizing enzymes (pectinases: hydrolases and lyases), and protopectinases. The first type catalyzes the de-esterification of the methoxyl group of pectin forming pectic acid (Alkorta et al., 1995).

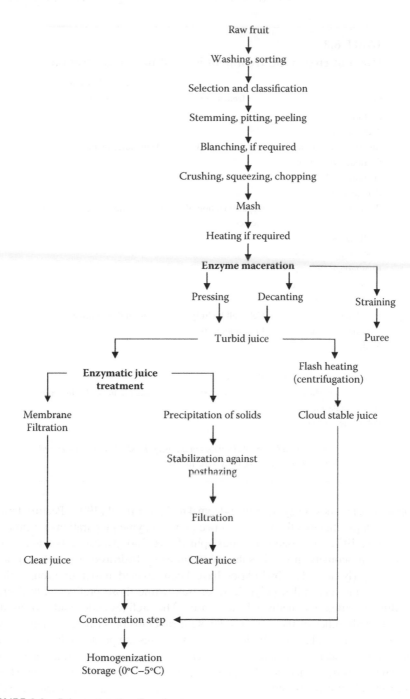

FIGURE 8.2　Juice extraction flowchart.

TABLE 8.3

Effect of Enzymatic Treatment in Fruit Juice Clarification

Enzyme	Treatment	Fruit and Process Application
Pectinlyase		
Arabanases		
Rhamnogalacturonase	Pressing of fruit	Apple juice extraction
Pectinacetylesterase		
Pectinmethylesterase		
Polygalacturonases		
Pectinlyase	Depectinization of juices	Clarification of apple, grape, and pear juices
Arabanases		
Arabinogalactanases		
Rhamnogalacturonases		
Pectinacetylestherases		
Endoglucanases		
Exoglucanases	Cell wall hydrolysis	Apple and pear juices
Cellobiohydrolase	Fruit liquefaction	
β-Glucosidase		
Xylanase		
Endopolygalacturonase	Pulp maceration	Purees
Galactomannanase	Gum hydrolysis	Pineapple juice clarification
Arabinogalactanases		
Polygalacturonases		

Source: Adapted from Aehle, W., *Enzymes in Industry. Production, Processes and Applications*, Wiley-VCH, Weinheim, 2007.

The optimal pH of these enzymes ranges from 4 to 5 (Serra et al., 1992). Pectinesterases are present in practically all commercial pectolytic enzyme preparations for processing (Voragen, 1972). The depolymerases split the α-(1,4)-glycosidic bonds between galacturonic monomers in pectic substances either by hydrolysis (hydrolases) or by β-elimination (lyases). The hydrolases have been divided into four groups: those preferring pectate are called polygalacturonases, while those preferentially degrading pectin are called polymethylgalacturonases. The prefixes endo- and exo- used in connection with either of these names denote a random- or terminal-action pattern, respectively (Serra et al., 1992). Endopolygalacturonases are produced by a wide variety of organisms such as numerous fungi, bacteria, a few yeasts, higher plants, and some plant parasitic nematodes. Exopolygalacturonases, however, have been shown to occur in different fruits and vegetables as well as fungi and some bacteria (Sakai et al., 1993). These enzymes, which hydrolyze the glycosidic bonds of pectate (endo- and exopolygalacturonate lyase) and pectin (endopolymethylgalacturonate lyase), are the only pectinases proven to hydrolyze pectin (Sakai et al., 1993). Finally, protopectinases, protopectin-solubilizing enzymes, which liberate water-soluble and highly polymerized pectin from protopectin, are classified into two types: one type reacts with the polygalacturonic acid region of protopectin (A type) and the other with the polysaccharide chains that may connect the polygalacturonic acid chain and cell wall constituents (B type). Most commercial preparations of pectic enzymes are obtained from fungal sources. In fact, although for obvious economic reasons it is very difficult to find reliable information about the commercial production of pectic enzymes, most producer strains are probably *Aspergillus* species.

8.2.4 CELLULASES AND HEMICELLULASES

Cellulases and hemicellulases catalyze thee degradation of cellulose and hemicellulose, respectively. Cellulases are components of industrial enzyme preparations and are a family of at least three groups of enzymes (Percival Zhang et al., 2006): endo-(1,4)-β-D-glucanase (EC 3.2.1.4), exo-(1,4)-β-D-glucanase (EC 3.2.1.91), and β-glucosidases (EC 3.2.1.21). The exoglucanase (CBH) acts on the ends of the cellulose chain and releases β-cellobiose as the end product; endoglucanase (EG) randomly attacks the internal O-glycosidic bonds, resulting in glucan chains of different lengths; and the β-glycosidases act specifically on the β-cellobiose disaccharides and produce glucose (Singh, 1999). Other enzymes that also are components in the industrial enzyme preparations for fruit juice treatments are hemicellulases, a mixture of hydrolytic enzymes including xylan endo-1,3-β-xylosidase, EC 3.2.1.32; xylan 1,4-β-xylosidase, EC 3.2.1.37; and α-L-arabinofuranosidase, EC 3.2.1.55. Mannanases are hydrolases that catalyze the endo-type of hydrolysis of β-1,4-mannosidic linkages in the main chain of naturally occurring mannan and heteromannans (McCleary, 1988). These enzymes include endo-β-1,4-mannanase (mannanase; EC 3.2.1.78) and β-mannosidase (EC 3.2.1.25). For complete hydrolysis of these mannans, other enzymes are necessary for cooperative actions such as α-galactosidases (EC 3.2.1.22) and acetyl esterases (EC 3.1.1.6) (Dekker, 1985). The polysaccharide araban (a polymer of the pentose sugar, arabinose) may cause a haze in fruit juice a few weeks after it has been concentrated. Although commercial pectinase preparations often contain arabanase, certain fruits (such as pears) are rich in araban and may require the addition of extra arabanase (Lozano, 2006). The adventitious presence of these enzymes in the enzymatic preparations is encouraged in order to reduce cellulose and hemicellulose levels.

8.2.5 OTHER ENZYMES IN ENZYMATIC MIXTURES FOR JUICE TREATMENT

Some fruits, such as apples, contain starch also, which is difficult to filter and causes membrane clogging and therefore slow filtration. Moreover, it can produce gelling after concentration and also haze and cloudiness in juices after processing. Enzymatic preparations must contain amylase enzymes in the right proportions to avoid these problems. Among the different types of amylases are the α-amylases (E.C.3.2.1.1), starch-degrading enzymes that catalyze the hydrolysis of internal α-1,4-O-glycosidic bonds in polysaccharides with the retention of α-anomeric configuration in the products; and β-amylase (E.C. 3.2.1.2), an exoenzyme that releases successive maltose units from the nonreducing end of a polysaccharide chain by hydrolysis of α-1,4-glucan or starch linkages. The shortest normal saccharide hydrolyzed is maltotetraose. Since it is unable to bypass branch linkages in branched polysaccharides such as glycogen or amylopectin, the hydrolysis is incomplete and a macromolecular dextrin limit remains. This problem is solved by amylo-α-1,6-glucosidase (E.C.3.2.1.33), which is a debranching enzyme separating the side chains of the amylopectine. The set of these amylases is completed with the amyloglucosidase enzyme (E.C.3.2.1.3). This enzyme catalyzes the hydrolysis of the α-1,4-O-glycosidic bonds from the reducing ends of the starch-releasing glucose molecules. To improve the clarification process and produce haze diminishment, enzymatic preparations can also contain fungal acid proteases. Pinelo et al. (2010) treated cherry juice with pectinases containing fungal acid protease (from *A. niger*, of 200,000 alkaline protease units [APU]) and found a significant reduction of immediate turbidity, but low clarification impact during the subsequent cold storage. In contrast, pectinase addition exerted a weak effect on immediate turbidity reduction, but effectively decreased the turbidity development during storage. Another enzyme that is not part of enzyme preparations but which may have utility in the fruit juice industry is glucose oxidase (E.C.1.1.3.4). This enzyme catalyzes the release of glucose to produce gluconic acid and hydrogen peroxide. This reaction utilizes molecular oxygen. Glucose oxidase (coupled with catalase to remove the oxygen peroxide) is therefore used to remove the oxygen from the head space in drink bottles, thereby reducing the nonenzymatic browning due to oxidation that otherwise occurs (Lozano, 2006). Other miscellaneous enzymes used are naringinase, for debittering of products from grapefruit and bitter oranges, and limoninase, desirable to reduce limonoid bitterness from grapefruits and Navel oranges.

8.2.6 Enzymatic Activity Determination for Enzymatic Mixtures for Juice Treatment

Typically, a sodium dodecyl sulfate–polyacrylamide gel electrophoresis (SDS-PAGE) (Laemmli, 1970) should be performed to assess the enzyme components of the industrial preparation and their molecular weights. Figure 8.3 shows an electrophoregram of an industrial enzymatic mixture to clarify juices, performed by Echavarría et al. (2012c). Currently, electrophoresis can be carried out more quickly using Bioanalizator® 2100 (Agilent Technologies, Palo Alto, CA) equipment To proceed with determination of the activity of each of the enzyme components of the enzymatic preparation, separation of the mixture is needed. Methods such as gel-filtration chromatography with Sephacryl® columns can separate enzymes without losing their activity, and they can then be analyzed using the methods shown below. This technique has the advantage that purification and separation of enzymes can be carried out at the same time. Another practical way would be to analyze globally in the enzyme preparation the two types of activities of carbohydrolases: endo- and exo-activity. Endo-activity can be determined by decreasing the kinematic viscosity through capillary viscometry using the adequate substrate at each experiment. The enzyme endo-activities are related to the initial reaction rate by the equation (Pagán et al., 2006):

$$r_i = (\eta_0 - \eta_\infty)k \tag{8.1}$$

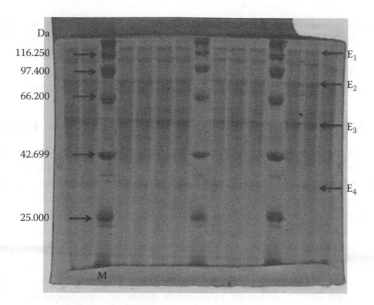

FIGURE 8.3 Electrophoregram of an enzyme preparation. M, protein markers. Bands: E_1, exopolygalacturonase (71 kDa); E_2, endopectate lyase (44 kDa); E_3, endopolygalacturonase (61 kDa); E_4, pectinesterase (23 kDa). (From Echavarría, A.P., Ibarz, A., Conde, J., and Pagan, J., *Journal of Food Engineering*, 111, 52–56, 2012. With permission.)

where:

r_i is the initial reaction rate
η_0 is the initial viscosity of substrate
η_∞ is the asymptotic value tending to the substrate viscosity
k is a first-order reaction kinetic constant

An endo-activity unit (U) is the amount of enzyme that decreases 50% of substrate viscosity per minute at optimal conditions of pH and temperature. Exo-activity can be determined through the increase of spectrophotometric absorbance related to the increase of the reducing sugars released in the hydrolysis reaction. The method used by Waffenschmidt and Jaenicke (1987) gives very precise results. An exo-activity unit (U) is the amount of enzyme that releases one micromole of reducing sugars each minute per gram of sample. Pectin esterase enzyme activity can be determined by a titrimetric assay (Rouse and Adkins, 1955) by measuring the pH decrease during a measured time in minutes to maintain the initial pH at 7.8 after addition of NaOH 0.02 N that causes the demethylation of pectin. The pectin-esterase activity (PE) is expressed as:

$$PE\ activity = \frac{mL\ NaOH\ 0.02\ N}{min \cdot g\ sample\ (°Brix/100)} 100 \tag{8.2}$$

The enzymatic activity of the glucose oxidase is the enzyme that catalyzes the oxidation of beta-D-glucose to hydrogen peroxide and D-glucono-1,5-lactone, which spontaneously hydrolyzes to gluconic acid. The enzymatic activity was measured by the method described by Bergmeyer et al. (1983): the increase of absorbance at 436 nm due to the oxidation of guaiacol in the reaction mixture containing peroxidase. Enzyme unit is defined as the amount of the enzyme that liberates one micromole of hydrogen peroxide per minute under the experiment conditions.

8.2.7   METHODS OF IMMOBILIZED PECTINOLYTIC ENZYMES IN FRUIT PROCESSING

Immobilization of enzymes consists in confining them in a defined region of space while keeping their catalytic activities, so they can be used repeatedly and continuously. To do this, the enzyme is associated with an insoluble matrix, and therefore it can be retained in the reactor for its reuse under the process conditions. Enzyme immobilization may provide several advantages: (a) some available binding sites and a very simple, mild, and time-saving process; (b) reuse and easier separation from the product (Pessela et al., 2003); (c) the reduction of immobilization costs; and (d) improved stability of the enzymatic activity. Demirel et al. (2004) reports data on immobilization of pectinolytic enzymes on different supports by various methods. Immobilization can be carried out by different methods: entrapment/microencapsulation, binding to a solid carrier, and cross-linking of enzyme aggregates, resulting in carrier-free macromolecules. Despite pectinase's excellent catalytic properties, the native enzymes as biocatalysts always present some drawbacks, such as poor stability under operational conditions, difficulty of product recovery, and impossibility of multiple reuses in an industrial process (Sheldon, 2007). There has been increased interest in the preparation of immobilized pectinase for the clarification and depectinization of fruit juices using a wide variety of carriers and methods. However, satisfactory results without any limitations have been rarely achieved and different methods have been developed for the preparation of immobilized pectinase that have their own advantages and disadvantages (Alkorta et al., 1996). Pectinase has been immobilized on various supports including polysulfone (Echavarría et al., 2012a), ion-exchange resin (Kminkova and Kucera, 1983), silk (Zhu et al., 1998), and chitin (Iwasaki et al., 1998) and in alginate by simple inclusion (Busto et al., 2006). In this last case, its residual activity was still slightly lower or had a lower stability, making it difficult to use on an industrial scale. An innovative method is the use of cross-linked enzyme aggregates (CLEAs) (Cao et al., 2000). The first step of the procedure is to precipitate the enzyme from an aqueous solution by adding a salt or a water-miscible organic solvent or polymer, such as poly(ethylene glycol). In the subsequent step, the physical aggregates of enzyme molecules are cross-linked with a bifunctional agent (Lopez-Serrano et al., 2002). An interesting feature of the CLEAs is that these preparations do not require extensive purification of the enzyme activities. The general protocol for the preparation of CLEAs consists of precipitating the enzyme activity by adding salt or an organic solvent (Schoevaart et al., 2004). This is followed by addition of a cross-linking reagent, which is generally glutaraldehyde. A CLEA method with substantial immobilization of pectinase, xylanase, and cellulase was prepared and characterized. Cellulase activity was most thermostable and its thermoinactivation was measured at 70°C. Pectinase was least stable and its thermoinactivation was measured at 50°C. The largest increase in stability was in the case of pectinase, in which the half-life increased from 17 to 180 min (Dalal et al., 2007). A particularly cheap and relatively inert matrix for immobilization of enzyme is nylon-6. The enzyme polygalacturonase from *A. niger* was immobilized by the covalent binding method on glutaraldehyde-activated nylon-6 and used for apple juice clarification (Shukla et al., 2010).

Immobilization of commercial pectinases has also been carried out. Pectinex® Ultra SP-L from Novozymes (Bagsvaerd, Denmark), a commercial pectinase, was immobilized onto an anion-exchange resin by a combined method. Combining the adsorption of a commercial pectinase onto Amberlite IRA900 Cl anion-exchange resin and the formation of cross-links between the adsorbed protein molecules, an immobilized enzyme product was prepared. The optimal pH value of the immobilized biocatalyst was found to be similar to that of the free enzyme but the immobilization increased the optimal temperature a little (Csanadi and Sisak, 2006).

8.2.7.1 Application of Native and Immobilized Pectinases in Ultrafiltration of Apple Juice

Commercial pectic enzymes or pectinases are used in apple juice manufacturing to depectinize pressed juices in order to remove turbidity and prevent cloud forming (Grampp, 1976). The application of ultrafiltration (UF) as an alternative to conventional processes for clarification of apple juice was demonstrated by Heatherbell et al. (1997). However, UF has not been completely accepted in the fruit processing industry because there are problems with its operation and fouling of membranes. During UF, two fluid streams are generated: the ultrafiltered solid-free juice (permeate) and the retentate with variable content of insoluble solids, which, in the case of apple juice, are mainly remains of cellular walls and pectin. Permeate flux results from the difference between a convective flux from the bulk of the juice to the membrane and a counter-diffusive flux or outflow by which solute is transferred back into the bulk of the fluid (Carrin et al., 2000).

To study the problem that causes clogging of UF filters, Echavarría et al. (2012b) performed experiments on a model process adding pectinases on a pectin gel layer cake, optimizing clogging removal. As a result of the mechanism of the mass transfer, pectin and other large solutes are brought to the membrane surface by convective transport during the hollow-fiber ultrafiltration (HFUF) of apple juice. Consolidation of this gel layer on the HFUF membrane has a drastic effect on the performance of the operation. In order to obtain a higher permeate flow, the fluids should be treated with pectinase enzymes recirculating through a tubular membrane (Echavarría et al., 2011b). Despite the different types of supports and reactor configurations proposed for a continuous performance of enzymatic reaction, immobilization of enzymes on micro- or ultrafiltration membranes appears to be an interesting alternative for treating cloudy fruit juices (Alkorta et al., 1995). Endopolygalacturonase and pectinlyase, among others, have been immobilized on different organic and inorganic supports, with uneven results (Spagna et al., 1995). The use of pectinase immobilized on UF membranes is expected to hydrolyze the pectin to lower-molecular-weight species (mainly anhydrogalacturonic acid, AGA) at the membrane–permeate interface, resulting in an increase of the permeate flux or at least an extension of the membrane operation without cleaning. Glutaraldehyde has been used as a cross-linking and spacing agent (Synowiecki et al., 1982).

8.2.7.2 Immobilized Pectinases in Mash Treatment and in Apple Juice Clarification

Enzymatic mash treatment is a well-known modern process for improving the yield of extracted juice from fruits and vegetables. According to the technique, cell wall and middle lamella pectin of the fruit are degraded by pectinase activities. Besides increasing press capacity and the yield of juice up to 20%, it also has a positive effect on carotene and dry matter content of the product. The immobilization process was carried out by using ion-exchange resin particles on carrot puree. The average yield increment was 30.23% with respect to the yield obtained from nonenzymic processed carrot juice (Demir et al., 2001).

Before concentration, pressed juice must be clarified. The catalytic behavior of a mixture of pectic enzymes, covalently immobilized on different supports (glass microspheres, nylon 6/6 pellets, and polyacrylonitrile [PAN] beads), was analyzed with an apple juice model system. The following parameters were investigated: the rate constant at which pectin hydrolysis is conducted, the time in which the reduction of 50% of the initial viscosity is reached, and the time required to obtain complete depectinization. The best catalytic system was proven to be PAN beads, and their pH and temperature behavior were determined. The yields of two bed reactors, packed or fluidized, using the catalytic PAN beads were compared to the circulation flow rate of real apple juice. The initial pectin concentration was the one that was present in the apple juice sample. No differences were observed at low circulation rates, while at higher recirculation rates, the time required to obtain complete pectin hydrolysis into the fluidized reactor was found to be 0.25 times shorter than in the packed bed reactor: 131 min for the packed reactors and 41 min for the fluidized reactors (Diano et al., 2008). A commercial pectinase, immobilized on appropriately functionalized γ-alumina spheres, was loaded in a packed bed reactor and employed to depolymerize the pectin contained in a model solution and in the apple juice. The activity of the immobilized enzyme was tested in several batch reactions and compared with the one of the free enzyme. Apple juice was successfully depectinized using the pectinase immobilized system (Dinella et al., 1996). An apple juice model system was also clarified using polysulfone membranes with immobilized pectinase improving the performance of the volumetric permeate flux (Echavarría et al., 2012a).

REFERENCES

Aehle, W. (2007). *Enzymes in Industry. Production, Processes and Applications*, 3rd edn. Weinheim: Wiley-VCH.

Alasalvar, C. and Shahidi, F. (eds) (2013). Composition, phytochemicals and beneficial health effects of dried foods: An overview. In *Dried Fruits, Phytochemicals and Health Effects*, pp. 1–18. Oxford: Wiley-Blackwell.

Albersheim, P., Mühlethaler, K., and Frey-Wyssling, A. (1960). Stained pectin as seen in the electron microscope. *Journal of Biophysical Biochemical Cytology* 8(2): 501–506.

Alkorta, I., Garbisu, C., Llama, M.J., and Serra, J.L. (1995). Viscosity decrease of pectin and fruit juices catalyzed by pectin lyase from *Penicillium italicum* in batch and continuous-flow membrane. *Journal of Chemical Technology and Biotechnology* 9(2): 95–100.

Alkorta, I., Garbisu, C., Llama, M.J., and Serra, J.L. (1996). Immobilization of pectin lyase from *Penicillium italicum* by covalent binding to nylon. *Enzyme Microbiology and Technology* 18: 141–146.

Ariel, R.V., Saladié, M., Rose, J.K.C., and Labavitch, J. (2007). The linkage between cell wall metabolism and fruit softening: Looking to the future. *Journal of the Science of Food and Agriculture* 87: 1435–1448.

Baker, R.A. (1997). Reassessment of some fruit and vegetable pectin levels. *Journal of Food Science* 62(2): 225–229.

Barros, S., Mendes, E., and Peres, L. (2004). Influence of depectinization in the ultrafiltration of West Indian cherry (*Malpighia glabra* L.) and pineapple (*Ananas comosus* juices). *Ciencia y Tecnologia Alimentaria* 24(2): 194–201.

Bergmeyer, H.U., Bergmeyer, J., and Grassl, M. (1983). *Methods of Enzymatic Analysis*. Weinheim: Verlag Chemie.

Bhat, M.K. (2000). Cellulases and related enzymes in biotechnology. *Biotechnology Advances* 18(5): 355–383.

Biely, P., Puls, J., and Schneider, H. (1985). Acetyl xylan esterases in fungal cellulolytic systems. *FEBS Letters* 186: 80–84.

Biscaro, D. and Cano, E. (2010). Purification and characterization of the exopolygalacturonase produced by *Aspergillus giganteus* in submerged cultures. *Journal of Industrial Microbiology and Biotechnology* 37: 567–573.

Bolwell, G.P. (1993). Dynamic aspects of the plant extracellular matrix. *International Review of Cytology* 146: 261–324.

Busto, M.D., García-Tramontín, K.E., Ortega, N., and Perez-Mateos, M. (2006). Preparation and properties of an immobilized pectinlyase for the treatment of fruit juices. *Bioresources Technology* 97: 1477–1483.

Cao, L., Van Rantwijk, F., and Sheldon, R.A. (2000). Cross-linked enzyme aggregates: A simple and effective method for the immobilization of penicillin acylase. *Organic Letters* 2: 1361–1364.

Carpita, N.C. and Gibeaut, D.M. (1993). Structural models of primary cell walls in flowering plants: Consistency of molecular structure with the physical properties of the walls during growth. *The Plant Journal* 3: 1–30.

Carrin, M.E., Ceci, L.N., and Lozano, J.E. (2000). Effects of pectinase immobilization during hollow fiber ultrafiltration of apple juice. *Journal of Food Process Engineering* 23: 281–298.

Carrin, M.E., Ceci, L.N., and Lozano, J.E. (2004). Characterization of starch in apple juice and its degradation by amylases. *Food Chemistry* 87: 173–178.

Coenen, G.C., Bakx, E.J., Verhoef, R.P., Schols, H.A., and Voragen, A.G.J. (2007). Identification of the connecting linkage between homo- or xylogalacturonan and rhamnogalacturonan type I. *Carbohydrate Polymers* 70: 224–235.

Cosgrove, D.J. (1997). Relaxation in a high-stress environment: The molecular basis of extensible walls and cell enlargement. *Plant Cell* 9(7): 1031–1041.

Csanadi, Z. and Sisak, C. (2006). Immobilization of pectinex ultra SP-L pectinase and its application to production of fructooligosacchride. *Acta Alimentaria* 35: 205–212.

Dalal, S., Sharma, A., and Gupta, M.N. (2007). A multipurpose immobilized biocatalyst with pectinase, xylanase and cellulase activities. *Chemistry Central Journal* 1: 16–22.

Darvill, A.G., McNeil, M., and Albersheim, P. (1978). Structure of plant cell walls. VIII. A new pectic polysaccharide. *Plant Physiology* 62: 418–422.

Dekker, R.F.H. (1985). Biodegradation of hemicelluloses. In Higuchi, T. (ed.), *Biosynthesis and Biodegradation of Wood Components*, pp. 505–533. Orlando: Academic Press.

Demir, N., Sarioglu, K., Acar, J., and Mutlu, M. (2001). The use of commercial pectinase in fruit juice industry. Part 3: Immobilized pectinase for mash treatment. *Journal of Food Engineering* 47: 275–280.

Demirel, D., Ozdural, A., and Mutlu, M. (2004). Performance of immobilized Pectinex Ultra SP-L on magnetic duolite-polystyrene composite particles. Part 1: A batch reactor study. *Journal of Food Engineering* 64: 417–421.

Diano, N., Grimaldi, T., Bianco, M., Rossi, S., Gabrovska, K., Yordanova, G., Godjevargova, T., et al. (2008). Apple juice clarification by immobilized pectolytic enzymes in packed or fluidized bed reactors. *Journal of Agriculture and Food Chemistry* 56: 11471–11477.

Dinella, C., Stagnia, A., Lanzarini, G., and Lausa, M. (1996). Immobilised pectinase efficiency in the depolymerisation of pectin in a model solution and apple juice. *Progress Biotechnology* 14: 971–978.

Donaldson, L. (2007). Cellulose microfibril aggregates and their size variation with cell wall type. *Wood Science and Technology* 41: 443–460.

Dourado, F., Bastos, M., Mota, M., and Gama, F.M. (2002). Studies on the properties of celluclast/eudragit L-100 conjugate. *Journal of Biotechnology* 99(2): 121–131.

Echavarría, A.P., Garcia-Valls, R., Torras, C., Pagán, J., and Ibarz, A. (2012a). Effect of pectinase immobilization in a polymeric membrane on ultrafiltration of fluid foods. *Separation Science and Technology* 47: 796–801.

Echavarría, A.P., Ibarz, A., Conde, J., Torras, C., and Pagan, J. (2012b). Optimizing by the response surface methodology the enzymatic elimination of clogging of a microfiltration membrane by pectin cake. *International Journal of Food Science and Technology* 47: 47–52.

Echavarría, A.P., Ibarz, A., Conde, J., and Pagan, J. (2012c). Enzyme recovery and effluents generated in the enzymatic elimination of clogging of pectin cake in filtration process. *Journal of Food Engineering* 111: 52–56.

Echavarría, A.P., Pagán, J., and Ibarz, A. (2011a). Effect of previous enzymatic recirculation treatment through a tubular ceramic membrane on ultrafiltration of model solution and apple juice. *Journal of Food Engineering* 102(4): 334–339.

Echavarría, A.P., Torras, C., Pagán, J., and Ibarz, A. (2011b). Fruit juice processing and membrane technology application. *Food Engineering Reviews* 3: 136–158.

Fernandes, A.N., Thomas, L.H., Altaner, C.M., Callow, P., Forsyth, V.T., Apperley, D.C., Kennedy, C.J., and Jarvis, M.C. (2011). Nanostructure of cellulose microfibrils in spruce wood. *Proceedings of the National Academy of Sciences USA* 108: 195–1203.

Fernández-González, M., Ubeda, F., Cordero-Otero, C., Thanvanthri Gururajanb, V., and Brionesa, A. (2005). Engineering of an oenological *Saccharomyces cerevisiae* strain with pectinolytic activity and its effect on wine. *International Journal of Food Microbiology* 102(2): 173–183.

Fry, S.C. (1986). Cross-linking of matrix polymers in the growing cell walls of angiosperms. *Annual Review of Plant Physiology* 37: 165–186.

Gibson, L.J. (2012). The hierarchical structure and mechanics of plant materials. *Journal of the Royal Society Interface* 9(76): 2749–2766.

Grampp, E.A. (1976). New process for hot clarification of apple juice for apple juice concentrate. *Flüssiges Obstadt* 43: 382–388.

Grassin, C. and Fauquembergue, P. (1996). Fruit juices. In Godfrey, T. and West, S. (eds), *Industrial Enzymology*, 2nd edn., pp. 226–264. London: MacMillan Press.

Harker, F.R., Redgwell, R.J., Hallett, I.C., Murray, S.H., and Carter, G. (1997). Texture of fresh fruit. In Janick, J. (ed.). *Horticultural Reviews*, vol. 20, pp. 121–224. New York: Wiley.

Heatherbell, D.A., Short, J.L., and Stauebi, P. (1997). Apple juice clarification by ultrafiltration. *Confructa* 22: 157–169.

Hori, R., Muller, M., Watanabe, U., Lichtenegger, H. C., Fratzl, P., and Sugiyama, J. (2002). The importance of seasonal differences in the cellulose microfibril angle in softwoods in determining acoustic properties. *Journal of Material Sciences* 37: 4279–4284.

Iwasaki, K., Inoue, M., and Matsubara, Y. (1998). Continuous hydrolysis of pectate by immobilized endo-polygalacturonase in a continuously stirred tank reactor. *Bioscience, Biotechnology and Biochemistry* 62: 262–267.

Jarvis, M.C. (1984). Structure and properties of pectin gels in the plant cell wall. *Plant Cell and Environment* 7: 153–164.

Karmakar, M. and Ray, R.R. (2011). Current trends in research and application of microbial cellulases. *Research Journal of Microbiology* 6(1): 41–53.

Kashyap, D., Vohra, P., Chopra, S., and Tewari, R. (2001). Applications of pectinases in the commercial sector: A review. *Bioresources Technology* 77: 215–227.

Kminkova, M. and Kucera, J. (1983). Comparison of pectolytic enzymes using different methods of binding. *Enzyme Microbiology and Technology* 5: 204–208.

Kuhad, R.C., Gupta, R., and Singh, A. (2011). Microbial cellulases and their industrial applications. *Enzyme Research* 2011: 1–10.

Laemmli, U.K. (1970). Cleavage of structural proteins during the assembly of the head of bacteriophage T4. *Nature* 277: 680–685.

Landbo, A. and Meyer, A. (2004). Effects of different enzymatic maceration treatments on enhancement of anthocyanins and other phenolics in black currant juice. *Innovative Food Science and Emerging Technologies* 5: 503–513.

Lau, J.M., McNeil, M., Darvill, A.G., and Albersheim, P. (1987). Treatment of rhamnogalacturonan I with lithium in ethylenediamine. *Carbohydrate Research* 168(2): 245–274.

Lin, T.-T. and Pitt, R.E. (1986). Rheology of apple and potato tissue as affected by cell turgor pressure. *Journal of the Texture Studies* 17: 291–313.

Lopez-Serrano, P., Cao, L., Van Rantwijk, F., and Sheldon, R.A. (2002). Cross-linked enzyme aggregates with enhanced activity: Application to lipases. *Biotechnology Letters* 24: 1379–1383.

Lozano, J.E. (2006). Processing of fruits: Ambient and low temperature processing. In *Fruit Manufacturing: Scientific Basis, Engineering Properties, and Deteriorative Reactions of Technological Importance* (Food Engineering Series), pp. 21–51. New York: Springer.

McCleary, B.V. (1988). Synthesis of β-D-mannopyranosides for the assay of β-D-mannosidase and exo-β-D-mannanase. *Methods in Enzymology* 160: 515–517.

Northcote, D.H. (1958). The cell wall of higher plants. *Biological Reviews* 33: 53–102.

O'Neill, M.A., Ishii, T., Albersheim, P., and Darvill, A.G. (2004). Rhamnogalacturonan II: Structure and function of a borate crosslinked cell wall pectic polysaccharide. *Annual Review of Plant Biology* 55: 109–139.

Pagán, A., Conde, J., Ibarz, A., and Pagán, J. (2006). Orange peel degradation an enzyme recovery in the enzymatic peeling process. *International Journal of Food Science and Technology* 41: 113–120.

Pap, N., Mahosenaho, M., Pongrácz, E., Mikkonen, H., Jaakkola, M., Virtanen, V., Myllykoski, L., Horváth-Hovorka, Z., Hodúr, C., and Vatai, G. (2012). Effect of ultrafiltration on anthocyanin and flavonol content of black currant juice (*Ribes nigrum* L.). *Food Bioprocess Technology* 5(3): 921–928.

Percival Zhang, Y.H., Himmel, M.E., and Mielenz, J.R. (2006). Outlook for cellulase improvement: Screening and selection strategies. *Biotechnology Advances* 24(5): 452–481.

Pessela, B.C.C., Fernandez-Lafuente, R., Fuentes, M., Vian, A., García, J.L., Carrascosa, A.V., Mateo, C., and Guisan, J.M. (2003). Reversible immobilization of a thermophilic β-galactosidase via ionic adsorption on PEI-coated Sepabeads. *Enzyme Microbiology and Technology* 32: 369–374.

Pinelo, M., Zeuner, B., and Meyer, A.S. (2010). Juice clarification by protease and pectinase treatments indicates new roles of pectin and protein in cherry juice turbidity. *Food and Bioproducts Processing* 88(2–3): 259–265.

Rai, P., Majumdar, G.C., Das Gupta, S., and De, S. (2007). Effect of various pretreatment methods on permeate flux and quality during ultrafiltration of mosambi juice. *Journal of Food Engineering* 78(2): 561–568.

Rees, D.A. (1977). Polysaccharide shapes and their interactions: Some recent advances. *Pure and Applied Chemistry* 53: 1–14.

Rouse, A.H. and Adkins, C.D. (1955). Pectinesterase and pectin in commercial citrus juices as determined by methods used at the Citrus Experimental Station. *University of Florida Agricultural Experiment Stations, Lake Alfred, Fla* 570: 1–19.

Saftner, R., Conway, W.S., and Sams, C.E. (1998). Effect of postharvest calcium chloride treatments on tissue water relations, cell wall calcium levels and postharvest life of 'Golden Delicious' apples. *Journal of the American Society of Horticultural Science* 123: 893–897.

Sakai, T., Sakamoto, T., Hallaert, J., and Vandamme, E.J. (1993). Pectin, pectinase, and protopectinase: Production, properties, and applications. In Neidleman, S. and Laskin, A.I. (eds), *Advances in Applied Microbiology*, vol. 39, pp. 213–294. San Diego: Academic Press.

Santón, M., Treiche, H., Valduga, E., Cabra, L., and Di Luccio, M. (2008). Evaluation of enzymatic treatment of peach juice using response surface methodology. *Journal of the Science of Food and Agriculture* 88: 507–512.

Scheller, H.V. and Ulvskov, P. (2010). Hemicelluloses. *Annual Review of Plant Biology* 61: 263–289.

Schoevaart, R., Wolbers, M.W., Golubovic, M., Ottens, M., Kieboom, A.P., van Rantwijk, F., van der Wielen, L.A., and Sheldon, R.A. (2004). Preparation, optimization and structures of cross-linked enzyme aggregates (CLEAs). *Biotechnology and Bioengineering* 87: 754–762.

Serra, J.L., Alkorta, I., and Llama, M.J. (1992). Aplicación industrial de las enzimas pécticas. *Alimentación, Equipos y Tecnología* October: 127–134.

Sheldon, R.A. (2007). Enzyme immobilization: The quest for optimum performance. *Advanced Synthesis and Catalysis* 349: 1289–1307.

Shukla, S.K., Saxena, S., Thakur, J., and Gupta, R. (2010). Immobilization of polygalacturonase from *Aspergillus niger* onto glutaraldehyde activated nylon-6 and its application in apple juice clarification. *Acta Alimentaria* 39: 277–292.

Singh, A. (1999). Engineering enzyme properties. *Indian Journal of Microbiology* 39(2): 65–77.

Spagna, G., Pifferi, P.G., and Gilioli, E. (1995). Immobilization of pectinlyase from *Aspergillus niger* for application in food technology. *Enzyme Microbiology and Technology* 17: 729–738.

Srimanta, P., Bharihoke, R., Chakraborty, S., Kumar, S., Sirshendu, D., and Sunando, D. (2008). An experimental and theoretical analysis of turbulence promoter assisted ultrafiltration of synthetic fruit juice. *Separation and Purification Technology* 62: 659–667.

Synowiecki, J., Sikorski, Z., and Naczk, M. (1982). Immobilization of amylases on krill chitin. *Food Chemistry* 8: 239–246.

Talbott, L.D. and Ray, P.M. (1992). Molecular size and separability features of pea cell wall polysaccharides: Implications for models of primary wall structure. *Plant Physiology* 98: 357–368.

Tong, C., Krueger, D., Vickers, Z., Bedford, D., Luby, J., El-Shiekh, A., Shackel, K., and Ahmadi, H. (1999). Comparison of softening-related changes during storage of 'Honeycrisp' apple, its parent, and 'Delicious'. *Journal of the American Society of Horticultural Science* 124: 407–415.

Vincken, J.-P., Schols, H.A., Oomen, R.J.F.J., McCann, M.C., Ulvskov, P., and Voragen, A.J.G. (2003). If homogalacturonan were a side chain of rhamnogalacturonan. I. Implications for cell wall architecture. *Plant Physiology* 132: 1781–1789.

Voragen, A.G.J. (1972). Characterization of pectin lyases on pectins and methyl oligogalacturonates. PhD Thesis, Agricultural University, Department of Food Science, Wageningen, the Netherlands.

Waffenschmidt, S. and Jaenicke, L. (1987). Assay of reducing sugars in the nanomole range with 2-2' bicinchoninate. *Analytical Biochemistry* 165: 337–340.

Zhan, D.F., Janssen, P., and Mort, A.J. (1998). Scarcity or complete lack of single rhamnose residues interspersed within the homogalacturonan regions of citrus pectin. *Carbohydrate Research* 308: 373–380.

Zhu, R.X., Lin, R., and Wang, J.O. (1998). Studies on immobilization of pectate lyase with silk fibroin. *Journal of Zhejiang University* 24: 74–78.

9 Advances in Fruit Juice Conventional Thermal Processing

José Lorente, Nuria Martí, and Domingo Saura

CONTENTS

9.1 Introduction 172
9.2 Pasteurization 172
    9.2.1 Microorganisms... 173
    9.2.2 Factors Affecting Pasteurization Level 174
        9.2.2.1 pH.. 174
        9.2.2.2 Water Activity... 174
        9.2.2.3 Oxygen 174
        9.2.2.4 Raw Material.. 175
        9.2.2.5 Rheological Properties of the Juice 175
    9.2.3 Most Common Contaminants in Juice 176
9.3 Common Thermal Pasteurization Technologies.. 176
    9.3.1 Current Pasteurization Technologies... 177
        9.3.1.1 Pasteurizer with Direct Heating/Cooling 177
        9.3.1.2 Pasteurizers with Indirect Heating/Cooling System......... 179
9.4 Indirect Heat Transfer Systems Description... 185
    9.4.1 Plate Heat Exchanger (PHE) 185
        9.4.1.1 General Description 185
        9.4.1.2 Plate Shape and Thickness... 188
    9.4.2 Tubular Heat Exchangers... 188
        9.4.2.1 General Description 188
        9.4.2.2 Tubes in Tube Design: For High-Viscosity
                Juices, Pulp, and Purees... 189
        9.4.2.3 Tubes in Shell Heat Exchangers 191
        9.4.2.4 Scraped Surface Heat Exchangers 193
References.. 195

9.1 INTRODUCTION

Pasteurization originated in the nineteenth century and is named for Louis Pasteur (Figure 9.1), a French chemist who developed studies on and discovered the lethal effect of heat on microorganisms and the thermal treatment effect in food preservation. His research and findings have had an enormous influence on food technology and preventing the spread of diseases.

Thermal treatment technology was initially applied in a crude way, and was extended to different applications, including domestic ones. Initially, it was shown that thermal treatment to preserve foods required a combination of temperature and time. In the twentieth century, the application evolved into a more accurate process related to the characteristics of the food to be preserved. Today, pasteurization is considered a technology that stabilizes a food and makes it possible to preserve and store it in order to be consumed later. This has also improved food safety and has enabled development in the food industry.

The current sophistication in food processing has made it possible to have high-quality foods available all year round and everywhere, even in places far away from production.

9.2 PASTEURIZATION

One of today's challenges for the food industry is to guarantee safe foods throughout the supply chain, while retaining similar properties to those present when the foods

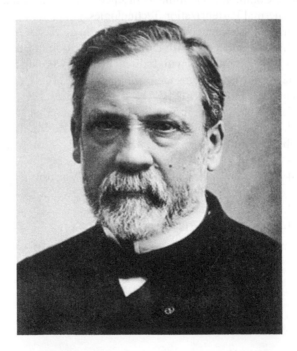

FIGURE 9.1 Louis Pasteur.

were freshly made. During distribution from food manufacturer to consumer, food products need to be protected against physical, chemical, and microbial deterioration.

Although new thermal technologies for pasteurization, such as microwave, radio-frequency, ultrasound, and ohmic treatment (Valero et al. 2007, 2010), are used in some new fruit and vegetable juice processing installations, conventional thermal processes are still in use in the majority of actual processing installations across the world (Plumey et al. 2013). Also, these conventional thermal technologies are being updated continuously and are presenting new profiles that include less treatment time and lower temperatures by using new exchanger designs (Lorente et al. 2012).

When pasteurizing a juice, the intention is to achieve a commercial aseptic state; according to the U.S. Food and Drug Administration (FDA-HHS 2001), this may be achieved:

- By applying heat to the food to eliminate the contamination of microorganisms, which are
  - Able to reproduce in the juice at normal conditions of distribution and storage without refrigeration
  - Vital microorganisms, including spores, that could damage consumers' health
- By controlling water activity combined with heat to make the microorganisms within juice unable to freely reproduce themselves in normal conditions of storage and transport without refrigeration

The thermal process applied to the juices has as a target (Tressler and Joslyn 1961; Nagy et al. 1977, 1992):

1. The inactivation of the natural enzymes to avoid juice stability degradation
2. The stabilization of the juice characteristics: color, turbidity, and aroma
3. The reduction of the microbial load of the juice to a very low level (industrial or commercial asepsis), the avoidance of juice spoilage, and the conservation of the juice in good conditions during its commercial life

9.2.1 Microorganisms

Microorganisms have many beneficial functions within the food industry. A few examples are yoghurt fermentation by *Lactobacillus* cultures, yeast leavening in bread manufacturing, and alcohol production using beer and wine yeast. Microorganisms are also responsible for food spoilage, and some are pathogenic.

For growth and multiplication, microorganisms need organic food (proteins, carbohydrates, fats), a convenient temperature, some moisture, in most cases some air, and a suitable pH. Knowledge about the conditions required for growth will also provide an insight into how to prevent microorganisms growing and therefore prevent food spoilage.

Pasteurization is required to maintain the storage stability of a juice. Heat input is required for the destruction of microorganisms and the inactivation of enzymes. It is easier to destroy microorganism cells than to inactivate enzymes. In a normal juice made from fruit or vegetables, the heat applied to inactivate the natural enzymes is enough to destroy the microorganisms.

The microorganisms that grow in a juice may consequently cause fermentation that could produce gas and off-flavors that degrade the quality of the juice.

9.2.2 FACTORS AFFECTING PASTEURIZATION LEVEL

There are several factors affecting the pasteurization level applied to a juice. The most important and their influences are (Nagy et al. 1977):

9.2.2.1 pH

Microorganism survival depends on the pH of the juice. A lower pH equals less microorganism resistance and a lower possible range of juice contamination (Figure 9.2).

9.2.2.2 Water Activity

When water activity increases, so does contamination. Microorganisms need water to grow: when the availability of water increases because of the increase in water activity, the microorganisms grow faster.

9.2.2.3 Oxygen

To grow and reproduce, microorganisms need oxygen. The presence of oxygen together with nutrients and water make growth possible. It is important to eliminate it from a stable juice.

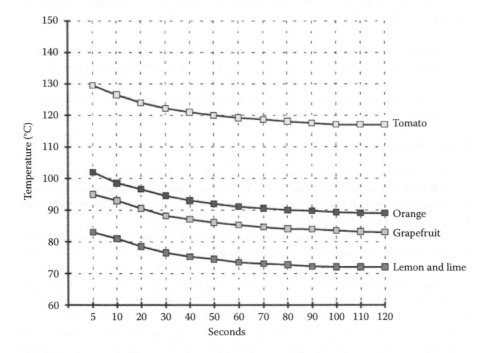

FIGURE 9.2 pH values versus pasteurization temperature in some juices.

9.2.2.4 Raw Material

The initial level of microorganisms found in nature will enter into the process via fruit, transport containers, or people. The number and diversity of microorganisms present in the fruit may be reduced by using good manufacturing practices in the process (Tetra Pak Processing Systems 2003, 2004):

- Good hygienic conditions in transport bins for fruit arriving in the plant.
- Correct storage conditions for fruit before processing.
- Good fruit grading process to eliminate all the defective and rotten fruit before processing.
- Complete fruit-washing process that will eliminate a large amount of contamination. There are specific procedures for each fruit and these should be designed according to the fruit's characteristics; for example, by using detergent soap to clean some fruits such as citrus fruits, melon, and watermelon.
- Application of a hygienic design to processing equipment (easy to clean and made of permanent materials) and keeping conditions hygienic to avoid recontamination after processing.
- Clean-in-place (CIP) to be integrated into the equipment and be part of the process, scheduling it according to the kind of product obtained, processed, and so on.
- Operating rules to be kept in accordance with hygiene and food safety legislation.

9.2.2.5 Rheological Properties of the Juice

Depending on the product's characteristics (viscosity, °Brix, etc.) the heat transmission within various juices is different. Juices could be considered, in general, as almost Newtonian fluids, although it is difficult for some of them to be considered as such: purees from stone fruits, juices with floating pulp such as citrus fruits and pineapple, and so on.

The determination of the rheology of juice is solely concerned with the modeling and optimization of the heat treatment processes. Juices are liquid derivatives of fruits, and their flow characteristics have been an extensive topic of study in recent years (Ibarz et al. 1996; Cepeda and Villarán 1999; Massa et al. 2010). The design and improvement of other operations, such as pumping, mixing, and heat exchange, also depend on them.

The rheological properties of most of the juices exhibit substantial changes during the processing stages because of their dependence on temperature and °Brix: orange juice (Rao et al. 1987; Crandall et al. 1990; Telis-Romero et al. 1999), fruit purees (Guerrero and Alzamora 1998; Hernández et al. 2010), and clarified fruit juices (Khalil et al. 1989; Ibarz et al. 1994).

To design a pasteurizer that is able to work with different kinds of juices means that it has to work with different pH levels, water activities, rheological properties, and contaminants. This requires different options for the temperature versus time equation in order to optimize juice quality and energy consumption results.

9.2.3 Most Common Contaminants in Juice

Although several microorganisms have been isolated from different juices, few of them cause spoilage. In a pasteurization process, it is necessary to have some reference microorganisms to calculate thermal treatment.

- Thermal death time (TDT): Necessary time to destroy all the microorganisms from sample, and at specific, temperature and conditions
- Decimal reduction time (D): Necessary time to destroy 90% of microorganisms in a sample at a specific temperature

These defined parameters may be used to measure the thermal efficiency of each microbial destruction treatment. The TDT is logarithmic and theoretically achieves complete microbial load destruction, but in reality this is simply impossible; it is better to choose the decimal reduction time D as the reference parameter to calculate the pasteurization level applied to a juice.

The reference microorganisms that will be considered to calculate pasteurization depend on the type of juice or fruit (Woodroof and Phillips 1981). An example: microorganisms in orange pulp (Valero et al. 2009) are (choosing two microorganisms per group, isolated from vegetal material):

- Gram-positive bacteria, which form endospores
  - *Alicyclobacillus acidoterrestris* (Colección Española de Cultivos Tipo, Universitat de València, Valencia, Spain [CECT] 7094)
  - *Bacillus subtilis* CECT 39 (Ehrenberg 1835; Cohn 1872)
- Lactic acid bacteria or acid-tolerant bacteria
  - *Lactobacillus brevis* (CECT 216)
  - *Leuconostoc mesenteroides* subsp. *dextranicum* (CECT 912)
- Pathogenic bacteria, rarely present in juices
  - *Salmonella enterica* subsp. *enterica* (CECT 443, serovar *Typhimurium*, ex Kauffmann and Edwards [1952]; Le Minor and Popoff [1987])
  - *Escherichia coli*
- Yeasts (the most frequent spoilage microorganisms)
  - *Saccharomyces cerevisiae*
  - *Pichia anomala* (CECT 1107)
- Filament molds (sensitive to heat treatments)
  - *Aspergillus niger*
  - *Penicillium digitatum*

Different programs to calculate the value of D—statistical parameters and heat treatment, based on the microbial count of different juice samples—could be used: for example, *TerMod* (JBT FoodTech R&D Alliance, Instituto de Biología Moelcular y Celular, Universidad Miguel Hernández de Elche).

9.3 COMMON THERMAL PASTEURIZATION TECHNOLOGIES

Pasteurization is achieved by a combination of heating to a specific temperature for a specific time. This temperature and time should be applied to the whole amount of juice. To achieve this homogeneous heat transmission within the juice more quickly, a lower temperature versus time can be applied and a better juice quality may be obtained (Figure 9.3).

The quality of the juice could be affected by the pasteurization process, mainly in organoleptic parameters (color, aroma, and taste), vitamin C content, and hydroxy-methylfurfural (HMF) formation.

Depending on the agitation system of the heat transfer equipment, pasteurization may be achieved at a different temperature/time rate. The inactivation of enzymes and pasteurization commence at different temperatures depending on the pH of the juice. The design of the heat transfer equipment is fundamental.

9.3.1 CURRENT PASTEURIZATION TECHNOLOGIES

We can select two different heating/cooling systems in a heat exchanger:

- Direct: no heat transfer plate between media and juice
  - Steam injection
  - Steam infusion
- Indirect: transfer plate between media and juice
  - Plates
  - Monotubular and multitubular, including shell
  - Scraped surface

9.3.1.1 Pasteurizer with Direct Heating/Cooling

In this case, the heat transfer is direct and is used in specific products, mainly concentrates:

- *Direct steam injection*: The steam is directly injected into the juice or concentrate (Figure 9.4). A good example is its use in flash cooler aseptic sterilizers (Figure 9.5), which are mainly used for tomato paste (con-

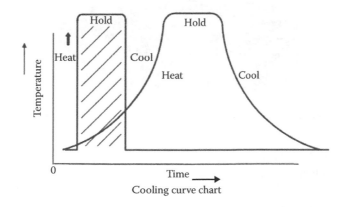

FIGURE 9.3   Heating/cooling rate in two different heaters.

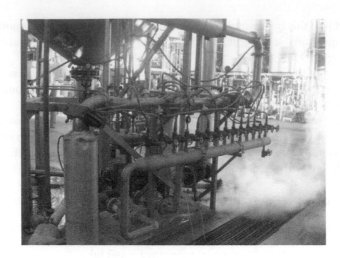

FIGURE 9.4   Heat injector. (Courtesy of JBT FoodTech in JBT FoodTech, pictures database.)

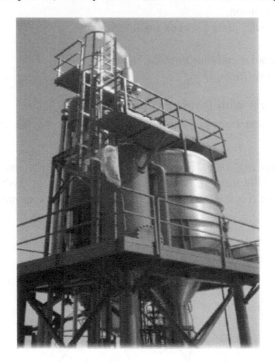

FIGURE 9.5   Fran Rica (JBT) flash cooler. (Courtesy of JBT FoodTech in JBT FoodTech, pictures database.)

centrate) after the evaporator and before aseptic filling, with significant quality advantages for juices and concentrates compared with a standard pasteurizer with indirect heating:

- Finished product has better color and flavor
- Does not reduce product consistency

- Heating by direct steam injection/cooling by flash in a vacuum chamber
- High capacity (up to 100 tons/h)
- Lower energy consumption
- Could run continuously for over 100 days
- In standby mode it does not lose sterility for 48 h
- Easy to operate, easy to maintain
- Permits a light evaporation to eliminate the excess of water incorporated when heating with direct steam

Steam injection may also be used in an indirect exchanger, to heat the water used as the heat transfer fluid.

- *Direct steam infusion*: The steam is incorporated into the same space in which the product is passing as a cloud. The product and steam are mixed and the heat is transferred from the steam to the product. The excess of steam is separated together with condensate (Figure 9.6). This action occurs under vacuum conditions.

9.3.1.2 Pasteurizers with Indirect Heating/Cooling System

A barrier exists between the product and the heating/cooling media. There is no direct contact between the media and the juice. This barrier could be in different materials, depending on the type of juice and the objective.

9.3.1.2.1 Materials and Heat Exchange, K Factor

The most common material used to construct the pasteurizer is stainless steel, which has good heat transfer characteristics.

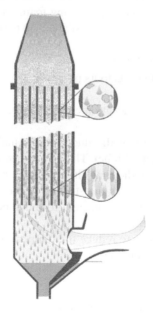

FIGURE 9.6 Steam diffusion.

The possibility also exists of using different materials such as heat-resistant plastics and alloys that have been newly developed for this purpose and are able to work properly at normal temperatures to achieve pasteurization.

The heat transfer coefficient K measures the quantity of heat transferred in 1 h through 1 m^2 of exchange surface per 1°C of temperature difference. The higher the value of K, the better the material is for use as a heat exchanger. K depends on:

- The pressure drop when the juice and the heat exchanger fluids enter into the heat exchanger. The higher this drop in pressure, the better the heat transfer.
- The viscosity of the juice and the heat transfer fluid.
- Material: It is necessary to have a good heat transfer material that accords with the legislation related to materials in contact with foods.
- Shape of the transfer wall: This has a specific shape to create turbulence, which is different depending on the characteristics of the juice to be pasteurized: viscosity, homogeneity, and so on.
- Thickness of the transfer wall: A thinner wall will transfer heat better but the thickness must be enough to support the pressure of the juice and the heat transfer fluid. Current new materials and alloys make it possible to reduce the thickness of the wall as compared with those in the past.

To improve the K factor, a reduction in the channel size through which the juice passes could be applied, decreasing the heat transfer distance and increasing the flow speed and turbulence. This would improve the heat transfer, but at the same time, products sensitive to agitation such as pulpy juices could be affected negatively (destroying part of the pulp) and the juice quality could be reduced by the oxidation of some compounds and the emulsification of part of the juice, promoting foam formation and making the heat transfer difficult. A deaeration step could partially help to solve this problem.

9.3.1.2.2 Main Steps to Consider

Pasteurization has three main parts to its process:

- *Heat transfer process*: to elevate the temperature to the required value for pasteurization.
- *Holding time*: the time that the juice must remain at this pasteurization temperature (in an external tube). The flow speed control, tube length, and diameter will determine the time that the juice remains at the fixed temperature. This holding tube is the starting point of the aseptic area in the pasteurizer, which is usually protected from that point on by steam barriers to preserve the aseptic environment.
- *Cooling transfer process*: to reduce the temperature of the juice from pasteurization to storage temperature.

9.3.1.2.3 Deaeration

In the different processing steps the juice is in contact with the air: extraction, refining/filtering, pumping, and so on. The air is partially dissolved in the juice and may also be dispersed in bubbles within it. This air can cause various problems in the juice quality (aroma, color, vitamin C, etc.) and create some difficulties in the process (foam production and difficulty in heat transmission). It is necessary to remove this air before pasteurizing the juice to improve its quality by avoiding oxidative reactions and making the pasteurization process more efficient.

9.3.1.2.3.1 Negative Influence of Oxygen Presence in Juice

1. *Enzymatic browning*, catalyzed by polyphenol oxidase, oxidation of phenols into slightly colored quinones, and further reactions leading to the formation of dark-brown pigments, decreasing the organoleptic quality and the nutritional value of the juice.

(1) $R-\underset{OH}{\overset{OH}{\bigcirc}} \xrightarrow{(O_2)} R-\bigcirc\overset{O}{\underset{O}{}} + H_2O_2$

(2) $H_2O_2 + CH_3\text{-}CH_2\text{-}OH \longrightarrow CH_3\text{-}CHO + 2H_2O$

2. Ascorbic acid is particularly vulnerable to oxidation, so vitamin C, which is naturally present in fruit, is quickly consumed due to the presence of oxygen (Figure 9.7).

9.3.1.2.3.2 Deaeration Process

Usually, deaeration is carried out after the fruit has been mashed and before the thermal treatment. When eliminating the air from the juice using a vacuum, some volatile compounds flow out together, and also some water. The volatile compounds could be recovered. The water eliminated could cause a small concentration of juice, which means that there would be some decrease in the juice yield.

The structure of the deaerator (Figures 9.8 and 9.9) is composed of:

- Tank with sharing product device
- Vacuum pump
- Condenser for the volatile aromas extracted, often let back into the product
- Inlet pump and extraction pump for the product
- Controls and instrumentation

The deaeration process (Holland 1981) is carried out by using a vacuum: the juice enters the deaerator tank in partial vacuum conditions, begins to expand, and the air bubbles, especially those that are close to the surface, leave the fluid.

To improve air removal from the juice it is important that the gas bubbles are close to the surface of the juice; this is achieved by distributing the product in thin layers.

The goal is to make a turbulent film to accelerate the rise of the bubbles until they leave the product.

Some studies show the importance of avoiding pulverization of the juice in the deaerator because the drops created by pulverization have a greater surface tension; then, the film makes it difficult for the air to exit from the juice.

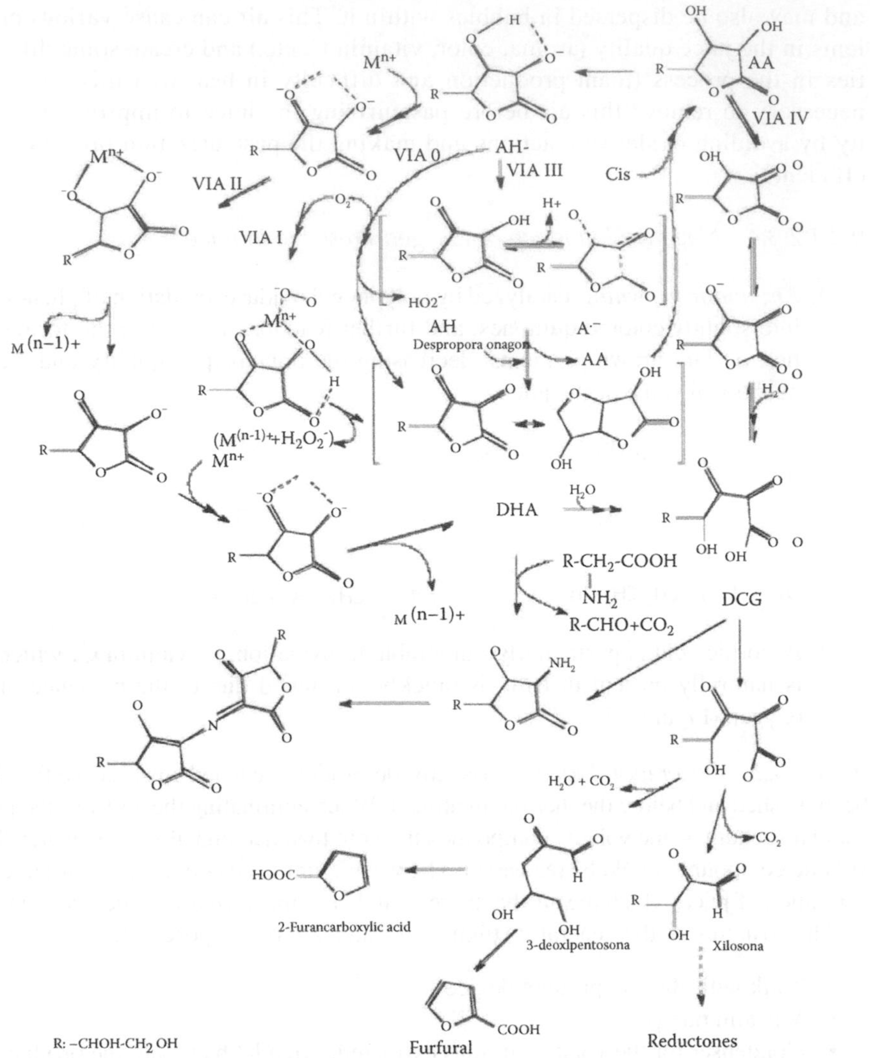

FIGURE 9.7 Ascorbic acid degradation pathways. (From Marti, N., et al., *Natural Products Communication*, 4 (5), 591–748, 2009.)

The most important items that influence deaeration are:

- Amount of gas (air) dissolved
- Temperature of the product
- Viscosity of the product
- Internal pressure of the deaerator (vacuum)
- Deaeration process characteristics

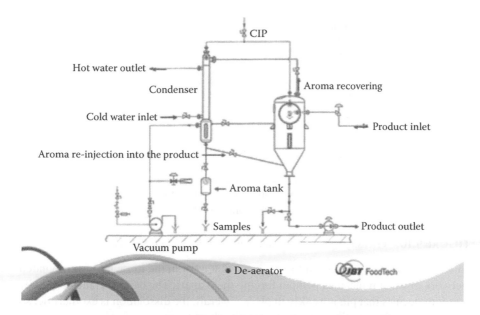

FIGURE 9.8   Deaerator schema. (Courtesy of JBT FoodTech in JBT FoodTech, manual and brochures.)

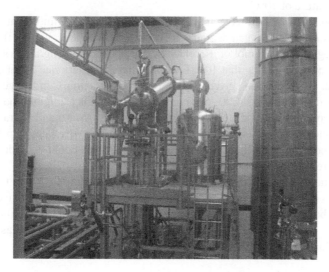

FIGURE 9.9   Deaerator installation. (Courtesy of JBT FoodTech in JBT FoodTech, pictures database.)

The viscosity of the product (which depends on temperature, as shown in Figure 9.10) and the degree of vacuum inside the deaerator are the most important parameters for the design of an effective process.

The solubility of oxygen is affected by the temperature and by the partial pressure of oxygen in the water. The solubility of oxygen is greater in colder water than

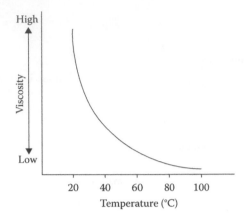

FIGURE 9.10   Viscosity versus temperature diagram for an orange juice.

in warm water. Oxygen slips into "pockets" that exist in the loose hydrogen-bonded network of water molecules without forcing them apart. The oxygen is then caged by water molecules that pin it weakly in place. Overall, the dissolution is exothermic, so cooling shifts the equilibrium toward the dissolved form.

The deaerator operates at a juice flow from 1000 to 1200 L/h, a pressure of 0.4 bar, and a temperature of 70°C.

The amount of dissolved oxygen at 70°C and 0.4 bar is 2.94 mmol/h (at a juice flow rate of 1000 L/h). Since oxygen degrades ascorbic acid in a mole ratio of 1:1, 2.94 mmol of oxygen degrades 2.94 mmol of ascorbic acid, or about 502.74 mg/h of vitamin C per 1000 L of juice. Considering that 1000 L of juice have to deteriorate about 0.503 mg of vitamin C per liter of juice and given the usual content of vitamin C in orange juice (400–700 mg/L) and in mandarins (200–600 mg/L), that amount is negligible and the process under these conditions can be considered very satisfactory (Martí and Saura 2013).

When removing the air, some aromas are also removed. In a later step, the aromas are condensed by cooling them with water. These aromas could be added back into the juice or recovered separately (Reed et al. 1992).

During the deaeration process (Megyesy 2001; Basmadjian 2007) there is also minimal loss of water, which in the operating conditions described above can be documented to be approximately 0.3%, using Raoult's and Dalton's laws and Antoine's equation (the latter with the equation of Capriste and Lozano), as well as the rule of Dühring (Martí and Saura 2013).

9.3.1.2.4   Flow in the Heat Exchanger

A different flow could be applied:

- *Parallel flow*: Both liquids enter the heat exchanger from the same side and flow in the same direction. This system permits heating of the product at a higher temperature than that obtained when mixing both liquids (the heating fluid and the juice).
- *Countercurrent flow*: The juice could be heated up to a temperature close to the entry temperature of the heating fluid (only 2°C–3°C lower).

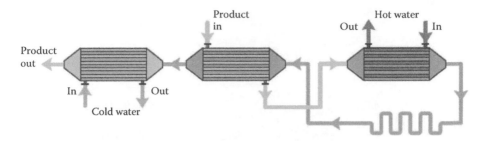

FIGURE 9.11 Simple regeneration: Product to product.

9.3.1.2.5 Energy Regeneration

This is a system that permits better use of energy. The heat from a juice as it leaves the pasteurization process is used to heat another liquid. There are two different ways to regenerate:

- Water to product: Circulate water between heating and cooling units and then transfer heat from the hot aseptic product to the water, then from the hot water to the cool raw product.
- Product to product: Transfer heat from the hot aseptic product to the cool raw product (Figure 9.11).

In both cases, the system maintains the following requirements:

- Up to 80% energy may be saved.
- There must be a pressure differential between the two juices.
- The juices must be fluid products and it is a requirement that the equipment can be thoroughly cleaned.

When regeneration is included in a pasteurizer, the total treatment time is longer and the quality may be slightly affected. A compromise is necessary between the percentage of regenerated energy and the final juice quality. There is a formula to calculate this regeneration R:

$$R = (t_1 - t) \times \frac{100}{t_0 - t}$$

where
  t_1 = temperature of the juice at the exit of the regeneration process
  t = temperature at the entry point of the juice
  t_0 = pasteurization temperature

9.4 INDIRECT HEAT TRANSFER SYSTEMS DESCRIPTION

9.4.1 PLATE HEAT EXCHANGER (PHE)

9.4.1.1 General Description

A PHE consists of a package of stainless steel plates attached to a frame. Several separate packages of plates, called sections, may be installed. Each section is dedicated

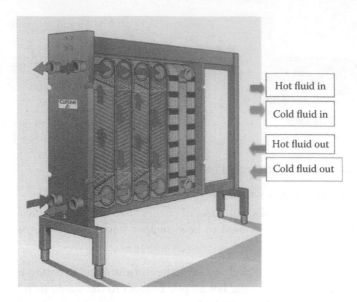

Hot fluid in

Cold fluid in

Hot fluid out

Cold fluid out

FIGURE 9.12   Plate heater/cooler. (Courtesy of Alfa Laval AB, Fusion Line Instruction Manual.)

to a different process: preheating, heating, or cooling. The heating medium is hot water and the cooling medium is cold water or glycol water (Figure 9.12).

The juice is passed between two plates creating a sandwich (medium–juice–medium) separated by the plates, which have a special design to maximize heat transfer. The internal face of the plate is different depending on the product to be treated; also, the separation between the plates depends on the application (Figures 9.13 and 9.14).

The plates are held together in the frame and have gaps between them creating channels to permit the juice to pass through, but this makes it impossible to process pulpy juices or juices with particles. Liquids pass between the plates through apertures in the plates' corners.

The system is closed by rubber joints between the plates at their perimeter.

To adjust the equipment correctly it is necessary to know the viscosity of the juice and the heating fluid. A higher viscosity means that less turbulence is generated when the juice flows through the exchanger.

Viscosity in juices depends on the temperature and, in some specific juices, the flow speed (Lapasin and Pricl 1995; Falguera et al. 2010; Falguera and Ibarz 2010): it is difficult to pass stone fruit purees and pulpy juices through plate exchangers.

This technology is specifically applied to:

- *Low-viscosity juices:* When the product has a high viscosity, the flow between the plates is difficult to manage. Specifically, when cooling the juice, the increase in viscosity is very high, making the flow very difficult to manage through the plates and the cooling transfer. Preferential pathways are created.
- *Homogeneous juices without floating pulp or fruit pieces:* The space between the plates is limited and when processing juices with floating pulp or pieces, these could be retained between the plates making the movement

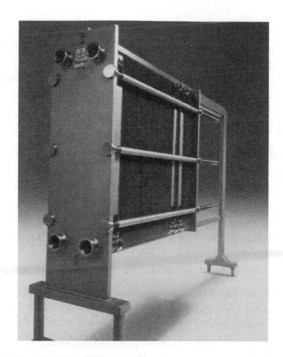

FIGURE 9.13   Plate heater/cooler photography.

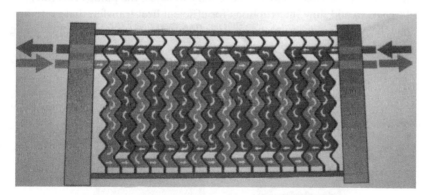

FIGURE 9.14   Plate heat exchanger schema.

of the juice difficult. The retained pulp may be overheated and create quality problems (cooked taste, black dots, color changes, etc.).

The application of plate exchangers has the following effects:

- High pressure drop in the line when the product enters between the plates.
- Large transfer surface area for heating and cooling, carrying this out very quickly.
- Hard to clean. To ensure that any retained piece/pulp is removed and will not create other problems, a thorough clean has to be carried out.
- High/low maintenance, depending on the use.

9.4.1.2   Plate Shape and Thickness

The wall of the plates is frequently corrugated to create a turbulent flow that will improve the heat transfer (Figure 9.15).

Other applications for PHEs are milk or soft drinks. In fruit-derived fluids, they are mainly applied in filtered juices, clarified juices, and low-density purees.

9.4.2   Tubular Heat Exchangers

9.4.2.1   General Description

Tubular heat exchangers (THE) use tubes for heat transfer: they consist of a set of tubes within a housing in different configurations, including product hold and process controls to ensure critical temperatures and an adequate holding time. They may be multi/monotubular or multitubular, enclosed within an outer shell. There are no universal arrangements for heat exchangers. The characteristics of the product must be taken into account. The juice passes through all the tubes (Figure 9.16).

Different tube diameters may be used. The main characteristics are as follows:

- There are no moving parts, the equipment is more compact and easy to operate in aseptic conditions, and maintenance is easier. It is also simple to inspect the tubes' integrity and clean them.
- Fluids and high-density products can be processed: has a bigger application range.
- High pressure drops with viscous products: causes a more efficient heat transfer.
- Important to consider velocity: necessary to adjust the pumps carefully.
- Possible to add flow interruptions for efficient heat transfer, that is, to agitate the juice and interrupt the laminar flow. Also ensures efficient cleaning with appropriate water pressure.

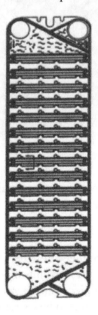 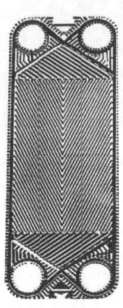

FIGURE 9.15   Different plate shapes for different applications.

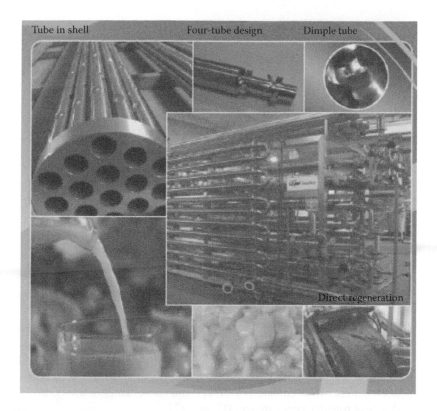

FIGURE 9.16 Different tubular pasteurizers. (Courtesy of JBT FoodTech in JBT FoodTech, manual and brochures.)

- No option for product retention: possible to operate with pulpy juices, purees, and juices with fruit pieces.
- Easy to operate with high temperatures or pressures (for low-acid products) (Glenna 2012).
- Path of least resistance compared with other systems.
- Different materials utilized for construction: stainless steel, special plastics, and alloys.

9.4.2.2 Tubes in Tube Design: For High-Viscosity Juices, Pulp, and Purees

Three concentric tubes are utilized, one inside the other as shown in Figure 9.17: the product moves through the yellow ring, covered on both sides by pipes containing heating fluid. The set of tubes, in total, comprises the length necessary to achieve pasteurization temperature, residence time, and cooling temperature (Figure 9.17).

To agitate the juice and improve heat transfer, it is possible to use different systems within the juice tube:

- *Fin deflectors*: These are mainly applied for viscous products and concentrates. Heat transfer effectively occurs from both sides (Figure 9.18). Scientifically arranged fins inside the annular space act as a static mixer, to

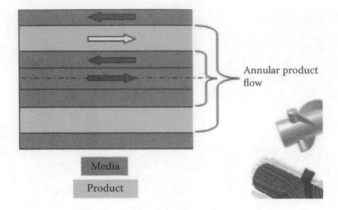

Annular product flow

Media

Product

FIGURE 9.17   Tube-in-tube design. (Courtesy of JBT FoodTech in JBT FoodTech, manual and brochures.)

ensure a more uniform and effective heat transfer by convection, also at low product speed. Used mainly for highly viscous products such as citrus pulp, fruit purees, tomato paste, and so on (Figure 9.19).

- *Dimpled tube*: Patented JBT FoodTech system (Figure 9.20) applied to low-viscosity products and also particulates and diced fruit. It incorporates smooth dimples on the internal surface in contact with the juice for gentle agitation of the product with minimal abrasion and shearing. This type of heat exchanger offers enhanced drainage and stable temperature control. It makes heat transfer very efficient (Figure 9.21).

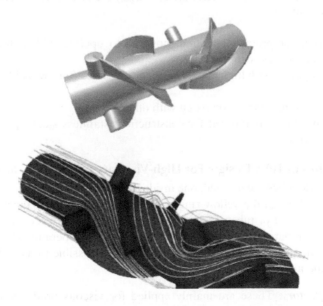

FIGURE 9.18   Fluid movement in a four-wing tube in-tube pasteurizer. (Courtesy of JBT FoodTech in JBT FoodTech, manual and brochures.)

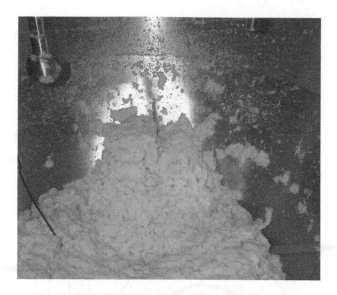

FIGURE 9.19   Orange pulp. (Courtesy of JBT FoodTech in JBT FoodTech, pictures database.)

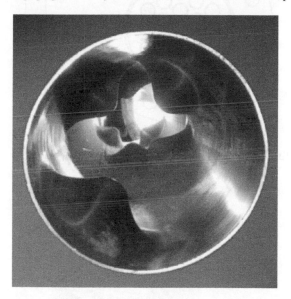

FIGURE 9.20   Dimple tube design: Front view. (Courtesy of JBT FoodTech in JBT FoodTech, pictures database.)

9.4.2.3   Tubes in Shell Heat Exchangers

This is a set of multiple single tubes inside a shell and housing. It is mainly used for low-viscosity products (Figures 9.22 and 9.23). The juice flows through the tubes and the heating/cooling fluid flows outside them, within a chamber in the space between the tubes. The turbulence for good heat transfer is achieved because of the shape

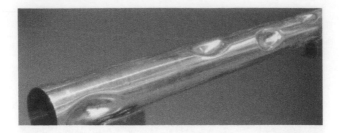

FIGURE 9.21 Dimple tube design: Lateral view. (Courtesy of JBT FoodTech in JBT FoodTech, pictures database.)

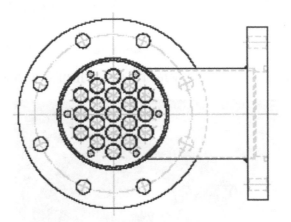

FIGURE 9.22 Tube disposal in a tube in shell equipment: schema.

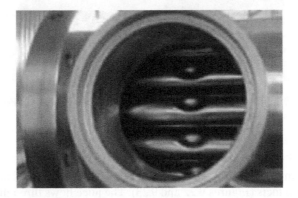

FIGURE 9.23 Tube disposal in a tube in shell equipment: view. (Courtesy of JBT FoodTech in JBT FoodTech, pictures database.)

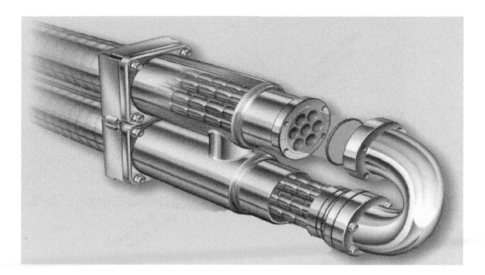

FIGURE 9.24   Multitubular heat exchanger with flange.

inside the tubes: corrugated, dimpled, and so on. The set of tubes is attached to a flat flange on both sides (Figure 9.24). The flange is sealed and permits the tubes to be easily disassembled for inspection and also to change them and make it possible to replace them with different tubes with a different setup for different applications. This floating design also allows thermal expansion to be absorbed.

Main characteristics of the system:

- Fluid products: able to work at high pressure and temperature
- Path of least resistance
- Velocity is a concern
- Decrease in the drop in pressure
- High surface area per linear meter
- Low maintenance
- CIP issues

9.4.2.4   Scraped Surface Heat Exchangers

This system is used to heat/cool viscous, sticky, and lumpy products, and also to crystallize some products. This technology is not very common in the juice industry: it is hardly used. It is used mainly for cooling in other industries.

The system (Figure 9.25) is a cylinder where the product is pumped countercurrent to the heater/cooler fluid circulating through the external jacket (Hernández et al. 2010). There are two rotors with different diameters that are interchangeable and three paddles with different profiles that permit the adaptation of the equipment to the treatment of different products. The smaller diameter is applied for larger particles (up to 25 mm). The larger diameter rotor permits a longer residence time.

The product enters the cylinder at the lower end and flows upward. The internal air will have been previously purged through the upper end. The product occupies the whole volume of the cylinder. The paddles scrape the product from the internal

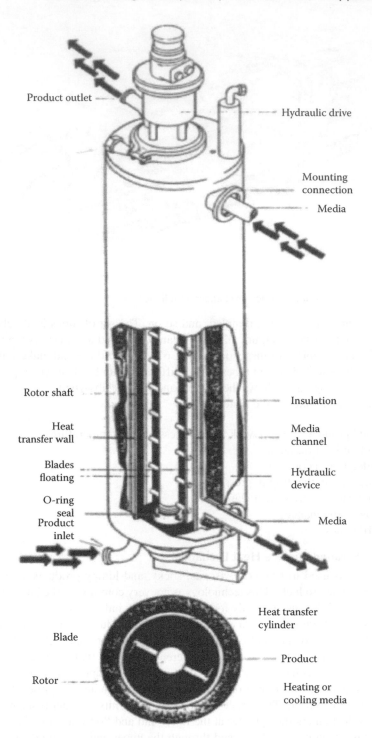

FIGURE 9.25   Scraped surface heat exchanger.

surfaces of the cylinder, optimizing heat transfer. The product exits from the upper part of the cylinder.

9.4.2.4.1 Main Characteristics of the System

- Viscous products such as jams, sweets, sauces, chocolate, etc., may be processed.
- Flow rate and speed change according to the type of product processed.
- Mechanically moves product from the heat exchange surface. These mechanical parts are externally moving and this may create problems when trying to ensure asepsis.
- Low pressure drop.
- High efficiency in heat transfer.
- Energy required for rotation.
- High maintenance.
- CIP easier.

REFERENCES

Basmadjian, D. 2007. *Mass Transfer and Separation Process: Principles and Applications.* Boca Raton, FL: CRC Press.

Cepeda, E. and Villarán, M.C. 1999. Density and viscosity of *Malus floribunda* juice as a function of concentration and temperature. *Journal of Food Engineering*, 41 (2), 103–107.

Cohn, F. 1872. Untersuchungen über bacterien. *Beiträge zur Biologie der Pflanzen*, 1 (1), 127–224.

Crandall, P.G., Davis, K.C., and Baker, R.A. 1990. Viscosity reduction of orange juice concentrate by pulp reduction vs. enzyme treatment. *Food Technology*, 3, 126–129.

Ehrenberg, C.G. 1835. Fortsetzung der mikrogeologischen studien. *Physikalische Abhandlungen der Koeniglichen Akademie der Wissenschaften zu Berlin aus den Jahren 1833–1835*, 145–336.

Falguera, V. and Ibarz, A. 2010. A new model to describe flow behaviour of concentrated orange juice. *Food Biophysics*, 5 (2), 114–119.

Falguera, V., Velez-Ruiz, J.F., Alins, V., and Ibarz, A. 2010. Rheological behaviour of concentrated mandarin juice at low temperatures. *International Journal of Food Science and Technology*, 45 (10), 2194–2200.

FDA-HHS (Food and Drug Administration, Department of Health and Human Services). 2001. 21 CFR Part 120: Hazard analysis and critical control point (HAACP): Procedures for the safe and sanitary processing and importing of juice: Final rule. *Federal Register: Rules and Regulations*, 66 (13), 6137–6202. January 19, 2001.

Glenna, M. 2012. Low acid products pasteurization. In: *JBT FoodTech: Manuals and Brochures,* Lakeland, FL.

Guerrero, S.N. and Alzamora, S.M. 1998. Effect of pH, temperature and glucose addition on flow behaviour of fruit purees: II. Peach, papaya and mango purées. *Journal of Food Engineering*, 37 (1–4), 77–101.

Hernández, E., Raventos, M., Auleda, J.M., and Ibarz, A. 2010. Freeze concentration of must in a pilot plant falling film cryoconcentrator. *Innovative Food Science and Emerging Technologies*, 11 (1), 130–136.

Holland, C.D. 1981. *Fundamentals of Multicomponent Distillation.* McGraw Hill Chemical Engineering Series. New York: McGraw Hill.

Ibarz, A., Garvin, A., and Costa, J. 1996. Rheological behaviour of sloe (*Prunus spinosa*) fruit juices. *Journal of Food Engineering*, 27 (4), 423–430.

Ibarz, A., Gonzalez, C., and Esplugas, S. 1994. Rheology of clarified fruit juices. III: Orange juices. *Journal of Food Engineering*, 21 (4), 485–494.

Kauffmann, F. and Edwards, P.R. 1952. Classification and nomenclature of *Enterobacteriaceae*. *International Bulletin of Bacteriological Nomenclature and Taxonomy*, 2, 2–8.

Khalil, K.E., Ramakrishna, P., Nanjundaswamy, A.M., and Patwardhan, M.V. 1989. Rheological behaviour of clarified banana juice: Effect of temperature and concentration. *Journal of Food Engineering*, 10 (3), 231–240.

Lapasin, S. and Pricl, S. 1995. *Rheology of Industrial Polysaccharides: Theory and Applications*. Glasgow: Blackie Academic and Professional.

Le Minor, L. and Popoff, M.Y. 1987. Request for an opinion. Designation of *Salmonella enterica* sp. nov., nom. rev., as the type and only species of the genus *Salmonella*. *International Journal of Systematic Bacteriology*, 37, 465–468.

Lorente, J., Valero, M., de Ancos, B., Martí, N., García, S., López, N., Ramos, S., et al. 2012. Capitulo 5. Aspectos industriales. In Urrecho, A., Garea, E., Miguelañez, R., Mena, A., González, C., Cámara, M., and Martí, N. (eds), *El Libro del Zumo*, pp. 79–116. Madrid: Asociación Española de Fabricantes de Zumos (Asozumos).

Martí, N. and Saura, D. 2013. Evaporative losses in de-aerators. Report for Refresco Holding BV, Mitra Sol Technologies, S.L. (unpublished results).

Marti, N., et al. 2009. *Natural Products Communications*, 4 (5), 591–748.

Massa, A., González, C., Maestro, A., Labanda, J., and Ibarz, A. 2010. Rheological characterization of peach purees. *Journal of Texture Studies*, 41 (4), 532–548.

Megyesy, E.F. 2001. *Manual de Recipientes a Presión: Diseño y Cálculo*. Mexico City: Limusa.

Nagy, S., Chen, C.S., and Shaw, P. 1992. *Fruit Juice Processing Technology*. Auburndale, FL: AGScience.

Nagy, S., Shaw, P.E., and Veldhuis, M.K. 1977. Citrus science and technology, volume 2. *Fruit Production, Processing Practices, Derived Products and Personnel Management*. Westport, CT: AVI Publishing.

Plumey, L., Braesco, V., and Bellisle, F. 2013. *Le Livre Blanc du Jus de Fruits*. Paris: Union Nationale Interprofessionnelle des Jus de Fruits (UNIJUS).

Rao, J.M., Aereo, J.E., Cooleu, H.J., and Ennis, R.N. 1987. Clarification of apple juice by hollowfiber ultrafiltration: Fluxis and retention of odor-active volátiles. *Journal of Food Science*, 52 (4), 375–377.

Reed, J.B., Hendrix, D.L., and Hendrix Jr., C.M. 1992. *Quality Control Manual for Citrus Processing Plants*, volume II. Auburndale, FL: AGScience.

Telis-Romero, J., Telis, V.R.N., and Yamashita, F. 1999. Friction factors and rheological properties of orange juice. *Journal of Food Engineering*, 40 (1), 101–106.

Tetra Pak Processing Systems. 2003. *Manual de Industrias Lácteas*. Lund: Tetra Pak Processing Systems.

Tetra Pak Processing Systems. 2004. *The Orange Book*. Lund: Tetra Pak Processing Systems.

Tressler, D.K. and Joslyn, M.A. 1961. *Fruit and Vegetable Juice Processing Technology*. Westport, CT: AVI Publishing.

Valero, M., Micol, V., Saura, D., Muñoz, N., Lorente, J., and Martí, N. 2010. Comparison of antimicrobial treatments for citrus juices. *CAB Reviews: Perspectives in Agriculture, Veterinary Science, Nutrition and Natural Resources*, 5 (020), 1–12.

Valero, M., Recrosio, N., Saura, D., Muñoz, N., Martí, N., and Lizama, V. 2007. Effects of ultrasonic treatments in orange juice processing. *Journal of Food Engineering*, 80 (2), 509–516.

Valero, M., Vegara, S., Martí, N., Saura, D., and Lorente, J. 2009. Pasteurization and microorganisms in orange pulp. In: *Manual and Brochures*. Elche, Spain: JBT FoodTech–IBMC R&D Alliance.

Woodroof, J.G. and Phillips, G.F. 1981. *Beverages: Carbonated and Noncarbonated*. Westport, CT: AVI Publishing.

10 Emerging Technologies in Fruit Juice Processing

*María Victoria Traffano-Schiffo, Nuria Balaguer,
Marta Castro-Giráldez, and Pedro J. Fito-Suñer*

CONTENTS

10.1 Introduction 197
10.2 Ohmic Heating... 198
    10.2.1 Theoretical Basis 198
    10.2.2 Applications of Ohmic Heating in Juice Processing 200
    10.2.3 Equipment..202
        10.2.3.1 Ohmic Heating System Design..202
10.3 Basic Principles in Electromagnetic Phenomena 203
    10.3.1 Dielectric Properties: Permittivity...204
    10.3.2 Penetration Depth 206
    10.3.3 Applications of Microwave Heating in Fruit Juices 206
    10.3.4 Microwave Equipment...208
    10.3.5 Applications of Radio-Frequency Heating in Juice Processing 209
    10.3.6 Radio-Frequency Equipment..209
10.4 Other Frequency Range Applications... 211
References.. 212

10.1 INTRODUCTION

Currently, one of the most important aspects concerning the juice industry is the preservation and improvement of the main organoleptic characteristics of its products, in order to cater to the most exigent consumer demands. As a result, optimizing heat treatments during the processing stages is essential for maintaining an equilibrium between food security and retaining the original nutritional quality of the raw material.

The traditional techniques used to apply heat are based on conduction and convection mechanisms. These mechanisms need hot fluids to transmit the energy by gradients of temperature. The main hot fluids are steam (vapor at high pressure), vapor, hot water, and hot air. These fluids are heated by the combustion of fuels or by electricity. Nevertheless, the use of these techniques has been commonly associated with considerable losses of heat on the surfaces of the equipment and installations, the reduction of heat transfer efficiency, and thermal damage by overheating, due to the time required to conduct sufficient heat into the thermal center of foods (Pereira and Vicente, 2010).

In order to address these problems, other techniques have been developed that do not depend on temperature gradients. Radiation technologies in food processing have gained industrial interest and have the potential to replace, at least partially, the traditional, well-established preservation processes (Vicente and Castro, 2007).

The benefits of the emerging heating techniques are mainly a result of internal heat generation. Electric energy exhibits unique properties, such as fast and differential heating, which can be an advantage, and improves the process efficiency and product quality (Ponne and Bartels, 1995). Among these new thermal techniques are ohmic (electric current) and dielectric heating (photon flux).

The aim of this chapter is to provide a general overview of the theoretical basis of new and emerging thermal technologies, emphasizing their potential applications in the juice industry.

10.2   OHMIC HEATING

Ohmic heating is one of the most innovative alternative processing techniques to have emerged since the end of the twentieth century. In general terms, by means of an electric current, certain products are susceptible to pasteurization, fermentation, or sterilization in a manner that is equally comparable, if not better, than the current methods of processing.

10.2.1   THEORETICAL BASIS

Ohmic heating, also known as joule heating, electrical resistance heating, direct electrical resistance heating, electroheating, and electroconductive heating, is based on the passage of an alternating electrical current (AC) through a body, which acts as a resistor, with the primary purpose of generating heat (Sastry and Barach, 2000). This technology provides rapid and uniform heating, and the absence of cold spots in the sample reduces thermal abuse to the product in comparison with conventional heating techniques (Leizerson and Shimoni, 2005a,b; Lee et al., 2012).

In contrast with microwave (MW) or radio-frequency (RF) heating, this technology requires the electrodes to be in direct contact with the food (see Figure 10.1). Another particularity of this process is the necessity of taking into account the fact that the food is an electrical component of the heater and because of this, its electrical properties must be matched to the capacity of the heater.

In this type of system, an AC voltage is supplied to both electrodes according to Ohm's law:

$$V = I \cdot R \tag{10.1}$$

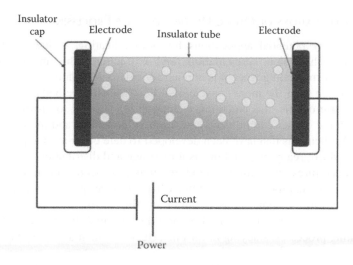

FIGURE 10.1   Schematic diagram showing the workings of an ohmic heating system.

This relation states that the potential difference (voltage) across an ideal conductor is proportional to the current through it, which is resistance (R), the constant of proportionality.

When an electron current flows through a conductor with resistance (as some foods), a part of the electric energy is transformed into thermal energy. Joule's law explains the thermal energy produced by an electric current as follows:

$$P = VI = RI^2 \qquad (10.2)$$

Foods whose main constituents are water and ionic components are capable of conducting electricity, simultaneously generating heat from the resistance when an electric current passes through the food.

Several factors must be considered when working with ohmic heating. One of the most important factors is the electrical conductivity of the product and its dependence on temperature variation. Therefore, in a multiphase system such as colloidal foods (e.g., milk and juice) the electrical conductivity of every phase must be considered. Related to this, if the electrical conductivities of the different components are equal, the product is expected to heat rapidly and uniformly to a high temperature, regardless of the particle size. This enables the sterilization of colloidal foods under ultrahigh-temperature (UHT) conditions while avoiding heat damage. In contrast, in the case of a colloid system in which the dispersed phase would have a higher temperature in comparison with the liquid phase, the heating would be faster, ensuring a more adequate process. Despite this, it is necessary to be aware of the possibility of heat channeling. This is an undesirable problem that may cause coupling between temperature and electric field distribution. Additionally, another important aspect to consider is the variation of the particle size and its orientation, since all of these effects coupled together could cause serious difficulties in the process as a whole.

10.2.2   Applications of Ohmic Heating in Juice Processing

There are many potential applications for ohmic heating, including blanching, evaporation, dehydration, fermentation, and extraction. This method provides rapid and uniform heating when it is applied for microbial control, resulting in less thermal damage than the more conventional heat transfer methods (Sarang et al., 2008). Because of this, this emerging technique is expected to provide food processors with the capacity to produce new, high value-added, and more shelf-stable products. Applications that have been developed to date cover aseptic processing of high value-added, ready-prepared meals for storage and distribution at ambient and chilled temperatures, preheating of food products prior to in-can sterilization, and heating of high-acid products such as tomato-based sauces prior to hot filling.

With regard to the applications of ohmic heating in the juice industry, a broad range of studies have mainly focused on proving its suitability for replacing traditional heating processes, studying in turn its effects on the maintenance of the vital nutrients in processed juices.

Related to this, Leizerson and Shimoni (2005a) examined the effects of ohmic heating on the stability of orange juice in comparison with conventional pasteurization. Specifically, the attributes that were analyzed to ensure the quality of orange juice were ascorbic acid concentration (vitamin C), pectin esterase (PE) activity (cloudiness), color, and five essential flavor compounds: decanal, octanal, limonene, pinene, and myrcene. The research showed that there was no significant difference between the different heating methods with regard to the degradation of vitamin C concentrations or residual PE activity, although the particle size of the cloud was noticeably less in the ohmically heated sample. In addition, the authors also observed that even though both thermal treatments prevented the growth of microorganisms for 105 days, the sensory shelf life of ohmic-treated orange juice was almost two times longer than that of conventionally pasteurized juice.

In a similar experiment, Leizerson and Shimoni (2005b) studied the effects of UHT ohmic heating on the quality of orange juice compared with juice obtained through a pasteurization process. The orange juice was treated at temperatures of 90°C, 120°C, and 150°C for 1.13, 0.85, and 0.68 s in an ohmic heating system and at 90°C for 50 s in a conventional pasteurizer. The ohmic treatment resulted in a higher-quality product with minimal sensory damage, since ohmic-heated orange juice maintained, again, higher amounts of the five representative flavor compounds than the heat-pasteurized juice.

In the same year, Vikram et al. (2005) carried out a comparative study of the kinetics of vitamin C degradation and changes in the visual color of orange juice after being sterilized using different methods of heating: MW, ohmic, IR, and conventional heating. The authors of the study determined that the destruction of vitamin C was influenced by the method of heating and the temperature of processing. It was also concluded that its degradation was highest during MW heating due to uncontrolled temperature generation during processing; nevertheless, MW heating was the system that caused the lowest degradation of color. On the other hand, ohmic heating provided better results, since it facilitated better vitamin retention at all temperatures.

Praporscic et al. (2006) analyzed the impact of ohmic heating on the juice extracted from potato and apple tissues. Two different experiments were carried out involving different treatment chambers: a textural and conductivity study of cylindrical samples and a juice yield test of tissue slices. The results showed that the degree of tissue disintegration and yield were dependent on the field intensity, temperature, treatment duration, and type of plant tissue. In particular, the best juice extraction was obtained when the plant tissue was electrically heated at a moderate temperature of 50°C. The combined effect of the possible electroporation and thermal softening of the tissues may explain the increased yield.

Içier et al. (2008) investigated the effects of ohmic heating on polyphenol oxidase (PPO) (one of the most important enzymes that contributes to browning, discoloration, and darkening in fruit and vegetables) at pasteurization temperature ranges in freshly squeezed grape juice. The main objectives were to measure the effect of the voltage gradient, temperature, and holding time on the PPO activity in grape juice ohmically heated to 70°C–90°C and to fit models to deactivation kinetics. The results obtained showed that the ohmic heating rate increased as the voltage gradient also increased. In fact, the critical deactivation temperature at 40 V was lower than the one managed at 20 and 30 V, probably because of the faster increase in electrical conductivity at higher voltage gradients, which could cause a higher deactivation of PPO.

Later, Yildiz et al. (2009) undertook research focused on determining the impact of ohmic heating on the color, total phenolic content, and rheological behavior of pomegranate juice and compared its efficacy in relation to conventional heating. The results obtained showed that there was practically no difference in the rheological properties and total phenolic contents of pomegranate juice between both types of heat treatment. Nevertheless, ohmic heating caused significantly less browning during heat treatment than conventional heating ($p < .01$).

With the aim of improving the maintenance of cloud stability in juices, Demirdöven and Baysal (2012) determined the efficacy of ohmic heating in the inactivation of the pectin methylesterase (PME) enzyme in orange juice. Related to this, they designed an experimental procedure in which orange juices were ohmically heated to different temperatures (34°C–76°C) at 50 Hz frequency, using different voltages (20–60 V). The juices obtained were compared with untreated control juices and conventionally heated juices in regard to PME inactivation and some quality characteristics such as their pectin and vitamin C content, total soluble matter (Brix), and color preservation. The results obtained showed that ohmic heating is the most effective system for PME inactivation and for improving the functional properties of orange juice. A recent study has attempted to inactivate *Escherichia coli* 0157.H7, *Salmonella typhimurium*, and *Listeria monocytogenes* in orange and tomato juices, since they are considered to be the most dangerous pathogens found in fruit and vegetables (Lee et al., 2012). To deal with this task, both juices were treated with electric field strengths in the range of 25–40 V for different treatment times. The authors concluded that the effects of inactivation were dependent on the applied electric field strength, treatment time, and electrical conductivity. In fact, a higher strength or longer treatment time resulted in a greater reduction of pathogens. Finally, they also observed that the concentration of vitamin C in the continuous ohmic-heated juice was significantly higher than in the conventionally heated juice ($p < .05$).

Considering all the favorable results obtained, it can be concluded that ohmic heating is, indeed, one of the most promising emerging thermal techniques destined to replace the heating techniques commonly used at industrial level. Nevertheless, it might be advisable to undertake further investigation to determine the optimum parameters for improving the shelf life and quality of the products.

10.2.3 EQUIPMENT

10.2.3.1 Ohmic Heating System Design

There are endless possibilities to design an ohmic heating system, but there are several key modules that must be present: a heater assembly, a power supply, and a control panel. In Figure 10.2, a typical diagram of a continuous-flow ohmic heating process is shown. This particular process was originally developed by the U.K. Electricity Council Research Centre and was then licensed to APV Baker, who has developed it into a commercial system. In this system, a colloidal food product is introduced into the continuous-flow ohmic heating system through a feed pump hopper. The product is then heated to the programmed temperature as it passes through electrodes, which are connected to a 50 Hz three-phase supply. Next, it enters the

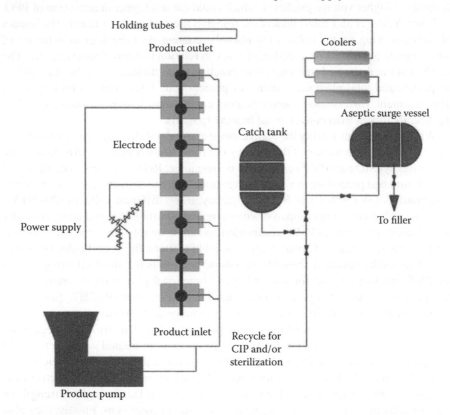

FIGURE 10.2 Flow sheet for an ohmic heating system. CIP, cleaning-in-place. (Adapted from Parrot, D.L., *Food Technology*, 96, 68–72, 1992.)

holding tubes for a fixed time in order to achieve the desired sterility. Finally, the product flows through tubular coolers and is stored in aseptic tanks until the filling and packaging stages take place (Parrot, 1992).

Due to the possible increase in the electrical conductivity of products as the heat increases, the holding tubes increase in length to maintain the same electrical impedance. A temperature control system constantly monitors the temperature, flow rate, heat capacity, and specific heat of the product to calculate the electrical power that is needed. Hence, the ohmic heaters must include the electrical components of the product to be heated, since the product itself is an electrical component. The resistance in an ohmic heater will therefore depend on the specific resistance of the product and the geometry of the heater.

It is important to emphasize that the design of the heater is tailored to products that have similar specific resistances and it cannot be used for other products without modification.

Contrary to conventional techniques, the rapid sterilization managed with ohmic heating is not lost during the packing process. The use of multiple electrodes provides a much greater degree of control, as well as a uniform electric field in the pipe sections. Special electrode material is used in order to eliminate polarization and contamination. The process allows food products, with particulates up to 25 mm, to be heated to sterilization temperatures of up to 140°C in less than 90 s, and to be cooled down within 15 min in the following stages.

10.3 BASIC PRINCIPLES IN ELECTROMAGNETIC PHENOMENA

In conventional thermal treatments, a material is heated by conduction or convection. Many materials, such as foods, can also be heated by applying a photonic energy flux.

Electric and magnetic phenomena at the macroscopic level are described by the Maxwell equations and, from a general point of view, by the particle standard model; the electromagnetic force is explained by the effect of photons flowing throughout a nonconductive medium. The physical properties that explain the effect of the electromagnetic force in a medium are included in the Maxwell equations (the laws of Gauss, Ampere, Faraday, and others; see Equations 10.3). In order to explain the main effect of the electric field, it is important to know that the engine of this force is a difference of voltage in the system; and in a magnetic field it is the intensity of the current charge.

$$\nabla \bar{E} = \frac{-\partial \bar{B}}{\partial t} - \bar{M} \tag{10.3a}$$

$$\nabla \bar{H} = \frac{\partial \bar{D}}{\partial t} + \bar{J} \tag{10.3b}$$

$$\nabla \bar{D} = \rho \tag{10.3c}$$

$$\nabla \bar{B} = 0 \tag{10.3d}$$

where:
  E is the electric field
  B is the magnetic flux density
  M is the magnetic current density
  H is the magnetic field
  D is the electric flux density (displacement)
  J is the electric current density
  ρ is the electric charge density

A dielectric medium produces resistance to the photon flux, and this resistance produces a displacement in the electric and magnetic fields (Equations 10.4).

$$\overline{D} = \varepsilon * \cdot \varepsilon_0 \cdot E = \left(\varepsilon' - j\varepsilon'' \right)\varepsilon_0 \cdot E \qquad (10.4a)$$

$$\overline{B} = \mu * \cdot \mu_0 \cdot H = \left(\mu' - j\mu'' \right)\mu_0 \cdot H \qquad (10.4b)$$

where the complex permittivity ($\varepsilon *$) represents the physical property that explains the response of the medium to an electric field and the complex permeability ($\mu *$) represents the physical property that explains the response of the medium to a magnetic field.

10.3.1 DIELECTRIC PROPERTIES: PERMITTIVITY

Dielectric heating is based on the electric energy transformation in thermal energy. This phenomenon depends on the capability of the material to absorb electric radiation and convert it into heat (Castro-Giráldez et al., 2010, 2011; Vicente and Pereira, 2010; Zhao, 2006). The real part of the complex permittivity is called the dielectric constant (ε'), and the imaginary part is called the loss factor (ε''). The dielectric constant is related to the material's ability to store electric energy in response to an applied electric field, and the dielectric loss factor is related to the dissipation of the electric energy into other kinds of energies such as thermal energy. The different dissipation effects of the loss factor spectrum are shown in Figure 10.3.

The MW heating effect is the result of two mechanisms: dipolar rotation and ionic conductivity. In foods, dipolar rotation is mainly caused by water, which is the most important dipole molecule; in the case of ionic conductivity, there is a wide variety of species with ionic capacity (cations, weak acids, and others). In America, commercial equipment operates at 915 MHz, where the main effect is the ionic conductivity, while in the rest of the world, such equipment operates at 2.45 GHz, where the main effect is the gamma dispersion (Marra et al., 2007).

When an electric field is applied to food, the polar molecules are forced to orientate themselves with the polarity of the force lines of the electric field. Heating occurs because the rotation and the translation produce friction. On the other hand, heating by ionic conductivity is produced by the translation of charged ions with the polarity of the force lines of the electric field.

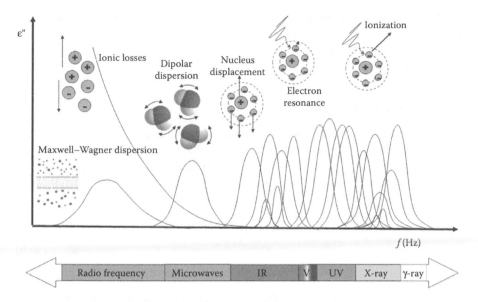

FIGURE 10.3 Dissipation effects of loss factor spectrum.

The RF heating effect is the result of the many mechanisms involved in the beta dispersion (ranging from kilohertz to megahertz). This dispersion covers all the mechanisms involved in the orientation of fixed charges on solid surfaces (membranes, walls, proteins, carbohydrates, etc.). One of the main effects is called the Maxwell–Wagner effect, and it is caused by the solid surface tension (e.g., pulp in fruit juices) (Feldman et al., 2003; Damez et al., 2007).

The thermal spectrum covers medium and near infrared (IR), visible, and ultraviolet (UV) nonionizing heating. The effect that produces this kind of heating is called electronic resonance and it is produced by the excitation of the electrons located at the external orbital (usually organic bond), producing an increase in the orbital level by photon absorption. The emission and absorption of photons are related to the relaxation of the excited electrons. The proportion of photon energy absorbed by the electrons represents the increase in the internal energy of the sample. The law that describes this effect is Planck's law (Equation 10.5) for a given wavelength (λ, m) and temperature (T, K).

$$E_{b,\lambda}\left(\lambda, T\right) = \frac{2\pi h C_0^2}{\lambda^5 \left[\exp\left(h C_0/\lambda k T\right) - 1\right]}$$

(10.5)

where:
$h = 6.6256 \times 10^{-34}$ is the Planck constant (J·s)
$k = 1.3805$ is the Boltzmann constant (J/K)
$C_0 = 2.998 \cdot 10^8$ is the speed of light in vacuum
T is the absolute temperature (K)

Above medium UV frequencies, the quantity of photon energy produces a displacement of the electrons outside the molecule, producing free radicals in the product and increasing the reactivity of the molecule (and its internal energy) and its oxidative capacity.

10.3.2 PENETRATION DEPTH

Another important concept for designing a dielectric heating system is the penetration depth (d_p), which is usually defined as the depth into a sample where the MW power has dropped to $1/e$ or 36.8% of its transmitted value. The penetration depth (d_p) can be calculated from the dielectric properties with the following equation:

$$d_p = \frac{\lambda_0 \sqrt{\varepsilon'}}{2\pi\varepsilon''} \tag{10.6}$$

where λ_0 is the free-space wavelength. The most common food products have $\varepsilon'' < 25$, which implies a penetration depth (d_p) of 0.6–1 cm (Venkatesh and Raghavan, 2004).

It is worth mentioning that as the wave travels through a material that has significant dielectric losses, its energy is attenuated. If the attenuation is high, the dielectric heating reduces quickly and the wave penetrates the material.

The power dissipated inside the material is proportional to ε''. The ratio $\varepsilon''/\varepsilon'$, called the loss tangent (tan δ), is used as an index of the material's ability to generate heat (Mudgett, 1986).

It is also important to analyze the rate of heating, which can be expressed by the power equation:

$$P_v = 2\pi f \varepsilon_0 \varepsilon'' |E|^2 \tag{10.7}$$

where:
P_v is the energy developed per unit volume in watts per cubic meter
f is the frequency in hertz
$|E|$ is the electric field strength inside the load in volts per meter (Ryynänen, 1995; Venkatesh and Raghavan, 2004)

10.3.3 APPLICATIONS OF MICROWAVE HEATING IN FRUIT JUICES

In the literature, many applications that are mainly used for juice pasteurization in order to extend the shelf life of the product can be found. The most commonly used parameters for the determination of correct pasteurization are inactivation of microorganisms and inactivation of enzymes.

MW heating of fruit juices provides a less invasive treatment, causing smaller changes in the quality attributes of fruit in comparison with conventional thermal fruit pasteurization.

MW pasteurization preserves the natural and organoleptic characteristics of the juice and reduces the treatment time, resulting in a lower loss of essential thermolabile nutrients (Cañumir et al., 2002).

With regard to the applications of MW heating in juice processing, there is sufficient information to demonstrate the benefits of this treatment, which is mainly focused on maintaining the organoleptic and nutritional characteristics of a fresh juice, thereby achieving its conservation over time.

Many studies have proved useful to demonstrate the inactivation of the PME enzyme. PME hydrolyzes ester bonds of pectin in citrus juices and, as a consequence, the juice loses its stability. This enzyme is more resistant to heat than microorganisms, so it is used to determine the adequacy of pasteurization.

Related to this, Nikdel et al. (1993), Tajchakavit and Ramaswamy (1997), Villamiel et al. (1998), Igual et al. (2010), and Cinquanta et al. (2010) concluded in all cases that MW treatment is effective for PME inactivation, preserving to a large extent the nutritional and organoleptic properties of fresh fruit juice and appreciably reducing the process time and the temperature used.

In similar experiments, the power of the MW to inactivate microorganisms was demonstrated. Cañumir et al. (2002) studied the effect of MW heating on the reduction of an *E. coli* population in apple juice and concluded that the quantity of microorganisms was lower in apple juice treated at 900 and 720 W power levels for 60 and 90 s. At these levels, no significant differences were found between a conventional thermal treatment and MW heating. Specifically, the reduction was within the range of 2–4 logs. In the same way, Tajchakavit et al. (1998) studied the benefits of MW heating in apple juice and determined the inactivation of *Saccharomyces cerevisiae* and *Lactobacillus plantarum*. *Lactobacillus* spp. imparts an undesirable buttermilk-type flavor to the juice due to the production of diacetyl and *Saccharomyces* generates fermented off-flavors associated with the production of carbon dioxide, ethanol, and traces of other fermentation products.

Gerard and Roberts (2004) undertook research that was more focused on determining the impact of MW heating on apple mash to improve juice yield and quality. One of the most important factors for determining the quality of juice is the concentration of phenolic and flavonoid components, which are drastically reduced after conventional processes. The aforementioned components, with bioactive activity, contribute to human health and may reduce the risk of cancer and cardiovascular heart disease. The results demonstrated that MW heating of mash increased juice yields and also increased the extraction of phenolics and flavonoids from apple mash; therefore, as a consequence, the final concentrations of these components in the final product were increased, with 60°C being the optimum temperature for improving the process. On the contrary, the yield did not increase at 70°C and had little effect on the final concentrations of total phenolics and flavonoids.

Other studies that have been developed have focused on the final concentrations of bioactive components in fruit juice after MW treatment, including carotenoids (Fratianni et al., 2010), with losses of violaxanthin and antheranthin (two carotenoids found in Valencia oranges) after 10 min of heating at 60°C and 70°C, while compounds with provitamin A activity (β-carotene, α-carotene, and β-cryptoxanthin) and lutein were more stable at the same temperatures. Several thermal effects were found at higher temperatures ($\geq 75°C$), especially on provitamin A, carotenoids, and lutein.

Igual et al. (2010) studied the effect of MW pasteurization on the main bioactive compounds of grapefruit juice and their stability over 2 months of frozen storage. The compounds studied were ascorbic acid, vitamin C, and organic acids (citric, tartaric, and malic acids). The results revealed that MW treatment preserved citric and ascorbic acids. Moreover, frozen MW pasteurized juices preserved total phenols and antioxidant capacity compared with the conventional process.

Later, Cendres et al. (2011) studied the possibility of extracting juice from fruits (plum, apricot, and grape) using MWs and gravity. The aims of this work were to optimize the extraction process in order to obtain better yields and to improve the maintenance of the organoleptic properties of juices. The process consists of applying MWs for the hydrodiffusion of the juice from inside to the exterior using earth's gravity to collect the fruit juice outside the MW cavity. The best results were obtained at optimized MW power and from frozen plums at 480 mL/kg, frozen apricots at 550 mL/kg, and frozen grapes at 620 mL/kg. The juices obtained with this new method were brightly colored and the endogenous enzymes such as PPO were inactivated.

Finally, Yousefi et al. (2012) investigated the effect on the evaporation rate and quality properties of pomegranate juice during concentration with different heating methods (comparing MW and conventional thermal treatment) at different operational pressures. The pomegranate (*Punica granatum* L.) is a tropical and seasonal fruit, and pomegranate juice is produced during August and September.

The pomegranate has a high anthocyanin content and antioxidant activity and it has been found to be effective in reducing heart disease risk factors, but processes such as concentration and drying are needed in order to preserve the fruit and its juice all year round. Another important quality attribute is its color. The main determining factors in the color of pomegranate juice are the anthocyanins, including 3,5-diglucoside of cyanidin, pelargonidin, delphinidin, and maldivian. The results of this investigation showed that the required time was affected by operational pressure as well as by the heating method. Moreover, the lowest time was obtained when low-pressure MW treatment was applied.

Regarding antocyanin content, it was increased when lower operational pressures (or lower temperatures) and MW heating were used. The results also showed that the degradation rate of anthocyanin (and antioxidant capacity) was more dependent on the process time than the temperature or pressure. In conclusion, the degradation of color, anthocyanins, and antioxidant activity were more important in conventional heating than in MW treatment.

10.3.4 MICROWAVE EQUIPMENT

Currently, due to the extensive use of MW heating on an industrial scale, more and more companies are focused on manufacturing MW heating equipment, developing different models according to the type of food.

For the fruit juice industry, in particular, there are companies around the world manufacturing MW heating equipment for liquid food, namely, Advance Microwave Technologies (AMT), Edinburgh; Tianshui Huayuan Pharmacy Equipment Science and Technology Co., Ltd., China; Jinan Adasen Microwave Equipment, China; and Kerone, India; among others.

10.3.5 Applications of Radio-Frequency Heating in Juice Processing

Many RF applications have been demonstrated throughout the history of electromagnetism. After World War II, possible RF heating applications for food processing, such as cooking processed meat products, heating bread, and dehydrating and blanching vegetables, were suggested.

Later, Demeczky (1974) showed that the content of juices (peach, quince, and orange) in bottles that were carried on a conveyer belt through an RF applicator had better bacteriological and sensorial qualities than juices treated with conventional thermal methods, so it was an important advance in proving the potential application of RF heating for the preservation of food safety and quality. Over the years, this development has been demonstrated.

Later, as a result of the reduced nutrient content in orange juice caused by thermal pasteurization, many consumers chose to drink unpasteurized juice. This led the Food and Drug Administration (FDA) to issue a warning to consumers against drinking unpasteurized orange juice because it could be a potential source of bacterial contamination since it had been associated with a human disease outbreak (FDA, 2005). Manzocco et al. (2008) studied the efficacy of the RF application for inactivating enzymes and reducing the loss of nutritional and organoleptic quality due to blanching caused by thermal treatment. Lipoxygenase and PPO enzymes (naturally present in foods) are responsible for food quality decay, such as changes in color, flavor, and nutritional value. RF was used as a blanching method, where the protein with enzymatic activity could undergo stereochemical modifications of its active site when subjected to an electromagnetic field, which would strengthen the thermal effect. With regard to the sensory point of view, the samples subjected to an electromagnetic treatment were not significantly different from the raw sample.

10.3.6 Radio-Frequency Equipment

The RF portion of the electromagnetic spectrum occupies a region between 1 and 300 MHz (Marra et al., 2007, 2009). This is an emerging and advanced technology for foodstuff application because of its advantages in relation to penetration depth, energy consumption, and heat distribution. Hence, RF is used to sterilize, pasteurize, disinfect, and heat food such as fruit juices.

RF heating is generated by applying a high-voltage AC signal to a set of capacitors (parallel electrodes) (Figure 10.4). One of these electrodes is grounded and the capacitor stores electric energy. The sample is set between the electrodes and the AC current flows through the medium. As a result, polar molecules align and rotate to match the applied AC electric field. The capacitor plates are alternatively charged from positive to negative many times per second depending on the frequency of the RF generator. For instance, if the system is operating at 27.12 MHz, the polarity of the electrodes changes 27.12 million times per second. Under these conditions, as previously mentioned, the polar molecules inside the food are forced to realign

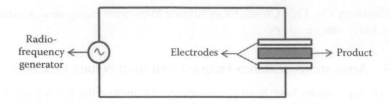

FIGURE 10.4 Schematic arrangement of RF heating. (Adapted from Marra, F., Zhang, L., and Lyng, J.G., *Journal of Food Engineering*, 91, 497–508, 2009.)

themselves with the polarity of the electrodes, producing heat because of the frictional losses as they rotate. When foods are placed between the applicator electrodes such as in RF heating, a complex electrical impedance is introduced into the electrical field (Jones and Rowley, 1997):

$$Z_c = \frac{1}{2\pi f C_0} \frac{\varepsilon' - j\varepsilon''}{\varepsilon''^2 + \varepsilon'^2} \tag{10.8}$$

where:
   Z_c is the capacitance of the material
   f is the frequency of the electric field
   ε' is the dielectric constant
   ε'' is the dielectric loss factor
   C_0 is the capacitance of the free space

RF heating offers advantages because it reduces cooking times and provides more uniform heating over the sample geometry since the low frequency of the incident electromagnetic radiation allows greater penetration depths than other forms of dielectric heating (McKenna et al., 2006). This treatment does not require direct contact with the product, so it is possible to apply the electromagnetic fields through packaged products, avoiding the risks of microbial contamination. No surface overheating occurs. This leads to minimum heat damage, reduces production floor-space requirements, is compatible with automated production batch and continuous flow processing, and is more energy efficient.

There are many different design alternatives for RF heating equipment, but all designs are based on the same principles. Since 1990, the food industry has developed RF heating equipment (Kock, 1990) that can work in a continuous process, avoiding stoppages throughout the production.

The equipment consists of a chamber where the electrodes (RF radiation source), the temperature sensors, and a conveyor belt are situated. The process is controlled by a computer, which is connected to the temperature sensor, the conveyor belt, and the RF generator. A schematic representation of the equipment is shown in Figure 10.5. The equipment provides for the uniform and rapid heating, pasteurizing, and sterilizing of food products that are packaged in closed or open containers.

The food containers are located on an endless conveyor belt which conveys them through an elongated treatment chamber. Electrodes are situated above and below

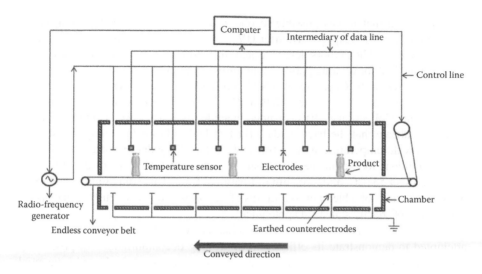

FIGURE 10.5 Schematic representation of a continuous radio-frequency electric field process. (Adapted from Kock, K., U.S. Patent No. 4,974,503, 1990.)

the treatment chamber, in a perpendicular direction to the product. Temperature sensors are arranged between the electrodes and are also connected to a computer through the intermediary of a data line with the aim of controlling the process. The computer program serves to compare the measured temperature with the specific constants of the product. As a result of this comparison, the computer controls the drive of the conveyor belt at predetermined time intervals, through the intermediary of a control line, by acting on the drive mechanism. Also, the computer can control the output of the RF generator, which is connected to electrode adjustment devices by control lines, within a frequency range of 13–440 MHz, so the product being radiated can be constantly controlled.

10.4   OTHER FREQUENCY RANGE APPLICATIONS

To date, the juice industry has been interested in the implementation of other alternative novel thermal techniques to improve the maintenance of the main organoleptic characteristics of their products, as well as to satisfy consumer demands by providing juices with improved functionalities (Rawson et al., 2011). As a result, the scientific community has studied UV, gamma, and IR heating to demonstrate their feasibility and suitability on an industrial level.

Recently, UV treatment has been used as an alternative tool to the common processes of pasteurization. Zhu et al. (2013) evaluated the viability of using monochromatic UV radiation at 253.7 nm for the reduction of patulin in fresh apple cider and juice, since patulin is a common micotoxin involved in fruit spoilage and in the development of undesirable health problems. To do this, Zhu et al. designed an experimental procedure with different types of test solutions: a model system and apple cider and apple juice with and without the addition of ascorbic acid. The results showed that it was possible to obtain a 56.5%, 87.5%, 98.6%, and 94.8% reduction of patulin, respectively, after UV exposure for 40 min at a UV irradiance of 3.00 mW/cm². The authors demonstrated, therefore, that UV radiation may be an effective method for treating patulin-containing apple cider and juice.

In other research, Gayán et al. (2013) utilized the UV system combined with mild temperatures to determine its lethal effect on the UV-resistant *E. coli* (Spanish Type Culture Collection 4201) suspended in apple juice. The results obtained in this research indicate that the bactericidal effect of UV light on *E. coli* synergistically increases with temperature up to a threshold value. They determined that the optimum conditions to exploit the synergistic effects were UV doses of 27.10 J/mL, a temperature of 55.0°C, and 3.58 min of treatment time. This study guaranteed more 5 $\log_{10}$ reductions of a blend of five strains of *E. coli* without affecting the pH, °Brix, and acidity of freshly squeezed apple juice.

On the other hand, as far as IR heating is concerned, several studies have attempted to demonstrate its efficacy in improving decontamination at processing stages. Hamanaka et al. (2011) investigated the application of single and sequential treatments of IR radiation heating and UV irradiation to decontaminate the surface of figs as a preliminary stage of juice production. The authors concluded that the sequential treatment was highly suitable for the decontamination of the fig fruit surface, since few undesirable effects were observed with regard to the surface color, hardness score, and respiration of fruits during storage. A single treatment with IR heating or UV irradiation had little impact on the inactivation of isolated *Rhodotorula mucilaginosa* cells. However, *R. mucilaginosa* cells were successfully inactivated by sequential treatment with IR heating and UV irradiation. The killing efficiencies appeared to be independent of the order in which IR heating and UV irradiation were applied to the samples. It was hypothesized that the DNA damage caused by UV irradiation and the inhibition of its repair might be enhanced by the thermal energy of IR heating to a sublethal level, since the temperature monitored during IR heating was considerably lower than the lethal level of *R. mucilaginosa* cells.

Finally, with regard to the gamma radiation technique, Alighourchi et al. (2008) studied the effects of gamma irradiation (0–10 kGy) on the stability of anthocyanins and the inhibition of microbial growth in pomegranate juice during storage. The results indicated that gamma irradiation can be satisfactorily applied to produce fruit juices with an improved shelf life. In fact, pomegranate juices irradiated at 0.5 and 10 kGy could retain approximately 80% and 10%, respectively, of their initial anthocyanin contents. Additionally, irradiation at doses greater than 2 kGy could completely inactivate the studied microorganisms and retard microbial growth during storage. However, higher doses had an undesirable effect on the total content of anthocyanins. It was concluded, therefore, that the optimal doses of irradiation applied should be lower than 2.0 kGy.

REFERENCES

Alighourchi, H., Barzegar, M., and Abbasi, S. (2008). Effect of gamma irradiation on the stability of anthocyanins and shelf-life of various pomegranate juices. *Food Chemistry* 110: 1036–1040.

Cañumir, J.A., Celis, J.E., Brujin, J., and Vidal, L. (2002). Pasteurization of apple juice by using microwaves. *Lebensmittel-Wissenschaft and Technologie* 35: 389–392.

Castro-Giráldez, M., Fito, P.J., Dalla Rosa, M., and Fito, P. (2011). Application of microwaves dielectric spectroscopy for controlling osmotic dehydration of kiwifruit (*Actinidia deliciosa cv* Hayward). *Innovative Food Science and Emerging Technologies* 12: 623–627.

Castro-Giráldez, M., Fito, P.J., and Fito, P. (2010). Application of microwaves dielectric spectroscopy for controlling pork meat (*Longissimus dorsi*) salting process. *Journal of Food Engineering* 97: 484–490.

Cendres, A., Chemat, F., Maingonnat, J.-F., and Renard, C.M.G.C. (2011). An innovate process for extraction of fruit juice using microwave heating. *LWT-Food Science and Technology* 44: 1035–1041.

Cinquanta, L., Albanese, D., Cuccurullo, G., and Di Mateo, M. (2010). Effect on orange juice of batch pasteurization in an improved pilot-scale microwave oven. *Journal of Food Science* 75: E46–E50.

Damez, J.-L., Clerjon, S., Abouelkaram, S., and Lepetit, J. (2007). Dielectric behavior of beef meat in the 1–1500 kHz range: Simulation with Fricke/Cole-Cole model. *Meat Science* 77: 512–519.

Demeczky, M. (1974). Continuous pasteurisation of bottled fruit juices by high frequency energy. In: Portela Marco, E. (ed.), *Proceedings of IV International Congress on Food Science and Technology Volume V*, pp. 11–20. Madrid: Instituto Nacional de Ciencia y Tecnología de Alimentos.

Demirdöven, A. and Baysal, T. (2012). Optimization of ohmic heating applications for pectin methylesterase inactivation in orange juice. *Journal of Food Science Technology* 49: 1–10.

Feldman, Y., Ermolina, I., and Hayashi, Y. (2003). Time domain dielectric spectroscopy study of biological systems. *IEEE Transactions on Dielectric and Electrical Insulation* 10 (5): 728–753.

Fratianni, A., Cinquanta, L., and Panfili, G. (2010). Degradation of carotenoids in orange juice during microwave heating. *Lebensmittel-Wissenschaft and Technologie* 43: 867–871.

Gayán, E., Serrano, M.J., Monfort, S., Álvarez, I., and Condón, S. (2013). Pasteurization of apple juice contaminated with *Escherichia coli* by a combined UV–mild temperature treatment. *Food and Bioprocess Technology* 6 (11): 3006–3016.

Gerard, K.A. and Roberts, J.S. (2004). Microwave heating of apple mash to improve juice yield and quality. *Lebensmittel-Wissenschaft and Technologie* 37: 551–557.

Hamanaka, D., Norimura, N., Baba, N., Mano, K., Kakiuchi, M., Tanaka, F., and Uchino, T. (2011). Surface decontamination of fig fruit by combination of infrared radiation heating with ultraviolet irradiation. *Food Control* 22: 375–380.

Içier, F., Yildiz, H., and Baysal, T. (2008). Polyphenoloxidase deactivation kinetics during ohmic heating of grape juice. *Journal of Food Engineering* 85: 410–417.

Igual, M., Gacía-Martínez, E., Camacho, M.M., and Martínez-Navarrete, N. (2010). Effect of thermal treatment and storage on stability of organic acids and the functional value of grapefruit juice. *Food Chemistry* 118: 291–299.

Jones, P.L. and Rowley, A.T. (1997). Dielectric dryers. In: Baker, C.G.J. (ed.), *Industrial Drying of Foods*, Chapter 8 pp. 156–178. London: Blackie Academic and Professional.

Kock, K. (1990). Apparatus for irradiating food products. U.S. Patent No. 4,974,503.

Lee, S.Y., Sagong, H.G., Ryu, S., and Kang, D.H. (2012). Effect of continuous heating to inactivate *Escherichia coli* O157:H7, *Salmonella typhimurium* and *Listeria monocytogenes* in orange juice and tomato juice. *Journal of Applied Microbiology* 112: 723–731.

Leizerson, S. and Shimoni, E. (2005a). Stability and sensory life of orange juice pasteurized by continuous ohmic heating. *Journal of Agricultural and Food Chemistry* 53: 4012–4018.

Leizerson, S. and Shimoni, E. (2005b). Effect of ultrahigh-temperature continuous ohmic heating treatment on fresh orange juice. *Journal of Agricultural and Food Chemistry* 53: 3519–3524.

Manzocco, L., Anese, M., and Nicoli, M.C. (2008). Radiofrequency inactivation of oxidative food enzymes in model systems and apple derivatives. *Food Research International* 41: 1044–1049.

Marra, F., Lyng, J., Romano, V., and McKenna, B. (2007). Radio-frequency heating of foodstuff: Solution and validation of mathematical model. *Journal of Food Engineering* 79: 998–1006.

Marra, F., Zhang, L., and Lyng, J.G. (2009). Radio frequency treatment of foods: Review of recent advances. *Journal of Food Engineering* 91: 497–508.

McKenna, B.M., Lyng, J., Brunton, N., and Shirsat, N. (2006). Advances in radio frequency and ohmic heating of meats. *Journal of Food Engineering* 77: 215–229.

Mudgett, R.E. (1986). Electrical properties of foods. In: Rao, M.A. and Rizvi, S.S.H. (eds), *Engineering Properties of Foods*, pp. 329–390. New York: Marcel Dekker.

Nikdel, S., Chen, C.S., Parish, M.E., MacKellar, D.G., and Friedrich, L.M. (1993). Pasteurization of citrus juice with microwave energy in a continuous-flow unit. *Journal of Agriculture and Food Chemistry* 41: 2116–2119.

Parrot, D.L. (1992). The use of ohmic heating for aseptic processing of food particulates. *Food Technology* 96 (12): 68–72.

Pereira, R.N. and Vicente, A.A. (2010). Environmental impact of novel thermal and non thermal technologies in food processing. *Food Research International* 43: 1936–1943.

Ponne, C.T. and Bartels, P.V. (1995). Interaction of electromagnetic energy with biological material: Relation to food processing. *Radiation, Physics and Chemistry* 45 (4): 591–607.

Praporscic, I., Lebovka, N.I., Ghnimi, S., and Vorobiev, E. (2006). Ohmically heated, enhanced expression of juice from apple and potato tissues. *Biosystems Engineering* 93 (2): 199–204.

Rawson, A., Patras, A., Tiwari, B.K., Noci, F., Koutchma, T., and Brunton, N. (2011). Effect of thermal and non thermal processing technologies on the bioactive content of exotic fruits and their products: Review of recent advances. *Food Research International* 44: 1875–1887.

Ryynänen, S. (1995). The electromagnetic properties of food materials: A review of the basic principles. *Journal of Food Engineering* 26: 409–429.

Sarang, S., Sastry, S.K., and Knipe, L. (2008). Electrical conductivity of fruits and meats during ohmic heating. *Journal of Food Engineering* 87: 351–356.

Sastry, S.H. and Barach, J.T. (2000). Ohmic and inductive heating. *Journal of Food Science* 65 (4): 42–46.

Tajchakavit, S. and Ramaswamy, H.S. (1997). Thermal vs. microwave inactivation kinetics of pectin methylesterase in orange juice under batch mode heating conditions. *LWT-Food Science and Technology* 30: 85–93.

Tajchakavit, S., Ramaswamy, H.S., and Fustier, P. (1998). Enhanced destruction of spoilage microorganisms in apple juice during continuous flow microwave heating. *Food Research International* 31 (10): 713–722.

Venkatesh, M.S. and Raghavan, G.S.V. (2004). An overview of microwave processing and dielectric properties of agri-food materials. *Biosystems Engineering* 88: 1–18.

Vicente, A.A. and Castro, I. (2007). Novel thermal processing technologies. In: Tewari, G. and Juneja, V. (eds), *Advances in Thermal and Non-thermal Food Preservation*, pp. 99–130. Oxford: Blackwell Publishing.

Vicente, A.A. and Pereira, R.N. (2010). Environmental impact of novel thermal and non-thermal technologies in food processing. *Food Research International* 43: 1936–1943.

Vikram, V.B., Ramesh, M.N., and Prapulla, S.G. (2005). Thermal degradation kinetics of nutrients in orange juice heated by electromagnetic and conventional methods. *Journal of Food Engineering* 69: 31–40.

Villamiel, M., Dolores del Castillo, M., San Martín, C., and Corzo, N. (1998). Assessment of the thermal treatment of orange juice during continuous microwave and conventional heating. *Journal of the Science of Food and Agriculture* 78: 196–200.

Yildiz, H., Bozkurt, H., and Icier, F. (2009). Ohmic and conventional heating of pomegranate juice: Effects on rheology, color and total phenolics. *Food Science and Technology International* 15: 503.

Yousefi, S., Emam-Djomeh, Z., Ali Mousavi, S.M., and Reza Askari, G. (2012). Comparing the effects of microwave and conventional heating methods on the evaporation rate and quality attributes of pomegranate (*Punica granatum L.*) juice concentrate. *Food and Bioprocess Technology* 4: 1328–1339.

Zhao, Y. (2006). Radiofrequency: Dielectric heating. In. Sun, D. (ed.), *Thermal Food Processing: New Technologies and Quality Issues*, pp. 469–492. Boca Raton, FL: Taylor & Francis.

Zhu, Y., Koutchma, T., Warriner, K., Shao, S., and Zhou, T. (2013). Kinetics of patulin degradation in model solution, apple cider and apple juice by ultraviolet radiation. *Food Science and Technology International* 19 (4): 291–303.

11 Emerging Nonthermal Technologies in Fruit Juice Processing

Olga Martín-Belloso, Ángel Robert Marsellés-Fontanet, Robert Soliva-Fortuny, and Pedro Elez-Martínez

CONTENTS

11.1 Introduction 217
11.2 Ultraviolet Light.. 218
    11.2.1 Fundamentals and Main Effects on Fruit Juice Components........... 218
    11.2.2 Engineering and Industrial Aspects 219
11.3 Pulsed Light... 220
    11.3.1 Fundamentals and Main Effects on Fruit Juice Components...........220
    11.3.2 Engineering and Industrial Aspects 221
11.4 Electric and Magnetic Fields 221
    11.4.1 Fundamentals and Main Effects on Fruit Juice Components.......... 221
    11.4.2 Engineering and Industrial Aspects 223
11.5 Sonication 225
    11.5.1 Fundamentals and Main Effects on Fruit Juice Components.......... 225
    11.5.2 Engineering and Industrial Aspects 226
11.6 High Hydrostatic Pressure 227
11.7 Other Technologies 230
11.8 Final Remarks.. 231
Acknowledgments.. 231
References.. 231

11.1 INTRODUCTION

Despite the consistent and long-term proven effects of thermal processing on the preservation of fruit juices at an industrial level, researchers are constantly looking for improvements that might help to overcome its major drawbacks (e.g., flavor and nutritive losses) without compromising customers' safety.

Since the nineteenth century, several attempts have been made to adapt technologies initially developed in other scientific fields to food processing and preservation applications. Many of the emerging technologies to preserve food that are currently under study and in industrial development are based on the physical properties of matter instead of its chemical properties. The basis of this approach could be the aversion of contemporary society to the mixture of the labels "chemistry" and "food."

The aim of this chapter is to provide an overview of the most important nonthermal emerging technologies, stating their effects on the composition of fruit juices as well as providing discussion about their benefits and main limitations from different points of view.

11.2 ULTRAVIOLET LIGHT

11.2.1 FUNDAMENTALS AND MAIN EFFECTS ON FRUIT JUICE COMPONENTS

Ultraviolet (UV) radiation is the region of the electromagnetic spectrum with wavelengths ranging from 10 to 400 nm. The fact that the energetic content of UV light coincides in part with the energetic range for electronic state transitions explains its absorption by matter. Only a small proportion of the UV light emitted by the sun reaches the surface of the earth. Most of this radiation corresponds to the UV range that is closest to visible light (300–400 nm), called near-UV radiation, which has the lowest energetic content. The highest energetic UV radiation, known as extreme-UV radiation (10–120 nm), and the region following, called far-UV radiation (120–200 nm), can break covalent bonds through a process called photoionization, thus generating ionized compounds (NASA Science Mission Directorate 2011; World Health Organization 2013). Ionized or radical species are very unstable and typically start a chemical reaction with a neighboring compound. It is assumed that radical reactions follow a specific pattern although the reaction outcome is rather unpredictable. Moreover, there is the possibility that the newly formed chemical products will start another cycle of radical reactions until the whole system becomes stable.

Some compounds are more susceptible than others to ionization as a consequence of their chemical structure. In particular, deoxyribonucleic acid (DNA) of living organisms is one of them. Only a UV light radiation of around 254 nm is absorbed and has the ability to cleave bonds between the chemical bases forming the strand of DNA. This fact hinders any biochemical process in this DNA region, such as DNA replication prior to cellular division, or DNA transcription to produce proteins (Matsumura and Ananthaswamy 2002). Longer UV wavelengths are less energetic, so instead of tearing electrons from atoms or molecules, the absorbed energy drives electrons to higher energetic states referred to as excited states. This situation is energetically unfavorable and, consequently, such atoms or molecules are abnormally reactive and tend to return to their initial state. The usual process, which is known as internal conversion, releases the acquired energy to the medium as heat, whereas fluorescent and phosphorescent molecules release it as light. Another pathway to achieve stabilization is reacting with a neighboring chemical compound, as described for ionized species (Wardle 2009).

Consequently, applications aimed at destroying microbial agents should control not only the wavelength of the UV irradiating source but also the exposure time, so that the damage overcomes the repair systems and eventually leads to cellular death (Table 11.1). On the other hand, an excessive exposure period could reduce the

TABLE 11.1

Examples of Use of UV and PL Technologies in Juices

Medium	Treatment Parameters	Microbial Species	Treatment Effects	Effects on Quality	Source
Apple cider	Continuous flow, 10 chambers UV light	*Escherichia coli* O157:H7	3.8-log		Wright et al. (2000)
Apple juice	Continuous flow, 450 kJ/m², 2 × 25 W UV lamps	*Saccharomyces cerevisiae*	1.34-log reductions	Small changes in	Guerrero-Beltrán and Barbosa-
		E. coli	5.10-log reductions	a* and b* color	Cánovas (2005)
		L. innocua	4.29-log reductions	coordinates	
Apple juice	Continuous flow, 4 J/cm² with pulsed light of 1.21 J/cm²/pulse, 3 Hz, 100–1100 nm	*E. coli*	4.0-log reductions		Pataro et al. (2011)
		L. innocua	2.98-log reductions		
Orange juice	Continuous flow, 4 J/cm² with pulsed light of 1.21 J/cm²/pulse, 3 Hz, 100–1100 nm	*E. coli*	2.90-log reductions		Pataro et al. (2011)
		L. innocua	0.93-log reductions		

quality of the irradiated products due to the extension of unspecific reactions of free radicals.

Other macromolecules in plant materials, such as natural polymers and fibers (e.g., pectin, celluloses, and tannins, among other components), can suffer the effects of UV irradiation up to a certain degree due to the formation of radicals and subsequent reactions. Furthermore, high enzyme inactivation rates can be attained in clarified juices with almost no modification of their physicochemical properties (Falguera et al. 2012). There are, though, reports about the effects of UV radiation on rheological properties (Shamsudina et al. 2013), induced off-flavors (Demirci and Krishnamurthy 2011), discolorations (Cuvelier and Berset 2005), and vitamin C loss (Falguera et al. 2012). The effects on particular components should be investigated on a case-by-case basis to obtain more accurate information.

11.2.2 Engineering and Industrial Aspects

As outlined above, the effects of UV treatments and their extension depend on the characteristics of the incident light, the nature of the agent that is being treated, and its surrounding environment such as the medium and its superficial shape. The engineering of the process only has a direct influence on the first factor by means of the spectral range and intensity, even though other parameters, such as the geometry of the treatment chamber(s), the physical arrangement of the UV source(s), the radiation path length, the product opacity, and the flow profile in continuous processing systems or the package characteristics in finished products, can also indirectly help to improve the homogeneity of the treatment (Koutchma 2000).

In this context, germicidal lamps are already available at a commercial level, and are extensively used to disinfect food-contact surfaces as well as water supplies. Fluorescent lamps containing low-pressure mercury vapor that emits UV light of 253.7 and 185 nm are among the most used (Atlantic Ultraviolet Corporation 2012). DNA absorbs the shortest wavelength better; however, the impurities of normal quartz tubes block it and leave only the longest wavelength.

Despite the fact that manufacturers usually give the radiant power (W) of the lamp, the appropriate measurement for a preserving technology that should be provided is fluence (J/m²), which is the absorbed energy power per area in a specific time interval, sometimes known as radiant exposure. In any case, a proper measure of this variable is necessary so that different processing designs can be compared.

The most important drawback of the technology is the short penetration range of UV light into the matter, which is roughly a few millimeters in solid foodstuffs. In fluid products, it depends on their transparency. The path length can be easily calculated using the Lambert–Beer law, provided that the absorption coefficient of the liquid is known (Shama 1999). So, the treatment chamber should be designed in such a fashion to allow the delivery of the minimum treatment required to the whole stream of product. There are already several commercial designs implemented for water treatment that could be adapted to flowing products that are not as transparent, such as fruit and vegetable juices. Critical decisions on the radiation source, reactor geometry, reaction medium properties, and their interaction need to be considered for successful industrial implementation. Falguera et al. (2011) present an outstanding review on the engineering aspects of radiation sources and different available photochemical reactors.

11.3 PULSED LIGHT

11.3.1 Fundamentals and Main Effects on Fruit Juice Components

Pulsed light (PL) involves the use of intense pulses of short duration and broad spectrum to decontaminate food and food-contact materials. This broad-spectrum radiation comprises UV and infrared radiations, together with white light, understood as the portion of the electromagnetic radiation spectrum found between the former that can be perceived by the human eye (400–700 nm). As previously discussed, UV light also interacts with matter since its energy coincides with different rotational and vibrational molecular states. Natural colorants have chemical groups called chromophores that are responsible for the absorption of specific wavelengths.

It has been suggested that the effectiveness of PL treatments on microorganisms is a response not only to photochemical but also to photothermal effects caused by the broad range of irradiated wavelengths (Oms-Oliu et al. 2010). Thus, light of short wavelengths would be responsible for damaging DNA microbial strands, whereas the longer-wavelength high-intensity radiation would account for thermal harm to microorganisms (Food and Drug Administration 2013). A summary of the main effects reported on fruit juices is shown in Table 11.1.

The susceptibility of other compounds found in foods of plant origin has been studied much less (Caminiti et al. 2012). It would not be illogical to suppose that the consequences in the irradiated region may be similar to those reported for thermal processing. However, as it is a localized treatment generally applied to solid or highly viscous products, the effects should have less extension and, consequently, the final nutritional and quality properties should be affected less. However, the application of high-intensity PL treatments has recently received more attention, as a feasible alternative to decontaminate fruit juices (Pataro et al. 2011; Palgan et al. 2011; Ferrario et al. 2013).

11.3.2 Engineering and Industrial Aspects

From the engineering point of view, PL processing is quite similar to UV light processing; hence the critical processing factors as discussed in the previous section. The most important difference is that lamps produce a broad spectrum of light from UV to infrared frequencies. Therefore, illuminated objects increase their superficial temperature due to the heat from lamps and the heat released from internal conversion. A way to overcome such an issue is to use very short pulses at a controlled repetition rate. The light sources are xenon lamps that allow the delivery of light pulses from 1 μs to 0.1 s with wavelengths from 170 to 2600 nm. Depending on the supporting electronics of the appliances, several pulses may be delivered in a short period of time, although this should be controlled to avoid unwanted thermal damage. Typical received energy doses range from 0.01 to 50 J/m² (MacGregor et al. 1998). Regulations in the United States state that the pulse length should be no longer than 2 ms and the whole treatment should not exceed 12 J/cm², using wavelengths ranging between 200 and 1100 nm (Food and Drug Administration 2008).

11.4 ELECTRIC AND MAGNETIC FIELDS

11.4.1 Fundamentals and Main Effects on Fruit Juice Components

Electric and magnetic fields are the components of the electromagnetic spectrum. Objects in a very near region of the emitter may perceive the effects of each field independently. Speaking specifically about the electric field, it may be defined as the space region where an electrically charged particle exerts its influence, which will be noticed as a force by another electrically charged particle placed inside this region. The forces exerted depend on the implied electrical charges and where they are located, as well as on the electrical properties of the medium. The described influence is also noticed by ionic- or dipolar-neutral species.

This is a rather simplistic view of the fundamentals of the electric field technology because only two different kinds of particles are being considered. Matter is composed of an uncountable number of charged compounds in the form of ionic species or dipolar molecules. In addition, unlike the technologies discussed until now, an electric field does not have a scalar but a vectorial nature, meaning that the variables may exhibit opposite directions, either positive or negative. Consequently, field direction, field sense, and field polarity are also important features to take into account, and have a determining influence on the effectiveness of the treatment. All these characteristics lead to more complex theoretical and calculation requirements for the development of technological applications. Regarding the application of pulsed electric fields (PEF) technology to foodstuffs, during the first decades of the twentieth century it was observed that the application of an electric current to milk and juices often induced not only microbial death but also the complete destruction of the product matrix. The subsequent refinements to reduce heat production due to the ohmic heating or joule effect led to the development of PEF treatments where the observed effects are attributed to the electric fields. Two hypotheses have been proposed in relation to the interaction of an external electric field with cell walls. This would compromise cellular homeostasis even though the possibility of thermal and electrochemical effects is still under discussion and cannot be completely discarded (Meneses et al. 2011; Jaeger et al. 2010).

It has been claimed that the external electric field induces a difference of voltage between both faces of the cell wall. The first hypothesis states that such a charge separation develops a pair of opposite forces at each cell wall face that push and deform this thin layer until they produce membrane pores in it (Zimmermann 1986). The other proposed mechanism suggests that the external electrical field destabilizes the membrane components responsible for controlling the exchange of materials between the internal medium and the environment, avoiding operational control of what enters and leaves the cell (Castro et al. 1993).

In this context, it is worth bearing in mind that PEF technology often implies delivering electric field pulses in a particular way so that the ohmic heating of the product can be kept under control. Hence, the membrane must cope not only with a perturbing external influence but also with a continuous variation of it in strength and time. Both mechanisms of action against the microorganisms described allow an explanation of the general behavior of microbial cells. For instance, the effectiveness of PEF treatments typically diminishes when the microbial cell size, the matrix electrical resistance, and the electric field strength are reduced. Regarding more resistant hazards such as spores and viruses, there have been no reports of a significant effect of PEF on them. Current research efforts are directed toward understanding how differences in equipment, the food matrix, and cells modify such a generic behavior and its extension (Martín-Belloso and Soliva-Fortuny 2011).

The same can be stated regarding nonliving components of fruit juices. It seems clear that electrical interactions between the generated external field and the internal electrical distribution of the chemical structures play a role. Modifications of the secondary structure of some enzymes have been reported, thus causing a modification of their activity (Zhong et al. 2005). However, a generic behavior in response to PEF treatments cannot be extrapolated to any protein. In some cases, their biological activity has been shown to be reduced, whereas others have exhibited an increase in their activity or have not shown any change (Ohshima et al. 2007; Yang et al. 2004). Neither is it obvious what happens with smaller entities such as single molecules, for example, sugars, amino acids, fatty acids, or vitamins (Martín-Belloso and Soliva-Fortuny 2011). It has been extensively suggested that PEF processing is milder than thermal pasteurization treatments as regards the bioactive natural composition of juices. However, the effects on each juice component should be examined case by case.

With regard to magnetic field technology, this is closely related to PEF, because any movement of a charged particle generates a magnetic field. Likewise, a magnetic field influences charged particles while they move. Consequently, any magnetic field generates a region of influence where any moving charged particle or magnetic dipole may notice it as a force, in a similar way to what was discussed in the case of electric fields. This force depends on the intensity of the magnetic field, the charge of the particle and its movement. Magnetic fields have also shown diverse effects on food sample components. Among the few scientific studies describing its effects, it seems that the influence on microorganism growth and reproduction depends on its own susceptibility, although researchers are reluctant to attribute a bactericidal action to it (Kohno et al. 2000; Abdelmelek et al. 2009). There are up to three postulated hypotheses that try to explain the biological effects of magnetic fields (Halgamuge et al. 2009). All of them claim that the external field disturbs the vibration frequency of ionic species in key compounds such as DNA and enzymes, and that this hampers their normal functions. Nevertheless, this technology has received much less attention and, consequently, more consistent results concerning its efficacy are needed to understand its whole potential as a preservative tool in the fruit juice industry. Table 11.2 presents some selected examples regarding the application of PEF and magnetic field treatments on juices and other liquid matrices.

11.4.2 ENGINEERING AND INDUSTRIAL ASPECTS

Obtaining electrical fields in a specific region of a space is relatively easy. A condenser is required to accumulate electrical charges, subsequently deliver them through a metallic conductor, and create an electrical field within the gap between two electrodes. The real challenge is to increase its extension so that a product can be placed inside while the electric field is kept homogeneous. As mentioned above, an electric field is a vectorial variable. Therefore, the relative position of a product inside the field must be taken into account when designing the treatment chambers (Altunakar and Barbosa-Cánovas 2011). Moreover, the strength of the electric field must be high enough to influence a certain agent. This means accumulating a high electric voltage, and such energy should be delivered as pulses of a specific shape for very short periods of time so that heating effects are kept below the desired threshold. This requires considerable numbers of electronic appliances as well as control systems. Currently, there are very few PEF device constructors of industrial equipment (Diversified Technologies 2009; DIL 2013).

PEF technology in the fruit juice industry has been proposed in two stages of the production process of fruit and vegetable juices. The first one implies using it as a preservative technology. Hence, the main targets are hazardous bacteria and enzymes. The magnitude of the electric field to be applied is in the range of megavolts per meter. Nevertheless, PEF may also be used as an extraction aid in order to increase juice yield. In this case, the strength of the electric field can be reduced by as much as 100 times because the size difference between vegetal and bacterial cells is of this order of magnitude (Toepfl and Heinz 2011).

TABLE 11.2

Examples of Use of PEF and Magnetic Field Technologies in Juices

Medium	Treatment Parameters	Studied Agent	Effects	Source
Apple juice	Continuous flow, 30 kV/cm, 43 pulses, 4 μs, 25°C	E. coli O157:H7	5-log reduction	Evrendilek et al. (1999)
Melon juice	Continuous flow, 35 kV/cm, 400 pulses, 4 μs, 39°C maximum	E. coli	3.8-log reduction	Mosqueda-Melgar et al. (2007)
		Salmonella enteritidis	4.3-log reduction	
		Listeria monocytogenes	3.9-log reduction	
Grape juice	Continuous flow, 35 kV/cm for 5 s with alternating squared pulses of 4 μs, 40°C maximum	Polyphenol oxidase	100% activity reduction	Marsellés-Fontanet and Martín-Belloso (2007)
		Peroxidase	50% activity reduction	
Strawberry juice	Continuous flow, 35 kV/cm for 1 s with alternating squared pulses of 4 μs, 35°C maximum	Polygalacturonase	28% activity reduction	Aguiló-Aguayo et al. (2009)
Tomato juice			62% activity reduction	
Buffer solution	Oscillating magnetic field, 4.0 T for 40 pulses	Horseradish peroxidase	67.7% activity reduction	Ma et al. (2011)
Culture medium	Static magnetic field, 100 mT for 24 h	Streptococcus mutans, Staphylococcus aureus, E. coli	Growth inhibition of S. mutans and S. aureus	Kohno et al. (2000)
Orange juice	Oscillating magnetic field, 40.0 T, 416,000 Hz (1 pulse)	Saccharomyces	3.6-log reduction	Hofmann (1985)

In either method, the accepted critical processing parameters are related to the shape of the electric field pulses and the way that they are delivered to the product matrix. Defining a PEF treatment requires information about pulse shape, pulse width, and field amplitude or strength. Regarding the way that the train of pulses is delivered, parameters such as pulse repetition rate, polarity, and effective treatment time are relevant in order to provide a characterization of the treatment. Even though PEF treatments last only a few milliseconds as a maximum, all these parameters should be optimized so that the unwanted joule effect is kept under control.

There are extensive reports on the effects of sinusoidal, exponential decaying, and triangle and square pulses. All of these have advantages and disadvantages, although the widespread use of square pulses suggest that they are the most effective. As already mentioned, field strengths and pulse widths vary upon application. Typical pulse widths range from 2 to 10 μs. The strength of electric fields in preservative treatments varies from 20 to 80 kV/cm, while common values for pressing purposes fall around 100 V/cm. A wide range of pulse trains has been tested. Some research-ers propose the use of alternate pulses as a way to avoid polarization issues occurring with pulses of the same polarity.

Even accepting that PEF technology allows feasible continuous processing of a stream of product, the attempts to develop industrial devices to apply electrical pulses to juice products still have to solve issues similar to those found in thermal processing. The most noteworthy is the difficulty of a homogeneous transmission of the physical agent, which in this case is an electric field, throughout the whole juice matrix being processed. Another is how to control such a process and guarantee its effectiveness when even the smallest local variation of the product conductivity may imply a risk. One last issue to take into consideration is the fact that even the tini-est electric current is often associated with electrochemical reactions of susceptible food components, the metallic electrodes, or both. So, the interface between the food matrix and the electrodes will suffer from electrode fouling because of corrosion and deposition (Kim and Zhang 2011).

Regarding the application of magnetic fields, the literature reports only the exis-tence of experimental laboratory-scale devices comprising a magnetic field generator and a temperature controller (Ma et al. 2011). The magnetic field generator is often a ferromagnetic coil connected to a transformer. The region inside the coil is typically the treatment chamber, although ferrite magnet plates have also been used (Kohno et al. 2000). Oscillating magnetic fields commonly follow the frequency of the distri-bution electrical network (50–60 Hz) even though there are studies describing more complex electrical appliances that can deliver frequencies of up to 500 kHz. Usual magnetic field strengths vary from just a few mT up to 50 mT for several minutes up to several days (Grigelmo-Miguel et al. 2011).

11.5 SONICATION

11.5.1 FUNDAMENTALS AND MAIN EFFECTS ON FRUIT JUICE COMPONENTS

Sonication treatments can be applied to fluids, causing agitation of their particles due to pressure changes. In this way, the microscopic bubbles of air present in the medium are forced to move, increase in volume, and quickly collapse. The rapid implosion of bubbles because of their instability in the environmental conditions of the fluid causes significant shock waves, which are considered to be the origin of the effects of sonication. In particular, intracellular cavitation has been suggested as the mechanism to disrupt bacterial cells in the laboratory (Hughes and Nyborg 1962). In any case, the ultrasound effect alone cannot guarantee the minimum safety requirements regarding microbial inactivation in complex matrices such as fruit and vegetable processing. It is acknowledged, though, that sonication treatments may enhance the effectiveness of other preservative treatments when combined (Feng and Yan 2011).

However, each particular application modulates sound properties to take advan-tage of the technology. Relatively gentle sonication intensities are used to homogenize mixtures and solutions, especially when the use of convective transport processes is not feasible. Mixing efficiency is favored because of the acceleration of diffusive effects caused by the movement of particles. Similar conditions are used in medicine to break down solid aggregates of insoluble material in the kidneys. Ultrasonication is also applied with the same function in the food industry in cutting, slicing, slitting, and chopping devices (Feng and Yan 2011).

For other hazardous agents such as spores, not only is the mechanism of action unclear but the effectiveness of the treatment is also under discussion. As far as the remaining components of the juices are concerned, some efforts have been made to understand the effect of ultrasounds when they are used as aids to extract proteins from raw plant and animal materials. The technology modifies typical protein functional properties such as emulsion and foam stabilization, gel formation, and enzyme activities. All of these are related to the tridimensional protein structure. Carbohydrates may undergo hydrolysis and cleavage, leading to polymer degradation, though the possible pathways of such processes remain under discussion (Weiss et al. 2011). Works providing examples of the application of ultrasounds to fruit juices are presented in Table 11.3.

11.5.2 ENGINEERING AND INDUSTRIAL ASPECTS

Ultrasounds are pressure waves with a frequency greater than the upper limit of the human hearing range. The advent of inexpensive and reliable generators of high-intensity ultrasound fostered the research in this field.

In a piezoelectric transformer an input voltage is applied across a short length of a bar of piezoceramic material, creating an alternating stress in the bar through the inverse piezoelectric effect and causing the whole bar to vibrate. The vibration

TABLE 11.3
Examples of Applications of Ultrasound Technology in Juices

Medium	Treatment Parameters	Microbial Species	Microbial Effects	Storage Conditions	Quality Effects	Source
Carrot juice	19.3 kHz, 700–800 W, 60 s, 60°C	*E. coli* K12	2.5-log reduction	35 days at 4°C	Improvement in surface color stability and L-ascorbic acid retention	Zenker et al. (2003)
Orange juice	500 kHz, 240 W, 15 min, 60°C	Total mesophilic aerobes	3.4-log reduction	14 days at 5°C	No detrimental effects on limonin content, brown pigments and color	Valero et al. (2007)
Orange juice	20 kHz, 500 W, 8 min, 10°C	Total mesophilic aerobes	1.38-log reduction	10 days at 4°C	Color and ascorbic acid content were affected during storage	Gómez-López et al. (2010)
		Yeast and mold	0.56-log reduction			

frequency is chosen to be the resonant frequency of the block, typically in the kilohertz to megahertz range. A higher output voltage is then generated across another section of the bar by the piezoelectric effect. Devices for food processing applications typically use frequencies in the range of 20–100 kHz and sound intensities from 10 to 1000 W/cm². Industrial devices of 16 kW are also available, allowing processing stream flow rates up to 10 m³/h and higher (Feng and Yan, 2011).

The process of bubble generation and subsequent implosion is known as cavitation, which is regarded as an undesirable event in propellers and pumps. The unique difference between sonication and a typical cavitation process is the way that the bubbles are generated. In a sonication process, bubbles are formed by the coalescence of microscopic air bubbles or the evaporation of fluid on the surface of such bubbles as a consequence of pressure differences generated by their rapid movement when trying to follow the external sonic perturbations. However, a combination of both processes should not be discarded. Therefore, the frequency and intensity of the sound waves and sonication time are key process parameters when using this technology.

The heating of the media is a side effect of this technology, since molecular vibration and cavitation eventually dissipate the received energy as heat. Therefore, a refrigeration system or a method of limiting the treatment time should be part of the device in order to constrain the temperature increase as far as possible.

11.6 HIGH HYDROSTATIC PRESSURE

The application of high hydrostatic pressure (HHP) to food applications is based on the fact that pressure is a scalar property of matter irrespective of its scale. This means that any pressure variation will be transmitted immediately throughout a product found within a fluid medium, regardless of the product size and geometry, even though pressure effects certainly depend on the product's dimensions and intrinsic architecture. Hence, when pressure is raised to a specific high value, large particles must support a quantitatively larger resultant force than small objects. As the force is always directed toward their interior, they require a more robust constitution than smaller particles to prevent them from collapsing. Such a principle is already known and used for juice extraction applications. Nevertheless, HHP technology subjects foodstuffs to pressures ranging from 100 MPa up to 1 GPa, which are between about 5 and 100 times the maximum pressure reached in industrial fruit juice presses. Since Chapter 12 will be entirely devoted to high-pressure treatments of fruit juices, in this section only a brief introduction about the topic will be given.

Assuming that the hazardous microorganisms of juices are prokaryotes that are roughly 10–100 times smaller than typical plant cells, it is probable that such high-pressure values will also affect them. Actually, within microorganisms the same pattern holds. For instance, vegetative yeast cells, which are larger than vegetative bacterial cells, are commonly less resistant to HHP processing (Black et al. 2011). Likewise, the effect of cell robustness has been studied, comparing similarly sized Gram-positive and Gram-negative bacteria. The former usually exhibit a higher resistance to HHP than the latter because of their thicker peptidoglycan layer (Ludwig and Schreck 1997). Hence, the list of microbial agents ordered by decreasing HHP susceptibility is: protozoa, vegetative microbial cells, spores, and viral particles. However, as combinations of size and structural strength provide a virtually unlimited range of possibilities, the selection of a specific HHP treatment for a particular product should be tested, taking into account the most resistant hazardous agent expected to be present.

The specific damage in microorganisms caused by HPP is diverse (Rendueles et al. 2011). Cell membrane disruption has been reported as a major cause of microbial destruction, together with intracellular organelle failure such as ribosomal breakdown, vacuole collapse, and inactivation of enzymes, as well as the failure of several transport systems. The described mechanism of action holds regardless of the type of object, whether living or not. Therefore, pressure drives proteins to lose their natural spatial arrangement. Concerning enzymes, denaturation leads to malfunction due to the strong relationship between their tridimensional layout and their function (Chauvin and Swanson 2011). The same process is thought to be the cause of viral inactivation, since their protective coat or envelope contains proteins (Kingsley et al. 2002).

Carbohydrates and lipids may be similarly affected by pressure (Jolie et al. 2012); fruits are a typical source of the former. This implies that HHP applied to the production of fruit- and vegetable-derived food systems will automatically have implications for their structural quality (texture, rheology, cloud stability). So, HHP technology can also be used to develop new products.

On the other hand, smaller molecules of food such as simple sugars and fatty and amino acids remain unchanged. They could even protect microorganisms from HHP effects in a similar way, as tissues and cells are protected from damage in freezing–thawing cycles (Molina-Hoppner et al. 2004). The specific effects of HHP on bioactive compounds and the sensory properties of fruit and vegetable juices have been reviewed by Sánchez-Moreno et al. (2009) and Oms-Oliu et al. (2012).

Leaving aside fruit and vegetable components, chemical reactions also suffer the consequences of pressure (Van der Plancken et al. 2012). According to Le Chatelier's principle, pressure in a closed system shifts the system equilibrium toward the state with the smallest volume. Thus, a greater pressure leads to an increase in the interaction among reactants, even though the energy delivered in HHP treatments is not enough to cleave covalent bonds of chemical compounds. In any case, the overwhelming complexity of the simplest juice advises investigation of the effect on specific chemical reactions. Some selected examples regarding the application of HHP to fruit juices are displayed in Table 11.4.

Many different high-pressure processing devices have been developed for application to different foodstuffs. Nevertheless, even if the product is a fluid, as in the case of juices, the required pressure is not achievable in an open arrangement. Consequently, product processing is a noncontinuous process by its nature. The batch cycle involves loading the product into a compartment, filling the chamber with a transmission fluid, which is commonly water, pressurizing it at the selected working pressure (typically from 200 up to 700 MPa), decompressing it after the holding time while the transmission fluid is recovered, and finally, unloading the product. The pressurization-releasing sequence may be repeated several times if needed.

TABLE 11.4

Examples of Use of HHP Technology in Juices

Medium	Treatment Parameters	Studied Microorganism	Reported Effect	Storage Conditions	Long-term Effects	Source
Guava puree	600 MPa, 15 min, 25°C	Yeast and mold and total aerobic count	<10 cfu/mL	4°C up to 60 days	Microbial, biochemical, and quality stability for 40 days	Gow-Chin and Hsin-Tang (1996)
Orange juice	500–700 Mpa, 60–90 s	Total aerobic count	<10 cfu/mL	4°C up to 16 weeks	Microbial, biochemical, sensory, and quality stability similar to thermally treated juice	Parish (1998)
Kiwifruit juice Pineapple juice	350 MPa, 60 s, 20°C	E. coli and L. innocua	>5-log reductions 2.5- and 3.5-log reduction	24 h, different temperature	Reduction of bacterial counts	Buzrul et al. (2008)
Apple juice	400 MPa, 60 s, 25°C	E. coli	8-log reduction			Ramaswamy et al. (2003)

Likewise, if a higher throughput is necessary, several devices could be combined to simulate a continuous processing stage.

However, what could be one of the major drawbacks of the technology from the industrial point of view can be regarded as one of its most attractive advantages. HHP technology allows the processing of a product already packed in its final format provided that the envelope meets a few requirements, such as not being too rigid, although hard enough to avoid disruptions (Mensitieri et al. 2013). This detail avoids posterior safety concerns as the inner part is no longer exposed to any source of contamination after the treatment. When processing packaged products, special care should be given to the design of the size and shape of the envelopes to take advantage of the technology. Nevertheless, flowing products may also be processed. In the case of bulk juices, a free-floating piston is usually used to transmit the pressure of the pressurizing fluid to the fluid food product, which is aseptically poured into containers after treatment.

In any case, HPP is one of the most successful nonthermal technologies, at least as far as the numbers of machinery manufacturers and industrial applications are concerned. Different engineering solutions have been developed and industrially applied to process diverse food products. Meat and seafood products, fluid foods such as dairy products, sauces, and vegetable and fruit juices are applications that have already been tested and are producing good results (Tonello 2011).

11.7 OTHER TECHNOLOGIES

Other nonthermal technologies with prospects regarding their application to fruit juice processing are cold atmospheric plasma and high-energy irradiation. For the sake of completeness, a few words about the fundamentals of each one are given.

Cold atmospheric plasma has started to develop as a food decontaminating technology, especially during the last decade, when technological advances have allowed the building of new plasma generators capable of working at atmospheric pressure and low flame temperatures. Plasma is regarded as the fourth state of matter. It consists of a mixture of neutral molecules, ionic species, and electrons forming a fluid-like haze, which is a rare state in mild environments like the earth. Actually, it only occurs naturally in the most distant atmospheric region when the wind from solar flares interacts with the earth's magnetic field, forming auroras.

Microbial destruction by cold plasma treatments is thought to be caused by interactions between cell membranes and radical species and UV light emitted due to gas excitation. These could also affect microbial DNA to a certain extent (Moisan et al. 2002). The technology is still experimental and knowledge about its effects on the nutritional and sensory characteristics of food products remains limited. Besides, plasma may be considered a fluid in terms of its flow behavior, which is a notable drawback when processing fluid products such as fruit and vegetable juices, since it would be rather challenging to apply it directly while guaranteeing a homogeneous treatment (Niemira and Gutsol 2011). Plasma has only been tested on the surfaces of inedible food components such as containers and packages or solid edible products such as sliced fruits and vegetables. Although it has shown some success in such cases, it is still a technology in a very early stage of study.

As far as irradiation is concerned, its use in fruit juice factories seems to be limited to packaging sterilization, despite its proven success on nearly all products on which it has been tested. However, the adverse implications of the term *radiation* do not allow the envisaging of a prosperous future for irradiation technology (Arvanitoyannis 2010). Irradiation acts by ionizing chemical components of matter, similarly to what has been described for UV radiation technology. Unlike this latter technology, though, irradiation treatments deliver far more energy. Consequently, a quicker effect can be expected, due to the massive damage caused to foodstuffs by direct radiation absorption and indirectly by chemically unstable species (Steward 2001). The foreseeable development of the technology is rather limited, since even taking for granted that residual radioactive compounds in the processed products are negligible due to the strict dosage control and rigorous security measures imposed by local governments and international institutions, a considerable initial investment is required, which does not help the establishment of this kind of facility.

Another nonthermal technology recently described for use in the fruit and vegetable juice industry is known as supercritical or dense phase processing. It consists of pressurizing carbon dioxide (CO_2) into foodstuffs. Carbon dioxide has an enhanced diffusivity in solids and liquids and a lipophilic character at supercritical conditions, which means above its critical values (31.1°C and 7.38 MPa) (García-González et al. 2007). These properties are suggested to be responsible for its effect on the reduction of microbial populations and spoilage enzyme activities, even though there is no consensus on the specific mechanisms. Until now, a reduction of the pH value, a precipitation of necessary cations as carbonates, and membrane rupture by the rapid expansion of carbon dioxide after pressure release are the possible explanations of the observed effects. This lack of information has not prevented the development of industrial devices for processing juices with apparently good results (Damar and Balaban 2011).

11.8 FINAL REMARKS

The majority of the technologies reviewed in this chapter share the property of submitting not only the unwanted components but the whole product to their effects. Hence, even assuming that the treatment is ideal—for example, that it is homogeneously applied to the whole production or batch—the response of each individual food component may be very specific depending on its own susceptibility and its particular local and temporal environment.

Moreover, it is assumed that the mechanisms that are the bases of these technologies are reproducible, even though only a few of them are already known and understood. In most cases, it is supposed that the extensions of their effects are also reproducible, although, due to the overwhelming complexity of the food matrices, this is quite difficult to evidence.

Consequently, research in nonthermal food processing should work to develop the necessary tools to produce this type of information to ensure that consumers' safety is not compromised. New materials, redesigned or rethought measuring sensors, mathematical models, or different analytical techniques are examples of the tools that may benefit the development of the nonthermal technologies in the food industry described here. These same tools should allow control of the processing stage when any of these technologies is eventually widely accepted for industrial use.

ACKNOWLEDGMENTS

The authors acknowledge the financial support of the Spanish Ministry of Economy and Competitiveness and the Spanish Institute of Agricultural and Food Research and Technology (INIA) through the projects AGL2010-21572 and RTA2010-00079-C02-02. Olga Martín-Belloso also acknowledges the ICREA Academia Award.

REFERENCES

Abdelmelek, H., R. Ben Aissa, A. Landoulsi, I. Maatouk, A. El May, and N. Ben Miloud. (2009). Effects of static magnetic field on cell growth, viability, and differential gene expression in *Salmonella*. *Foodborne Pathogens and Disease* 6(5): 547–552.

Aguiló-Aguayo, I., R. Soliva-Fortuny, and O. Martín-Belloso. (2009). Changes on viscosity and pectolytic enzymes of tomato and strawberry juices by high-intensity pulsed electric fields. *International Journal of Food Science and Technology* 44: 2268–2277.

Altunakar, B. and G.V. Barbosa-Cánovas. (2011). Engineering aspects of pulsed electric fields. In: H.Q. Zhang, G.V. Barbosa-Cánovas, V.M. Balasubramaniam, C. Patrick Dunne, D.F. Farkas, and J.T.C. Yuan (eds), *Nonthermal Processing Technologies for Food*, pp. 176–189. Chichester: Wiley-Blackwell and IFT Press.

Arvanitoyannis, I.S. (2010). *Irradiation of Food Commodities*: *Techniques, Applications, Detection, Legislation, Safety and Consumer Opinion.* London: Academic Press.

Atlantic Ultraviolet Corporation. (2012). Ster-L-Ray® ultraviolet germicidal lamps. http://www.ultraviolet.com/lamp/sterlray.htm (accessed May 2013).

Black, E.P., C.M. Stewart, and D.G. Hoover. (2011). Microbiological aspects of high-pressure food processing. In: H.Q. Zhang, G.V. Barbosa-Cánovas, V.M. Balasubramaniam, C. Patrick Dunne, D.F. Farkas, and J.T.C. Yuan (eds), *Nonthermal Processing Technologies for Food*, pp. 51–71. Chichester: Wiley-Blackwell and IFT Press.

Buzrul, S., H. Alpas, A. Lageteaua, and G. Demazeau. (2008). Inactivation of *Escherichia coli* and *Listeria innocua* in kiwifruit and pineapple juices by high hydrostatic pressure. *International Journal of Food Microbiology* 124(3): 275–287.

Caminiti, A.M., F. Noci, D.J. Morgan, D.A. Cronin, and J.G. Lyng. (2012). The effect of pulsed electric fields, ultraviolet light or high intensity light pulses in combination with manothermosonication on selected physico-chemical and sensory attributes of an orange and carrot juice blend. *Food and Bioproducts Processing* 90(C3): 442–448.

Castro, A.J., G.V. Barbosa-Cánovas, and B.G. Swanson. (1993). Microbial inactivation of foods by pulsed electric fields. *Journal of Food Processing and Preservation* 17: 47–73.

Chauvin, M.A. and B.G. Swanson. (2011). Biochemical aspects of high-pressure food processing. In: H.Q. Zhang, G.V. Barbosa-Cánovas, V.M. Balasubramaniam, C. Patrick Dunne, D.F. Farkas, and J.T.C. Yuan (eds), *Nonthermal Processing Technologies for Food*, pp. 72–87. Chichester: Wiley-Blackwell and IFT Press.

Cuvelier, M. and C. Berset. (2005). Phenolic compounds and plant extracts protect paprika against UV-induced discoloration. *International Journal of Food Science and Technology* 40: 67–73.

Damar, S. and M.O. Balaban. (2011). Effects of dense phase CO_2 on quality attributes of beverages. In: H.Q. Zhang, G.V. Barbosa-Cánovas, V.M. Balasubramaniam, C. Patrick Dunne, D.F. Farkas, and J.T.C. Yuan (eds), *Nonthermal Processing Technologies for Food*, pp. 324–358. Chichester: Wiley-Blackwell and IFT Press.

Demirci, A. and K. Krishnamurthy. (2011). Pulsed ultraviolet light. In: H.Q. Zhang, G.V. Barbosa-Cánovas, V.M. Balasubramaniam, C. Patrick Dunne, D.F. Farkas, and J.T.C. Yuan (eds), *Nonthermal Processing Technologies for Food*, pp. 249–261. Chichester: Wiley-Blackwell and IFT Press.

DIL (Deutsches Institut für Lebensmitteltechnik). (2013). Process technology. DIL http://www.dil-ev.de/en/leistungen/prozesstechnologie.html (accessed June 2013).

Diversified Technologies. (2009). Food and wastewater processing. Diversified Technologies http://www.divtecs.com/food-and-wastewater-processing/ (accessed June 2013).

Evrendilek, G.A., Q.H. Zhang, and E. Richter. (1999). Inactivation of *Escherichia coli* O157:H7 and *Escherichia coli* 8739 in apple juice by pulsed electric fields. *Journal of Food Protection* 62(7): 793–796.

Falguera, V., J. Pagán, S. Garza, A. Garvín, and A. Ibarz. (2011). Ultraviolet processing of liquid food: A review. Part 1: Fundamental engineering aspects. *Food Research International* 44(6): 1571–1579.

Falguera, V., S. Garza, J. Pagán, A. Garvín, and A. Ibarz. (2012). Effect of UV-Vis irradiation on enzymatic activities and physicochemical properties of four grape musts from different varieties. *Food and Bioprocess Technology* 5(1): 1–7.

Feng, H. and W. Yan. (2011). Ultrasonic processing. In: H.Q. Zhang, G.V. Barbosa-Cánovas, V.M. Balasubramaniam, C. Patrick Dunne, D.F. Farkas, and J.T.C. Yuan (eds), *Nonthermal Processing Technologies for Food*, pp. 135–154. Chichester: Wiley-Blackwell and IFT Press.

Ferrario, M., S.M. Alzamora, and S. Guerrero. (2013). Inactivation kinetics of some microorganisms in apple, melon, orange and strawberry juices by high intensity light pulses. *Journal of Food Engineering* 118(3): 302–311.

FDA (Food and Drug Administration). (2008). 21 CFR 179.41. Pulsed light for the treatment of food. FDA.

FDA (Food and Drug Administration). (2013). Kinetics of microbial inactivation for alternative food processing technologies—pulsed light technology. FDA http://www.fda.gov/Food/FoodScienceResearch/SafePracticesforFoodProcesses/ucm103058.htm (accessed May 20, 2013).

García-González, L., A.H. Geeraerd, S. Spilimbergo, K. Elst, and L. Van Ginneken. (2007). High pressure carbon dioxide inactivation of microorganisms in foods. *International Journal of Food Microbiology* 117: 1–28.

Gómez-López, V.M., L. Orsolani, A. Martínez-Yépez, and M.S. Tapia. (2010). Microbiological and sensory quality of sonicated calcium-added orange juice. *LWT—Food Science and Technology* 43(5): 808–813.

Gow-Chin, Y. and L. Hsin-Tang. (1996). Comparison of high pressure treatment and thermal pasteurization effects on the quality and shelf life of guava puree. *International Journal of Food Science and Technology* 31: 205–213.

Grigelmo-Miguel, N., R. Soliva-Fortuny, G.V. Barbosa-Cánovas, and O. Martín-Belloso. (2011). Use of oscillating magnetic fields in food preservation. In: H.Q. Zhang, G.V. Barbosa-Cánovas, V.M. Balasubramaniam, C. Patrick Dunne, D.F. Farkas, and J.T.C. Yuan (eds), *Nonthermal Processing Technologies for Food*, pp. 222–235. Chichester: Wiley-Blackwell and IFT Press.

Guerrero-Beltrán, J.A. and G.V. Barbosa-Cánovas. (2005). Reduction of *Saccharomyces cerevisiae*, *Escherichia coli* and *Listeria innocua* in apple juice by ultraviolet light. *Journal of Food Process Engineering* 28(5): 437–452.

Halgamuge, M.N., B.R.R. Perssont, L.G. Salford, P. Mendis, and J. Eberhardt. (2009). Comparison between two models for interactions between electric and magnetic fields and proteins in cell membranes. *Environmental Engineering Science* 26(10): 1473–1480.

Hofmann, G.A. (1985). Deactivation of microorganisms by an oscillating magnetic field. U.S. Patent 4,524,079.

Hughes, D.E. and W.L. Nyborg. (1962). Cell disruption by ultrasound. *Science* 38: 108s–114s.

Jaeger, H., N. Meneses, J. Moritz, and D. Knorr. (2010). Model for the differentiation of temperature and electric field effects during thermal assisted PEF processing. *Journal of Food Engineering* 100(1): 109–118.

Jolie, R.P., S. Christiaens, A. De Roeck, I. Fraeye, K. Houben, S. Van Buggenhout, A.M. Van Loey, and M.E. Hendrickx. (2012). Pectin conversions under high pressure: Implications for the structure-related quality characteristics of plant-based foods. *Trends in Food Science and Technology* 24(2): 103–118.

Kim, M. and H.Q. Zhang. (2011). Improving electrode durability of PEF chamber by selecting suitable material. In: H.Q. Zhang, G.V. Barbosa-Cánovas, V.M. Balasubramaniam, C. Patrick Dunne, D.F. Farkas, and J.T.C. Yuan (eds), *Nothermal Processing Technologies for Food*, pp. 201–211. Chichester: Wiley-Blackwell and IFT Press.

Kingsley, D.H., D.G. Hoover, E. Papafragkou, and G.P. Richards. (2002). Inactivation of hepatitis A virus and a calicivirus by high hydrostatic pressure. *Journal of Food Protection* 65: 1605–1609.

Kohno, M., M. Yamazaki, I. Kimura, and M. Wada. (2000). Effect of static magnetic fields on bacteria: *Streptococcus mutans*, *Staphylococcus aureus*, and *Escherichia coli*. *Pathophysiology* 7(2): 143–148.

Koutchma, T. (2000). Advances in ultraviolet light technology for non-thermal processing of liquid foods. *Food and Bioprocess Technology* 2(2): 138–155.

Ludwig, H. and C. Schreck. (1997). The inactivation of vegetative bacteria by pressure. In: K. Heremans (ed.), *High Pressure Research in the Bioscience and Biotechnology*, pp. 221–224. Leuven: Leuven University Press.

Ma, H., L. Huang, and C. Zhu. (2011). The effect of pulsed magnetic fields on horseradish peroxidase. *Journal of Food Process Engineering* 34(5): 1609–1622.

MacGregor, S.J., J.G. Anderson, R.A. Fouracre, O. Farish, L. McIlvaney, and N.J. Rowan. (1998). Light inactivation of food-related pathogenic bacteria using a pulsed power source. *Letters in Applied Microbiology* 27: 67–70.

Marsellés-Fontanet, A.R. and O. Martín-Belloso. (2007). Optimization and validation of HIPEF processing conditions to inactivate oxidative enzymes of grape juice. *Journal of Food Engineering* 83: 452–462.

Martín-Belloso, O. and R. Soliva-Fortuny. (2011). Pulsed electric fields processing basics. In: H.Q. Zhang, G.V. Barbosa-Cánovas, V.M. Balasubramaniam, C. Patrick Dunne, D.F. Farkas, and J.T.C. Yuan (eds), *Nonthermal Processing Technologies for Food*, pp. 157–175. Chichester: Wiley-Blackwell and IFT Press.

Matsumura, Y. and H.N. Ananthaswamy. (2002). Short-term and long-term cellular and molecular events following UV irradiation of skin: Implications for molecular medicine. *Expert Reviews in Molecular Medicine* 4(26): 1–22.

Meneses, N., H. Jaeger, and D. Knorr. (2011). Minimization of thermal impact by application of electrode cooling in a co-linear PEF treatment chamber. *Journal of Food Science* 76(8): E536–E543.

Mensitieri, G., G. Scherillo, and S. Iannace. (2013). Flexible packaging structures for high pressure treatments. *Innovative Food Science and Emerging Technologies* 7: 12–21.

Moisan, M., J. Barbeau, M. Crevier, J. Pelletier, N. Phillip, and B. Saoudi. (2002). Plasma sterilization. Methods and mechanisms. *Pure and Applied Chemistry* 74: 349–358.

Molina-Hoppner, A., V. Doster, R.F. Vogel, and M.C. Ganzle. (2004). Protective effect of sucrose and sodium chloride for *Lactococcus lactis* during sublethal and lethal high-pressure treatments. *Applied and Environmental Microbiology* 70(4): 2013–2020.

Mosqueda-Melgar, J., R.M. Raybaudi-Massilia, and O. Martín-Belloso. (2007). Influence of treatment time and pulse frequency on *Salmonella enteritidis*, *Escherichia coli* and *Listeria monocytogenes* populations inoculated in melon and watermelon juices treated by pulsed electric fields. *International Journal of Food Microbiology* 117(2): 192–200.

NASA Science Mission Directorate. (2011). Tour of the electromagnetic spectrum. NASA Science Mission Directorate. March 23, 2011. http://missionscience.nasa.gov/ems/index.html (accessed May 2013).

Niemira, B.A. and A. Gutsol. (2011). Nonthermal plasma as a novel food processing technology. In: H.Q. Zhang, G.V. Barbosa-Cánovas, V.M. Balasubramaniam, C. Patrick Dunne, D.F. Farkas, and J.T.C. Yuan (eds), *Nonthermal Processing for Food*, pp. 271–288. Chichester: Wiley-Blackwell and IFT Press.

Ohshima, T., T. Tamura, and M. Sato. (2007). Influence of pulsed electric field on various enzyme activities. *Journal of Electrostatics* 65(3): 156–161.

Oms-Oliu, G., O. Martín-Belloso, and R. Soliva-Fortuny. (2010). Pulsed light treatments for food preservation: A review. *Food and Bioprocess Technology* 3(1): 13–23.

Oms-Oliu, G., I. Odriozola-Serrano, R. Soliva-Fortuny, P. Elez-Martínez, and O. Martín-Belloso. (2012). Stability of health-related compounds in plant foods through the application of non thermal processes. *Trends in Food Science and Technology* 23(2): 111–123.

Palgan, I., I.M. Caminiti, A. Muñoz, F. Noci, P. Whyte, D.J. Morgan, D.A. Cronin, and J.G. Lyng. (2011). Combined effect of selected non-thermal technologies on *Escherichia coli* and *Pichia fermentans* inactivation in an apple and cranberry juice blend and on product shelf life. *International Journal of Food Microbiology* 151(1): 1–6.

Parish, M.E. (1998). Orange juice quality after treatment by thermal pasteurization or isostatic high pressure. *LWT—Food Science and Technology* 31(5): 439–442.

Pataro, G., A. Muñoz, I. Palgan, F. Noci, G. Ferraria, and J.G. Lyng. (2011). Bacterial inactivation in fruit juices using a continuous flow pulsed light (PL) system. *Food Research International* 44(6): 1642–1648.

Ramaswamy, H.S., E. Riahi, and E. Idziak. (2003). High-pressure destruction kinetics of *E. coli* (29055) in apple juice. *Journal of Food Science* 68(5): 1750–1756.

Rendueles, E., M.K. Omer, O. Alvseike, C. Alonso-Calleja, R. Capita, and M. Prieto. (2011). Microbiological food safety assessment of high hydrostatic pressure processing: A review. *LWT—Food Science and Technology* 44(5): 1251–1260.

Sánchez-Moreno, C., B. De Ancos, L. Plaza, P. Elez-Martínez, and M.P. Cano. (2009). Nutritional approaches and health-related properties of plant foods processed by high pressure and pulsed electric fields. *Critical Reviews on Food Science and Nutrition* 49(6): 552–576.

Shama, G. (1999). Ultraviolet light. In: R.K. Robinson, C. Batt, and P. Patel (eds), *Encyclopedia of Food Microbiology*, pp. 2208–2214. London: Academic Press.

Shamsudina, R., C.S. Linga, N.M. Adzahanb, and W.R.W. Daud. (2013). Rheological properties of ultraviolet-irradiated and thermally pasteurized Yankee pineapple juice. *Journal of Food Engineering* 116(2): 548–553.

Steward, E. (2001). Food irradiation chemistry. In: R. Molins (ed.), *Food Irradiation: Principles and Applications*, pp. 37–76. New York: Wiley.

Toepfl, S. and V. Heinz. (2011). Pulsed electric field assisted extraction: A case study. In: H.Q. Zhang, G.V. Barbosa-Cánovas, V.M. Balasubramaniam, C. Patrick Dunne, D.F. Farkas, and J.T.C. Yuan (eds), *Nonthermal Processing Technologies for Food*, pp. 191–200. Chichester: Wiley-Blackwell and IFT Press.

Tonello, C. (2011). Case studies on high-pressure processing of foods. In: H.Q. Zhang, G.V. Barbosa-Cánovas, V.M. Balasubramaniam, C. Patrick Dunne, D.F. Farkas, and J.T.C. Yuan (eds), *Nonthermal Processing Technologies for Food*, pp. 36–50. Chichester: Wiley-Blackwell and IFT Press.

Valero, M., N. Recrosio, D. Saura, N. Muñoz, N. Martí, and V. Lizama. (2007). Effects of ultrasonic treatments in orange juice processing. *Journal of Food Engineering* 80(2): 509–516.

Van der Plancken, I., L. Verbeyst, K. De Vleeschouwer, T. Grauwet, R.L. Heiniö, F.A. Husband, M. Lille, et al. (2012). (Bio)chemical reactions during high pressure/high temperature processing affect safety and quality of plant-based foods. *Trends in Food Science and Technology* 23(1): 28–38.

Wardle, B. (2009). *Principles and Applications of Photochemistry.* Chichester: Wiley.

Weiss, J., I. Gulseren, and G. Kjartansson. (2011). Physicochemical effects of high intensity ultrasonication on food proteins and carbohydrates. In: H.Q. Zhang, G.V. Barbosa-Cánovas, V.M. Balasubramaniam, C. Patrick Dunne, D.F. Farkas, and J.T.C. Yuan (eds), *Nonthermal Processing Technologies for Food*, pp. 109–133. Chichester: Wiley-Blackwell and IFT Press.

WHO (World Health Organization). (2013). Ultraviolet radiation and the INTERSUN Programme. WHO. http://www.who.int/uv/en/index.html (accessed May 2013).

Wright, J.R., S.S. Summer, C.R. Hackney, M.D. Pierson, and B.W. Zoecklein. (2000). Efficacy of ultraviolet light for reducing *Escherichia coli* O157:H7 in unpasteurized apple cider. *Journal of Food Protection* 63(5): 563–567.

Yang, R.J., S.Q. Li, and Q.H. Zhang. (2004). Effects of pulsed electric fields on the activity of enzymes in aqueous solution. *Journal of Food Science* 69(4): FCT241–FCT248.

Zenker, M., V. Heinz, and D. Knorr. (2003). Application of ultrasound-assisted thermal processing for preservation and quality retention of liquid foods. *Journal of Food Protection* 66(9): 1642–1649.

Zhong, K., X. Hu, G. Zhao, F. Chen, and X. Liao. (2005). Inactivation and conformational change of horseradish peroxidase induced by pulsed electric fields. *Food Chemistry* 92: 473–479.

Zimmermann, U. (1986). Electrical breakdown, electropermeabilization and electrofusion. *Reviews in Physiology Biochemistry and Pharmacology* 105: 175–256.

12 Pressure Treatments in Juice Processing

Homogenization Pressures Applied to Mandarin and Blueberry Juices

*Juan Manuel Castagnini, Ester Betoret,
Noelia Betoret, and Pedro Fito-Maupoey*

CONTENTS

12.1 Origin and Evolution of Pressure Treatments Applied to Food
Processing 238
12.2 Types of Pressure Treatments: Mode of Action and Variables Affected 238
12.2.1 Static Pressure Treatments 239
12.2.2 Dynamic Pressure Treatments 241
12.3 Pressure Effects on Microorganism Content 242
12.4 Pressure Effects on Enzyme Inactivation 244
12.5 Pressure Effects on Bioactive Compounds 247
12.5.1 Effect of Pressure Processing on Bioactive Compounds of Juices
When Compared with Fresh Juices, Thermally Treated Juices,
and Juices Treated by Other Techniques 247
12.5.2 Effect of Pressure Processing on Bioactive Compounds of Juices
and Their Storage Stability 249
12.5.3 Effect of Pressure Processing on Bioactive Compounds of Juices
and Their *In Vitro* and *In Vivo* Bioaccessibility 250
12.6 Case Studies 252
12.6.1 Low Homogenization Pressure Applied to Enhance Functional
Properties of Mandarin Juice 252
12.6.2 High Homogenization Pressure Applied to Enhance Functional
Properties of Blueberry Juice 254
References 255

12.1   ORIGIN AND EVOLUTION OF PRESSURE TREATMENTS APPLIED TO FOOD PROCESSING

The development of pressure treatment as a tool in the food industry has emerged recently. As well described by Rivalain et al. (2010), high-pressure treatment to kill bacteria such as *Escherichia coli* and *Staphylococcus aureus* was first studied by Roger (1895). Hite et al. (1914) applied hydrostatic pressure for the inactivation of some micro-organisms in order to preserve fruits and vegetables. Between 1932 and 1956, James and Jacques Basset in collaboration with others (Basset and Macheboeuf 1932; Macheboeuf and Basset 1934; Basset et al. 1956) studied high-pressure effects in order to inactivate different microorganisms in food processing development and biological applications. During the last 50 years, an increase in the interest of researchers in studying biology at high pressure has allowed the introduction of a large range of applications, increasing the number of those related to food processing. Over the 1960s and 1970s, the research focused on pressure effects on microorganisms in raw milks (Timson and Short 1965), on the sterilization of low-acidic foods using pressure and pasteurization temperatures (Wilson 1974), and on the use of pressure for the long-term refrigerated storage of foods (Charm et al. 1977). During the 1980s, research involving high pressure and food processing had evolved into high-pressure effects on enzymes (Morild 1981) and on proteins and other biomolecules (Heremans 1982), into the biological effects of high hydrostatic pressure (HHP) on food microorganisms (Hoover et al. 1989), and into the applications of high-pressure homogenization (HPH) for food preservation (Popper and Knorr 1990).

Intense efforts to set up new food processes were conducted in Japan in particular (Hayashi 1989, 1990; Horie et al. 1991; Ogawa et al. 1990; Tanaka and Hatanaka 1992), and the first food product stabilized under high pressure reached the Japanese market in 1993. Over the last 15 years, high-pressure technology in food processing has steadily increased. Several such products are now available on the market in different countries: fruit juices, jam, tofu, ham, shellfish, and biopolymers (such as proteins or starches) (Rivalain et al. 2010).

It is possible to classify food pressure applications into three main areas:

1. Microbial inactivation
2. Enzyme inactivation
3. Effects on bioactive components and functional applications

Thus, it can be observed that the trend of the research articles published between 2000 and now has changed considerably. In 2000, the main articles published concerning pressure effects on food products related to enzyme inactivation followed by microbial inactivation. However, by 2012, this topic had been replaced by those related to functional applications (Figures 12.1 and 12.2).

12.2   TYPES OF PRESSURE TREATMENTS: MODE OF ACTION AND VARIABLES AFFECTED

Two types of pressure treatments can be applied to food products: static and dynamic. Depending on the different treatment principles, certain phenomena and generated

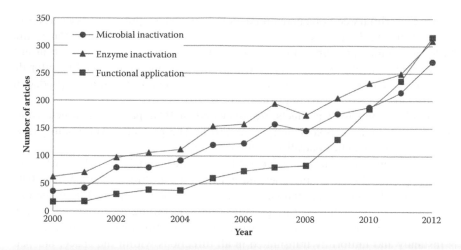

FIGURE 12.1 Tendency of research articles related to pressure effects and food applications over the years. (From www.sciencedirect.com. With permission.)

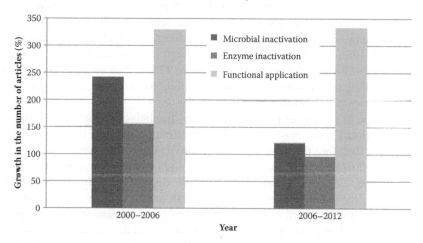

FIGURE 12.2 Growth in the number of articles over the years. Growth expressed as the percentage difference in articles in the final and initial years divided by the number of articles existing in the initial year.

$$\text{Growth} = \frac{(\text{articles in the final year-articles in the initial year})}{\text{articles in the initial year}} \times 100$$

forces occur and explain the changes to the physicochemical and functional properties and the safety of the particular food product.

12.2.1 STATIC PRESSURE TREATMENTS

Static pressures are applied in treatments where a constant pressure value is maintained during a period of time. This technology is called high-pressure processing

(HPP). The primary equipment required for HPP includes a pressure vessel, a closure mechanism to seal the vessel, a device to hold the closure mechanism in place while the vessel is under pressure, a high-pressure intensifier pump, the pressure-transmitting medium (usually water in the food area), a system to control and monitor the pressure and temperature, and a product-handling system to transfer the product to and from the pressure vessel (da Cruz et al. 2010).

Liquid or solid food products are processed in their packaging which avoids microbial recontamination (Dumay et al. 2010). The pressure level, holding time, and temperature can be controlled within the process.

Two principles explain the effects of this treatment: firstly, Le Chatelier's principle, according to which any phenomenon (phase transition, chemical reactivity, change in molecular configuration, chemical reaction) accompanied by a decrease in volume will be augmented by pressure. Also, according to Arrhenius' law, an increase in temperature results in an increase of the reaction rate. Secondly, pressure is instantly and uniformly transmitted in all directions within the space, independent of the size and the geometry of the food. This is known as isostatic pressure. Pressure induces some compression of aqueous samples, but there is no shearing effect, because the sample is not subjected to a flow or biomolecule covalent bond compression at the pressure levels applied in the food area, due to the low energy resulting from pressure (Dumay et al. 2013). Federighi et al. (1995) explain the susceptibility of different chemical interactions to high-pressure treatments by defining a $\Delta V_{dissociation}$ (milliliters per mole) related to the Gibbs free energy. The pressure effect on covalent interactions tends to stabilization, in contrast to the destabilization effect on hydrophobic interactions.

From the point of view of protein stability, hydrophobic interactions are those of weak interactions, stabilizing the protein conformation that has the most negative ΔV value and therefore the most pressure sensitive. These interactions play a major role in the stabilization of the tertiary structure and in protein–protein interactions.

The stability of proteins under high pressure depends mainly on their conformational stability to compensate the loss of weak interactions, but also on the size of the cavities within which water molecules can penetrate and modify the hydration degree (Rivalain et al. 2010). This modification can be explained by two main effects. First, the opening up of the cavities allows a solvent to occupy an internal volume that was previously excluded from interactions with this solvent. Second, the surface area in contact with the solvent is larger for unfolded proteins than for native ones (Smeller 2002; Heremans 2005; Royer 2005; Winter and Dzwolak 2005; Silva and Foguel 2009).

Another effect induced by the pressure applied is an increase in the temperature of the product. Indeed, adiabatic compression of water increases the temperature by about 3°C/100 MPa (Knorr 1999).

As a consequence, the mode of action of HPP depends on the food system and the pressure level (Figure 12.3). In the case of microorganisms, cellular death is caused by coupled effects induced by high-pressure treatments. The effect of pressure starts at pressures that can influence gene expression and protein synthesis (between 30 and 50 MPa); at pressures around 100 MPa the nuclear membrane of yeasts is affected, and at more than 400–600 MPa further alteration occurs in the

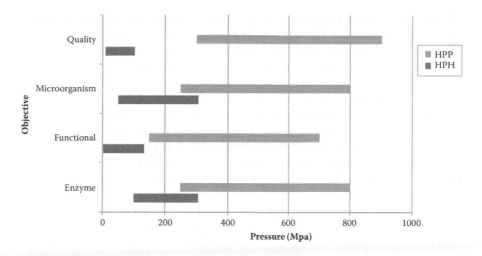

FIGURE 12.3 Types of pressure treatments most applied in juice industry. Pressure levels and objectives. Quality: improvement or modification of physical or sensory properties. Microorganism: inactivation or disruption of microorganism cells. Functional: improvement of probiotic characteristics or enhancement of functional properties. Enzyme: inactivation of enzymes.

mitochondria and the cytoplasm. A perturbation of the bacterial membrane and a decrease of intracellular pH is almost always involved during pressure treatment (Smelt 1998).

High-pressure treatments may also have beneficial effects on probiotics and the digestibility of food products. For example, in the dairy industry, high-pressure treatments can increase the compression of the food matrix, helping to protect probiotic bacteria along their pathway through the human body; the treatments minimize the loss of probiotic bacteria during whey removal and increase sensory performance because of the growth of the probiotic bacteria and their role in secondary proteolysis (da Cruz et al. 2010). Also, it is often proposed that partial proteolysis of food products, in particular milk proteins, under high pressure increases their digestibility and reduces their allergenicity (Chicón et al. 2008; Masson et al. 2001; Zeece et al. 2008).

12.2.2 Dynamic Pressure Treatments

Dynamic pressures concern high pressures developed over a short length of time, applied to liquids, and usually associated with an increase of temperature as a secondary effect. Depending on the pressure level applied, the technology is called standard homogenization (20–60 MPa) or high-pressure homogenization (HPH: up to 150–400 MPa). Essentially, HPH equipment consists of a positive displacement pump and a homogenizing valve. The liquid is brought to high pressure in a unit called a pressure intensifier and is then forced through the valve gap of a few micrometers in width.

In the case of HPH, the pressure drop (ΔP) generates intense mechanical forces and elongational stress in laminar flow at the valve entrance and in the valve gap, and turbulence, cavitation, and impacts with solid surfaces at the gap outlet. During the passage of the liquid through the homogenizer, a short-term heating phenomenon occurs. Firstly, the fluid temperature increases with the homogenization pressure by 2°C–3°C/100 MPa due to the heat of compression generated in the pressure intensifier. Then, when the pressurized fluid is forced through the high-pressure valve, its velocity is increased due to the pipe-size reduction accompanied by the pressure drop (ΔP). The fluid temperature measured immediately at the high-pressure valve outlet increases linearly with the homogenization pressure by 14°C–18°C/100 MPa, due to shear effects and partial conversion of mechanical energy into heat. A total jump in temperature by 17°C–21°C/100 MPa was therefore measured when processing whole milk or oil/water emulsions processed at an initial temperature of 4°C–24°C (Cortés-Muñoz et al. 2009; Picart et al. 2006; Thiebaud et al. 2003).

HPH is a continuous method applied to liquid products. The major parameters determining its efficiency are operating pressure, number of passes through the valve, temperature, and homogenizer valve design (Moore et al. 1990; Stang et al. 2001), while the scale of operation does not appear to influence the extent of homogenization (Siddiqi et al. 1997).

Microorganisms may be considered as microparticles that can be ruptured by shearing effects in combination with a jump in temperature (Dumay et al. 2013). Indeed, high pressure and velocity gradients, shear stresses, turbulence, shocks, and cavitation phenomena occurring through the high-pressure valve may induce mechanical disruption, or at least cause alteration of cell membranes (Middelberg 1995; Gogate and Pandit 2008; Kleinig and Middelberg 1998). The efficiency of HPH for microorganism inactivation was found to increase with the pressure level, the extent of the recycling through the homogenizer, and the temperature of the inlet fluid (Thiebaud et al. 2003; Picart et al. 2006; Donsì et al. 2009; Maresca et al. 2011). The food matrix (water, fat content, pH, viscosity) and the type of microorganism (Gram-positive bacteria showed a higher resistance) also influenced the degree of inactivation by HPH. Enzyme inactivation may result from protein unfolding followed by aggregation (Dumay et al. 2013). The combination of mechanical forces as pressure increases and drops, high-velocity gradients, shearing effects, and short-term temperature jumps induces protein structural changes at pressures above 200 MPa (Dumay et al. 2013). From the point of view of functional compounds, the specific assemblies produced by HPH (submicron emulsion, modified assemblies of phosphocaseins) are potentially suitable to trap and protect bioactive components that are poorly water soluble from unfavorable environmental conditions during processing until consumption and digestion (Dumay et al. 2013).

12.3   PRESSURE EFFECTS ON MICROORGANISM CONTENT

The food industry continues to be interested in the use of minimal processing and nonthermal technologies as a way of meeting consumer demand to extend shelf life, without the need for chemical preservatives and without compromising the wholesomeness and safety of foods (McKay et al. 2011). The retention of fresh-like characteristics, nutritional quality and safety are particularly important in certain foods such as fruit juices, and can be used in the marketing strategy for premium added-value products.

High-pressure treatment is a proven method for the inactivation of different kinds of microorganisms which may be present in fruit juices (Brinez et al. 2006; Campos and Cristianini 2007; McKay 2009; Tahiri et al. 2006). Its application in the food industry has been widely studied since the development of HPH and HHP technology in the 1980s.

The advances in the field of HPH in the inactivation of microorganisms in food applications have been studied, analyzed and reviewed over the years in various books and articles. Donsì et al. (2009) refer to specific applications for the treatment of a wide range of microorganisms in liquid substrates, as well as the role of the main physical and operating parameters regulating microbial inactivation and the different hypotheses about the mechanisms of inactivation. Also, Diels and Michiels (2006) describe different approaches for modeling cell disruption/inactivation, factors affecting microbial inactivation as process parameters (pressure, temperature, number of passes, and type of equipment), microbial physiological parameters (type of microorganism [bacteria, yeast, spores, viruses], cell concentration, and growth phase of microorganism), and the characteristics of fluids that affect high-pressure inactivation (viscosity, additives, and liquid matrix).

HHP is one of the most promising nonthermal treatment methods. This technology is already used commercially around the world for a variety of foods, including cooked meats, shellfish, fruit and vegetable juices, sauces, and dips (Norton and Sun 2008; Sampedro et al. 2010; Gassiot and Masoliver 2010); and in 2001, the European Commission authorized the sale of fruit juice pasteurized by high pressure (Commission of the European Communities 2001). Fruit juices are normally treated at 400 MPa or greater for a few minutes at 20°C or below. This is sufficient to significantly reduce the numbers of spoilage microorganisms, such as yeasts, molds, and lactic acid bacteria, and extend refrigerated shelf life to more than 30 days (Patterson 2005). In the scientific field, various reviews have collated the research and the advances over the years. The improvements are related to the understanding of HHP on microorganism inactivation and how different process parameters, such as degree of pressure, temperature, and time, are implied in cell death. The multiplicity of damage accumulated in different parts of the cell due to changes in proteins, cell membrane permeability, ribosome, protein synthesis, and enzyme activity is responsible for microorganism inactivation. The type of microorganism, the composition of the cell wall, the cell membrane unsaturated fatty acids composition, and the growth phase of the microorganism also influence the degree of inactivation reached by HHP treatment.

The high-pressure treatment of juices is a wide field of research where several authors have studied different juices: mandarin (Carreño et al. 2011); orange (Tahiri et al. 2006; Maresca et al. 2011; Erkmen, 2011; Belloch et al. 2012; Velázquez-Estrada et al. 2012); apple (Bevilacqua et al. 2012; McKay 2009, 2011; Pathanibul et al. 2009; Suárez-Jacobo et al. 2012); apricot (Patrignani et al. 2009, 2010, 2013); cashew apple (Lavinas et al. 2008); grapefruit (Uckoo et al. 2013); pineapple (Maresca et al. 2011); pomegranate (Varela-Santos et al. 2012); carrot (Pathanibul et al. 2009; Patrignani et al. 2009, 2010; Patterson et al. 2012); and tomato (Dede et al. 2007; Daryaei and

Balasubramaniam 2013), among others. In addition, the inactivation of various bacteria has been studied (*E. coli, Listeria innocua, Lactobacillus plantarum, Frateuria aurantia, Salmonella typhimurium*), yeasts (*Saccharomyces bayanus, S. cerevisiae*), and bacterial spores (*Bacillus* spp., *Clostridia* spp). Currently, investigations are related to the use of combined factors that are characteristic of the operations: for example, the HPH effect on the microbial disruption may be powered by modification of the outlet temperature and the retention time at that temperature after homogenization (Belloch et al. 2012); the number of homogenization passes also has an effect on the microbial inactivation (Tahiri et al. 2006). In the case of HHP, the exposure time, the temperature of treatment, and the adiabatic heating (2.5°C/100 MPa) (McKay et al. 2011) have consequences for microbial inactivation.

In addition, the combination of high-pressure treatment with other operations and the combination of high pressure with antimicrobial compounds have been studied, such as citral and HPH on apricot juice (Patrignani et al. 2013), nisin and HPH on apple and carrot juices (Pathanibul et al. 2009), or high carbon dioxide pressure and HHP on carrot juice (Park et al. 2002).

The comparison of resistance of different bacteria to HPH (100–300 MPa) and HHP (200–400 MPa) showed significant differences between the two techniques in terms of resistance and the inactivation mechanisms involved (Wuytack et al. 2002). According to Wuytack et al. (2002), there are large differences in terms of resistance to HHP, but not to HPH. Also, within the group of Gram-negative bacteria, a different arrangement exists with regard to resistance to HPH as opposed to HHP. For example, they found that *Yersinia enterocolitica* is very resistant to HPH while it is very sensitive to HHP. Another example is *E. coli* mutant LMM1010, which is much more resistant to HHP than its parental strain, but equally resistant to HPH. Finally, as other authors found (Hauben et al. 1996; García-Graells et al. 1998; Kalchayanand et al. 1994, 1998; Ritz et al. 2001), HPH does not cause sublethal injury, in contrast to HHP (Wuytack et al. 2002).

Different microorganisms can be used to compare different inactivation treatments. *L. plantarum* has been used by several authors to study the impact of thermal treatment, as well as nonthermal technologies such as pulsed electric fields (PEF), HPP, and HPH, in acidic products such as orange juice, orange–carrot juice, and orange juice–milk beverage. The Weibull distribution function-based model is the most widely applied distribution to explain microorganism inactivation kinetics after nonthermal processing. Applying Weibullian equations, different thermal and nonthermal treatments can be compared (Carreño et al. 2011).

12.4 PRESSURE EFFECTS ON ENZYME INACTIVATION

Enzymes related to food quality (pectin methylesterase [PME], peroxidase [POD], PG, polyphenol oxidase PPO, pectate lyase) can be deactivated by pressure (Seyderhelm et al. 1996). The pressure required depends on the enzyme: some enzymes may be deactivated at room temperature by a few hundred megapascals, while others can withstand thousands of megapascals (Macheboeuf and Basset 1934; Heinisch et al. 1995; Cano et al. 1997). In a few cases, enzymes may be activated due to pressure treatment (Cano et al. 1997; Cheftel 1995).

In terms of HPP, enzyme inactivation is related to the effect of high pressure on the protein structure. The biological activity of an enzyme arises from an active site and through a three-dimensional configuration of the molecule (Hendrickx et al. 1998). Small changes in the active site can lead to a loss of enzyme activity (Tsou 1986). The functionality of an enzyme can be changed due to conformational changes associated with protein denaturation.

Enzyme inactivation by HPH is principally related to the inherent increase of temperature due to the passing of the fluid through the valve gap, producing protein unfolding followed by aggregation and, in consequence, loss of activity. The HPH-induced effect depends significantly on processing parameters (homogenization pressure level, inlet temperature, time of processed fluid at outlet temperature level), sensitivity of the enzyme under study to high pressure, shear, temperature, and the matrix environment (Dumay et al. 2013).

The pressure range within which enzyme inactivation occurs is strongly dependent on the type of enzyme, pH, medium composition, temperature, and the addition of salts, sugars, or other compounds (Cheftel 1991; Balny and Masson 1993; Hendrickx et al. 1998).

Enzyme activation can be explained in terms of pressure-induced decompartmentalization (Butz et al. 1994; Gomes and Ledward 1996). In intact tissues, enzymes and substrates are often separated into compartments, which can be destroyed upon application of low pressure (Jolibert et al. 1994; Butz et al. 1994). Pressure-induced membrane damage and the resulting leakage of enzymes and substrates result in enzyme–substrate contact. The enzymatic reaction resulting from this contact can, in turn, be accelerated or decelerated by pressure, depending on the reaction volume of the enzyme-catalyzed reaction (Morild 1981).

PME is an enzyme that is responsible for cloud destabilization of juices, gelation of concentrates, and loss of consistency in juice products. Because of its technological relevance in fruit juice processing and its thermal stability, PME is used as the standard when evaluating pressure effects on enzyme inactivation in fruit juices. In this sense, the effect of high pressure may be twofold: stability (through protein denaturation) as well as catalytic activity can be affected, depending on the pressure level involved (Aertsen et al. 2009; Balny 2004; Cheftel 1992; Knorr et al. 2006). Comparatively low pressures (around 100 MPa) have been shown to activate some enzymes (Asaka et al. 1994; Curl and Jansen 1950; Jolibert et al. 1994). This stimulation effect is, however, only observed for monomeric enzymes.

Since the pioneering study by Ogawa et al. (1990), numerous studies on the pressure stability of PME, including detailed kinetic studies, have been performed. Irreversible inactivation of a wide range of PMEs (e.g., citrus fruit, tomato, apple, carrot, strawberry, banana, plum, and bell pepper) has been investigated, in model systems and in real food matrices (recently reviewed by Duvetter et al. [2009]). Generally speaking, PME can be regarded as a rather barotolerant enzyme (>600 MPa at room temperature). However, considerable variation in pressure stability exists between PMEs from various sources, ranging from moderately pressure sensitive (e.g., orange and carrot PME) (Balogh et al. 2004; Goodner et al. 1998; Nienaber and Shellhammer 2001b; Polydera et al. 2004; Van den Broeck et al. 2000; Vervoort et al. 2011) to extremely pressure stable (e.g., tomato PME, strawberry PME, and fungal *Aspergillus aculeatus* PME) (Crelier et al. 2001; Dirix et al. 2005; Fachin et al. 2002; Ly Nguyen et al. 2002). Researchers have shown that HHP treatments below 400 MPa have little effect on the activity of PME in orange juice (Cano et al. 1997; Basak and Ramaswamy 1996; Nienaber and Shellhammer 2001a).

Lacroix et al. (2005) suggest that at comparable pressure (170–200 MPa), HHP would be more effective than HPH at inactivating PME in orange juice. The involvement of physical forces in HPH treatment does not thus appear to compensate for its comparatively short exposure time. This should not be overlooked; however, the HPH treatment produced relatively stable suspensions despite the higher residual enzyme activity. Modification or breakdown of the pectin structure may have occurred as a result of mechanical forces present in homogenization, making the pectin less accessible to the enzyme (Lacroix et al. 2005). On the other hand, HPH could have additional advantages in terms of juice quality. Lacroix et al. (2005) found that prewarmed (50°C during 10 min) orange juice treated by HPH improves its flavor. This suggests that homogenization increases cell and organelle destruction, liberating additional flavoring substances into the medium and thereby improving the scores obtained for freshness and texture (Lacroix et al. 2005).

Different authors have evaluated the effect of high pressure on different enzymes and food products. Krebbers and Matser (2003) found that HPP at ambient temperature caused an approximate decrease of 70% in PG activity. However, increasing the pressure from 300 to 700 MPa had no significant additional effect, demonstrating the pressure resistance of PG. In apricot nectars, Huang et al. (2013) found that PPO and POD were activated after HPP treatment at all pressure levels (300–500 MPa for 5–20 min). Similar results were reported by Rovere et al. (1994) in apricot puree; Bayındırlı et al. (2006) obtained a significant initial enhancement of PPO activity after treating apple juice at 450 MPa at 25°C. In banana juice, a complete inactivation of pectate lyase was obtained at a pressure level greater than 200 MPa ($T_{in} = 4$°C; $T_{out} > 55$°C) (Calligaris et al. 2012). Finally, according to Cano et al. (1997), in strawberry puree, POD was increasingly inactivated up to 300 MPa for treatments at 20°C for 15 min. Above 300 MPa, POD activity was slightly increased. Above 45°C, a decrease in activity was found for all pressures (50–400 MPa). At room temperature, the activity of orange POD decreased up to 400 MPa (processing time 15 min). The highest inactivation rate (50%) was found at 32°C.

Combined treatments may enhance the effects of nonthermal processing and reduce the severity of nonthermal treatment needed to obtain a given level of enzyme inactivation. Thus, the processing conditions required are generally less severe than those used for either treatment alone.

Thus, the only occasion that HPH did not affect the activity and stability of β-galactosidase was when the process was carried out at neutral pH; for the other conditions, HPH resulted in partial inactivation of the enzyme.

Corwin and Shellhammer (2002) and Boff et al. (2003) found a synergistic effect of combined HHP and CO_2 treatments in the inactivation of PME, and that enzyme activity decreased with increasing pressure. Hu et al. (2013) reviewed the effect of different pressure levels in combination (or not) with CO_2 on different enzymes in orange and carrot juices.

12.5 PRESSURE EFFECTS ON BIOACTIVE COMPOUNDS

The nutritional quality of processed foods is of great interest to the consumer and food processing industry due to its direct and indirect impact on consumer health (Buckow et al. 2010). As consumers demand minimally processed and fresh food products, the application of nonthermal techniques is gaining popularity (Cao et al. 2012). Furthermore, consumers are increasingly more aware of the influence of food on their health. Thus, the presence of natural or enriched foods high in bioactive compounds adds value to producers who see the permanence of these products in the market. Several commercial juices, that is, mandarin, grapefruit, apple, orange, and carrot juices, and broccoli–apple juice mixture treated by pressure are currently available on the market (Buzrul et al. 2008; Barba et al. 2013). The changes produced in food compounds by pressure treatments assist in the knowledge of how these modifications affect the nutritional quality, bioavailability, or stability of bioactive compounds. In addition, evaluating the influence of process variables on the stability of bioactive compounds, as well as antioxidant activity and physicochemical parameters of juices, is a key factor in defining treatment conditions to avoid the loss of these important properties of foods and to obtain a food beverage with high benefits for the consumer's health (Barba et al. 2013).

Intense efforts to elucidate the effects of pressure treatments on bioactive compounds of fruit and vegetable juices are being made. The number of research papers related to these effects are increasing steadily. Essentially, they are focused on three main aspects:

- The effect of pressure processing on bioactive compounds of juices when compared with fresh juices, thermally treated juices, and juices treated by other techniques (e.g., PEF processing)
- The effect of pressure processing on bioactive compounds of juices and their storage stability
- The effect of pressure processing on bioactive compounds of juices and their *in vitro* and *in vivo* bioaccessibility

12.5.1 EFFECT OF PRESSURE PROCESSING ON BIOACTIVE COMPOUNDS OF JUICES WHEN COMPARED WITH FRESH JUICES, THERMALLY TREATED JUICES, AND JUICES TREATED BY OTHER TECHNIQUES

The effect of pressure processing on bioactive compounds has been evaluated in a lot of juices, predominantly blueberry, tomato, carrot, and citrus juices, but also in others such as strawberry, apple, grapefruit, and pomegranate juices. The main bioactive compounds studied in all reported papers are anthocyanin, vitamin C, α-carotene, β-carotene, lycopene, and flavonoids. The total antioxidant activity is evaluated in most cases, as well as some other physicochemical properties that have a great influence on the juices' final quality, such as viscosity, suspended pulp, cloudiness, particle size, color, and so on.

In all papers, the reported antioxidant activity values obtained from juices after pressure treatments are, in most cases, not statistically significant when compared with fresh juices and, in those cases in which differences are significant, the anti-oxidant activity values obtained from treated juices are always higher than those from thermally treated juices. The same occurs with bioactive compounds: higher values occur in pressure-treated juices than in thermally treated juices, and in some cases these values are higher than those obtained from fresh juices. Evaluating the influence of process variables on the stability of bioactive compounds, as well as the antioxidant capacity, is important in order to obtain a beverage with functional properties. In addition, the evaluation of physicochemical parameters is a key factor defining treatment conditions, thus determining consumer acceptance. According to the results obtained, it is possible to say that pressure treatments positively affect the color of juices, resulting in a brighter appearance than fresh juices. In the same way, reducing the particle size with homogenization pressure is a good way to improve the stability of suspended pulp, an important quality parameter in citrus juices.

For example, Bull et al. (2004) studied the quality of HPP Valencia and Navel orange juices compared to fresh and thermally pasteurized juices. The juices were pressure processed at 600 MPa/20°C for 60 s, and it was determined that orange juice quality parameters such as °Brix, viscosity, titratable acid content, alcohol-insoluble acids, browning index and color, and ascorbic acid and β-carotene concentrations were not significantly affected by HPP. Velázquez-Estrada et al. (2013) evaluated the effect of HPH treatments on the bioactive compounds and antioxidant activity of orange juice. Freshly squeezed orange juice was prewarmed at two inlet temperatures (10°C and 20°C) and processed at 100, 200, and 300 MPa. The remaining content of vitamin C in the HPH-treated samples at any pressure was significantly higher than in the thermally pasteurized one. The flavanone content, more specifically the amount of hesperidin, increased with the HPH treatments, achieving its highest concentration in the samples treated at 200 and 300 MPa. No significant differences were observed in the total polyphenol content and antioxidant capacity values between the fresh and the HPH-treated orange juice samples, while these values were significantly lower in the thermally pasteurized sample. Ferrari et al. (2010) investigated the application of HPP on the quality of pomegranate juice. The experiments clearly demonstrate that high-pressure treatment at room temperature improves the quality of pomegranate juice, increasing the intensity of the red color of the fresh juice and preserving the content of the natural anthocyanin. Barba et al. (2013) studied the impact of HPP at different pressures (200, 400, and 600 MPa) and treatment times (5, 9, and 15 min) on the ascorbic acid, total phenolic, and anthocyanin stability and the total antioxidant capacity, pH, °Brix, and color of blueberry juice. HPP treatments resulted in more than 92% vitamin C retention at all treatment intensities. The total phenolic content in the juice was increased, mostly after HPP at 200 MPa for all treatment times. The total and monomeric anthocyanin was similar or higher than the value estimated for the fresh juice, reaching its maximum level at 400 MPa/15 min (a 16% increase). Antioxidant capacity values were not statistically different for treatments at 200 MPa/5–15 min in comparison with fresh juice. No significant changes were observed in pH and °Brix. Color changes were not visually noticeable in pressurized beverages for all pressures and times. Suárez-Jacobo et al. (2011) evaluated the effect of HPH treatments (100, 200, and 300 MPa) on the quality characteristics of apple juice such as its antioxidant capacity, polyphenol composition, vitamin C, and provitamin A content, in comparison with raw and pasteurized (90°C/4 min) apple juice. HPH processing did not change the antioxidant capacity of apple juice. Vitamin C concentrations did not change in HPH-treated samples, retaining the same values as in raw juice. However, significant losses were observed for provitamin A content, but lower than in pasteurized samples. The authors conclude that HPH treatments at 300 MPa can be an alternative to thermal treatment in order to preserve the quality of apple juice.

Pressure treatments have also been compared with other techniques such as PEF processing. For example, Vervoort et al. (2011) compared the impact of thermal, high-pressure, and PEF processing for mild pasteurization of orange juice. Examining the effect on specific chemical and biochemical quality parameters directly after treatment and during storage at 4°C revealed significant differences in residual enzyme activities only. POD was completely inactivated by heat pasteurization and was much less susceptible to high-pressure and PEF processing. All other quality parameters investigated, including the sugar profile, the organic acid profile, bitter compounds, vitamin C, and the carotenoid profile, experienced no significantly different impact from the three pasteurization techniques.

Current knowledge thus indicates that the use of pressure treatments in juice processing has been established as a new nonthermal technology that is able to maintain and improve the nutritional and quality properties of juices as compared to thermal treatments. This technology represents a rapid, efficient, and reliable alternative to improve the quality of food but there is also the potential to develop new products with a unique functionality. There are no studies on the differences observed by using IIPP or IIPII. All reported papers show that there are no differences in the results obtained with these two treatments. Considering the content of bioactive compounds treatment at 200 or 400 MPa seems to be a determining factor in some cases (Barba et al., 2013). Taking into account the pressure levels and treatment conditions established, it is not possible to establish or define a critical pressure level.

12.5.2 Effect of Pressure Processing on Bioactive Compounds of Juices and Their Storage Stability

Despite the fact that pressure processing minimally affects the quality of fruit products, they change during storage due to coexisting chemical reactions such as oxidation and biochemical reactions when endogenous enzymes are incompletely inactivated (Oey et al. 2008); thus, it is necessary to analyze the quality changes of pressure-treated products during storage (Cao et al. 2012). The storage temperatures analyzed are 4°C and 25°C, and the period studied varies a great deal. Thus, we can find storage assays from 21 days to 6 months in the literature. The main compounds analyzed are anthocyanin and ascorbic acid. Total antioxidant activity and total phenolic content parameters are also determined in most cases.

Uckoo et al. (2013) studied the effects of HPP and thermal processing on the levels of bioactive compounds in grapefruit juice. In general, HPP treatment maintained the levels of phytochemicals in grapefruit juice comparably to thermal processing treatment during storage at 4°C. HPP technology also maintained the color of the juice, resulting in a fresh-like appearance for 21 days, unlike thermal processing.

Zhao et al. (2013) evaluated the effects of HHP at 400 MPa/4 min and 500 MPa/2 min and thermal pasteurization at 85°C/15 s with 100 IU/mL of nisin on natural microbial flora, chlorophyll a and b, color, lipoxygenase activity, and the four C9 key odorants of (E,Z)-2,6-nonadienal, (E,Z)-3,6-nonadien-1-ol, (E)-2-nonenal, and (Z)-6-nonenal in cucumber juice drinks over 50 days of storage at 4°C. Yeast and molds were completely inactivated by all treatments, and their levels were below the detection limit during storage. Nisin with HHP or thermal pasteurization had a synergistic effect on the inactivation of total aerobic bacteria. For all the quality attributes studied in this article, their retention was significantly better in the HHP-treated samples than in the thermally pasteurized samples during storage. The samples treated by 500 MPa/2 min with 100 IU/mL of nisin exhibited a longer shelf life as compared with other treated samples.

Some authors have modeled the degradation kinetics of those bioactive compounds in order to determine their storage stability. Buckow et al. (2010) studied the degradation kinetics and storage stability of total anthocyanin in blueberry juice. In the same way, Cao et al. (2012), Cerdán-Calero et al. (2013), and Dede et al. (2007) evaluated the quality parameters of strawberry, orange, tomato, and carrot juices, respectively, during storage, trying to shed light on the degradation kinetics mechanisms of bioactive compounds. All reported papers point toward industrial applications in order to extend the shelf life of processed juices. The mechanisms by which bioactive compounds degrade are numerous, complex, and sometimes unknown. High-pressure treatments modify the mechanism of bioactive degradation by affecting the molecules involved in the kinetics of reaction, such as enzymes. The residual activity of the enzymes along with a small concentration of dissolved oxygen can cause the degradation of the bioactive compounds during the storage of the processed juice, as widely supported by studies reported in the current scientific literature (Suthanthangjai et al. 2005; Zabetakis et al. 2000). A better understanding of the complex physicochemical mechanism of action of nonthermal processing technologies and their effects on the technological and functional properties of fruits and their products would also contribute to reinforce the presence of their applications (Rawson et al. 2011).

12.5.3 Effect of Pressure Processing on Bioactive Compounds of Juices and Their In Vitro and In Vivo Bioaccessibility

Nutrient bioaccessibility, defined as the fraction of an ingested nutrient released from the matrix and available for intestinal absorption (Parada and Aguilera 2007), is a prerequisite for its bioavailability (Holst and Williamson 2008) and depends on nutrient localization in the food matrix (Colle et al. 2010). The food matrix in which the bioactive compound is incorporated and which can be altered by food processing greatly influences its bioaccessibility (Castenmiller and West 1998). Recently, the relationship between food microstructure and nutritional food properties has attracted a lot of attention (Ellis et al. 2004; Parada and Aguilera 2007; Lemmens et al. 2009; Singh et al. 2007; Ferrua et al. 2011). In this relationship, the intactness (Ellis et al. 2004) and the pectin properties (Lemmens et al. 2009) of the plant cell walls seem to play an important role. Therefore, it is also very likely that pressure treatment, which has an impact on the microstructure of juices, will influence the bioaccessibility of bioactive compounds and therefore its bioavailability. The changes introduced into the cell walls, such as breakdown or permeability increase, can cause the liberation of compounds, making them more bioaccessible, but can also promote their reaction with others, resulting in novel bioactive compounds. In this case, it is important to consider that the bioactive compound should be in a form available to interact with the physiological target within the organism, but at the same time be protected in order not to deteriorate during processing or storage. The effect of pressure treatments on bioactive compounds of juices has emerged recently and there are a few papers reporting the bioaccessibility of these compounds after pressure processing. The lycopene, carotene, and probiotic microorganisms are the most studied (Castro et al. 2012; Colle et al. 2010; Plaza et al. 2012; Svelander et al. 2011; Uckoo et al. 2013; Tabanelli et al. 2012; Chaikham et al. 2012).

Eylen et al. (2008) studied the effect of thermal and high-pressure/high-temperature treatments on the stability and activity of endogenous myrosinase in broccoli, as well as on cell permeability. The conversion of glucosinolates into active compounds by myrosinase occurs after cell disruption, for example, by mastication or processing. However, as myrosinase is heat sensitive, cooking or blanching will result in myrosinase inactivation before the beneficial compounds can be formed. High-pressure/high-temperature treatments can induce cell permeabilization at moderate conditions (Ade-Omowaye et al. 2001), which can be useful to bring myrosinase into contact with glucosinolates. At the end of the study, it was observed that pressure only had a limited effect on activity. Some high-pressure and high-temperature conditions were chosen to verify whether it was possible to obtain glucosinolate conversion, which is necessary to create health-promoting hydrolysis products, through high-pressure/high-temperature processing. The optimal temperature at atmospheric pressure was 40°C while at elevated pressure the highest activity was found at 45°C and 100 MPa.

Svelander et al. (2011) showed that HPH using a split-stream approach is a feasible way to produce nutritionally improved fruit and vegetable products while maintaining a high nutrient retention. However, while pressure homogenization affected the carrot and tomato matrices, the effect of HPP on the *in vitro* accessibility of carotenes depended on carotene speciation. The cell wall disruption by HPP increased the *in vitro* bioaccessibility of α- and β-carotene from carrot, but not of lycopene from tomato. In the same way, Colle et al. (2010) studied the effect on the microstructure, the lycopene content, and the lycopene *in vitro* bioaccessibility of tomato pulp of HPH followed by thermal processing. As hypothesized by Colle and others, the homogenization pressure resulted in the breakdown of the tomato cell aggregate structures, but improved the strength of a fiber network, which may trap the lycopene and reduce its bioavailability, as indicated also in a review by McClements et al. (2009). Thermal processing (30 min at 90°C), subsequent to HPH, was not able to sufficiently decrease the strength of the fiber network of homogenized tomato pulp in order to improve the lycopene *in vitro* bioaccessibility.

HPP and HPH technologies have also been used to enhance the survival of probiotic strains or to modify their overall functionality in a positive way. When HPH was applied to milk, it showed good potential for the formulation of functional foods, mainly probiotic products. In fact, in the functional dairy sector, HPH has been proposed to manufacture probiotic fermented milks and cheeses with enhanced sensorial or functional properties, that is, improving their strain viability over refrigerated storage and accelerating fermentation kinetics (Burns et al. 2008; Patrignani et al. 2009). Lanciotti et al. (2007) showed that HPH is able to modify, in relation to the strain and to the treatment applied, both the fermentation kinetics and the enzymatic activities of lactic acid bacteria without detrimental effects on cell viability. When low levels of pressure were applied directly to cells of probiotic bacteria, strain-dependent effects were observed in relation to the capacity to enhance functional properties of interest in these cultures. Tabanelli et al. (2012) observed that a 50 MPa HPH treatment increased *Lactobacillus paracasei* A13 hydrophobicity and resistance to simulated gastric digestion. Tabanelli et al. (2012) assessed the *in vivo* effects of HPH treatment applied to probiotic lactobacilli on their interaction capacity with the gut and on their ability to induce immunoglobulin A (IgA) cell proliferation in the intestines of mice. IgA is the most abundant immunoglobulin at the mucosal surfaces, whose main function is to exert immune exclusion of invading pathogens or foreign proteins (Macpherson et al. 2001). HPH treatment was able to modify some features linked to the cell wall and, consequently, altered the interaction of probiotic lactobacilli with the small intestine. HPH-treated cells induced a higher IgA response compared to untreated ones, in a strain- and feeding period-dependent way. HPH treatment could increase some *in vivo* functional characteristics of probiotic strains, highlighting the potential of this technique for the development of probiotic cultures.

12.6 CASE STUDIES

The authors have studied the effect of pressure homogenization on two fruit juices, mandarin and blueberry juices, at different levels, taking into account the most important problems associated with each juice.

12.6.1 LOW HOMOGENIZATION PRESSURE APPLIED TO ENHANCE FUNCTIONAL PROPERTIES OF MANDARIN JUICE

In the case of mandarin juice, the processing industry has made a lot of efforts aimed at preserving the characteristics of fresh juices and trying to avoid the typical "cooked flavor" of processed citrus juices. This characteristic cooked flavor occurs as a result of high treatment temperatures applied in order to stabilize the juice and inactivate PME (the cell wall enzyme associated with the pulp [Rouse and Atkins 1955]). For this reason, Izquierdo et al. (2007) developed a patented procedure (WO/2007/042593) entitled "Method of obtaining refrigerated pasteurized citrus juices." The procedure consists of separating the citrus juice into two fractions, one fraction rich in pulp, and the other with low pulp content (1%) denominated serum. A different thermal treatment is applied to each fraction. A temperature-time of 85°C/15 s is applied to the pulp-rich fraction where the enzymes are located. A temperature-time of 63°C/15 s is applied to the low pulp content fraction where the most flavor and functional compounds are located. The patented procedure aims to join both fractions at the end of the process, resulting in a juice with sensorial properties very similar to fresh juices.

Additionally, the serum fraction may be suitable for some applications such as developing functional foods. But in some cases, low pulp content represents a disadvantage since it results in a juice with less color and cloudiness: both important quality characteristic parameters. This problem can be easily avoided by converting part of the suspended pulp into a background pulp by a homogenization operation. This operation has already been applied to citrus juices, increasing their yield (Lortkipanidze et al. 1972) and improving some of their quality factors such as viscosity (Crandall and Davis 1991), color (Lee and Coates 2004), cloudiness (Baker 1977), and stability of suspended solids (Carle et al. 1998). Evidently, technological processes applied to orange juices can significantly modify their chemical composition, mainly affecting heat-sensitive compounds or those directly linked to the pulp of juices such as volatile constituents (Cerdán-Calero et al. 2013). Compositional modifications affect the flavor and functional characteristics of the resultant products and have a key role in their acceptability to consumers.

We studied the effect of low homogenization pressures on the physicochemical and functional properties of mandarin juice (*cv. Ortanique*). More concretely, we applied pressures of 0, 5, 10, 15, 20, 25, and 30 MPa to the low-pulp juice obtained by the patented procedure described above, and its particle size, color, cloudiness, antiradical activity, and flavonoid content were evaluated. The obtained results have recently been published in Betoret et al. (2009, 2012b).

Generally, the homogenization pressure affected the particle size distribution and color of the citrus juices, making it possible to define different sample groups on the basis of the applied pressure. Above 10 MPa, the low transmittance values indicated a high level of cloudiness and suspended pulp in low-pulp juice that increased with homogenization pressure. This effect was explained by taking into account that the homogenization pressure converted sensible pulp to background pulp (Kupper et al. 1987) and the cloud particles were more stable. The 2,2′-azino-bis(3-ethylbenzothiazoline-6-sulfonic acid) (ABTS) test indicated minor significant differences between samples. However, a slight increase in antiradical activity was observed as the homogenization pressure increased. The 2,2-diphenyl-1-picrylhydrazyl (DPPH) test and modeling showed no significant differences in the values obtained at any level of the homogenization pressure applied. Moreover, the antiradical activity of the low-pulp juice was no smaller than that of an industrial, pasteurized mandarin juice. In the same way, the content of the flavonoids narirutin, hesperidin, and didymin were not affected by the homogenization pressures applied. Homogenization pressure is a mechanical process that does not affect the content of flavonoids in the juice overall, but it may produce changes in the content of the flavonoids suspended in the juice cloud. We observed a tendency to an increase in the flavonoid content suspended in the cloud as homogenization pressure increased. This is important when homogenization pressure is applied prior to other operations or processes in which the suspended solids affect the efficiency and the yield of the process or the quality of the final product. This occurs, for example, in the case of vacuum impregnation operations. We found that the application of homogenization pressure led to greater incorporation of low-pulp juice into the structural matrix of apple juice and that the functional compounds were stable in the juice cloud, due to pulp stability and particle size reduction.

12.6.2 High Homogenization Pressure Applied to Enhance Functional Properties of Blueberry Juice

In the case of blueberry juice, an HPH process was applied after thermal pasteurization in order to study the effects of homogenization on the physicochemical and functional properties of the juice.

Blueberries are an important source of antioxidant compounds because of their high content of total phenolics, mainly anthocyanin. Blueberry juice represents an important alternative for direct consumption or for use as an ingredient in functional foods development. From the nutritional quality point of view, information is limited on how different processing methods affect the content of bioactive compounds in the final product (Brownmiller et al. 2008). Besides, significant losses were observed in the content of anthocyanin during juice processing (Lee et al. 2002; Rossi et al. 2003; Srivastava et al. 2007). Furthermore, studies on the flow behavior of juices made from small fruits such as blueberry (*Vaccinium corymbosum*) and red raspberry (*Rubus idaeus*) are scarce (Nindo et al. 2005). A study on how HPH affects the physicochemical, rheological, and functional properties was carried out. The results show that homogenizing the juice at 150 MPa at 25°C inlet temperature produces changes in the size of the suspended particles, moving down the size distribution down from a D[4,3] value of 147.21 ± 6.04 to 30.6 ± 0.9 μm. This consequently causes changes in the stability of the suspended pulp and cloudiness. Homogenization increases the stability of the suspended pulp and the cloudiness of the juice. The importance of an increase in these two characteristics is because the suspended pulp and cloud contain a number of important functional components (Garau et al. 2007; Betoret et al. 2012b).

The homogenization operation also causes color changes. If the homogenized and nonhomogenized juice are compared with a fresh blueberry smash, the CIE L*a*b* coordinates of the homogenized juice approaches the control coordinates. After HPH, the global color difference of the nontreated juice was reduced from 8.48 ± 0.19 to 5.40 ± 0.03.

The reduction of the particle size decreases the interaction between the particles and causes changes in the flow behavior. In this respect, the consistency index of the Ostwald–de Waele model decreases from 0.57 ± 0.03 to 0.33 ± 0.06 Pa.s^n and the flow behavior index increases from 0.33 ± 0.02 to 0.38 ± 0.06 for the nonhomogenized and homogenized juice, respectively, turning the behavior of the juice more Newtonian.

Finally, the HPH reduces the total phenolic content and the antioxidant activity by 15% and 20%, respectively, due to the thermal effect of homogenization. However, the total monomeric anthocyanin increases by 17%. This could be attributed to the lower size of the suspended particles that could aid a higher extraction of anthocyanin.

In the case of the vacuum impregnation operation, we found that the application of homogenization pressures led to greater incorporation of low-pulp juice into the structural matrix of apple juice and that the functional compounds were stable in the juice cloud, due to pulp stability and particle size reduction.

REFERENCES

Ade-Omowaye, B.I.O., Rastogi, N.K., Angersbach, A., Knorr, D. (2001). Effects of high hydro-static pressure or high intensity electrical field pulse pre-treatment on dehydration characteristics of red paprika. *Innovative Food Science and Emerging Technologies* 2: 1–7.

Aertsen, A., Meersman, F., Hendrickx, M.E.G., Vogel, R.F., Michiels, C.W. (2009). Biotechnology under high pressure: Applications and implications. *Trends in Biotechnology* 27(7): 434–441.

Asaka, M., Aoyama, Y., Nakanishi, R., Hayashi, R. (1994). Purification of a latent form of polyphenoloxidase from La France pear fruit and its pressure-activation. *Bioscience, Biotechnology, and Biochemistry* 58: 1486–1489.

Baker, R.A. (1977). Process to control juice cloud. Symposium of the international society of citriculture. *Proceedings of the International Society of Citriculture* 3: 751–755.

Balny, C. (2004). Pressure effects on weak interactions in biological systems. *Journal of Physics: Condensed Matter* 16(14): S1245–S1253.

Balny, C., Masson, P. (1993). Effects of high pressure on proteins. *Food Reviews International* 9(4): 611–628.

Balogh, T., Smout, C., Nguyen, B.L., Van Loey, A.M., Hendrickx, M.E. (2004). Thermal and high-pressure inactivation kinetics of carrot pectin methylesterase: From model system to real foods. *Innovative Food Science and Emerging Technologies* 5(4): 429–436.

Barba, F.J., Esteve, M.J., Frigola, A. (2013). Physicochemical and nutritional characteristics of blueberry juice after high pressure processing. *Food Research International* 50(2): 545–549.

Basak, S. and Ramaswamy, H.S. (1996). Ultra high pressure treatment of orange juice: A kinetic study on inactivation of pectin methyl esterase. *Food Research International* 29(7): 601–607.

Basset, J., Lepine, P., Chaumont, L. (1956). Effects of high pressures on the poliomyelitis virus (Lansing strain). *Annales de l'Institut Pasteur (Paris)* 90: 575–593.

Basset, J., Macheboeuf, M.A. (1932). Etude sur les effets biologiques des ultra-pressions: Résistance des bactéries, des diastases et des toxines aux pressions très élevées. *Comptes Rendus Hebdomadaires des Seances de l'Academie des Sciences* 195: 1431–1433.

Bayındırlı, A., Alpas, H., Bozoğlu, F., Hızal, M. (2006). Efficiency of high pressure treatment on inactivation of pathogenic microorganisms and enzymes in apple, orange, apricot and sour cherry juices. *Food Control* 17(1): 52–58.

Belloch, C., Gurrea, M.C., Tárrega, A., Sampedro, F., Carbonell, J.V. (2012). Inactivation of microorganisms in orange juice by high-pressure homogenization combined with its inherent heating effect. *European Food Research and Technology* 234(5): 753–760.

Betoret, E., Betoret, N., Carbonell, J.V., Fito, P. (2009). Effects of pressure homogenization on particle size and the functional properties of citrus juices. *Journal of Food Engineering* 92(1): 18–23.

Betoret, E., Betoret, N., Arilla, A., Bennár, M., Barrera, C., Codoñer, P., Fito, P. (2012a). No invasive methodology to produce a probiotic low humid apple snack with potential effect against *Helicobacter pylori*. *Journal of Food Engineering* 110(2): 289–293.

Betoret, E., Sentandreu, E., Betoret, N., Fito, P. (2012b). Homogenization pressures applied to citrus juice manufacturing. Functional properties and application. *Journal of Food Engineering* 111(1): 28–33.

Bevilacqua, A., Campaniello, D., Sinigaglia, M., Ciccarone, C., Corbo, M.R. (2012). Sodium-benzoate and citrus extract increase the effect of homogenization towards spores of *Fusarium oxysporum* in pineapple juice. *Food Control* 28(2): 199–204.

Boff, J.M., Truong, T.T., Min, D.B., Shellhammer, T.H. (2003). Effect of thermal processing and carbon dioxide-assisted high-pressure processing on pectin methylesterase and chemical changes in orange juice. *Journal of Food Science* 68(4): 1179–1184.

Brinez, W.J., Roig-Sagues, A.X., Herrero, M.M.H., Lopez, B.G. (2006). Inactivation by ultra high-pressure homogenization of *Escherichia coli* strains inoculated into orange juice. *Journal of Food Protection* 69: 984–989.

Brownmiller, C., Howard, L.R., Prior, R.L. (2008). Processing and storage effects on monomeric anthocyanins, percent polymeric color, and antioxidant capacity of processed blueberry products. *Journal of Food Science* 73(5): H72–H79.

Buckow, R., Kastell, A., Terefe, N.S., Versteeg, C. (2010). Pressure and temperature effects on degradation kinetics and storage stability of total anthocyanins in blueberry juice. *Journal of Agricultural and Food Chemistry* 58(18): 10076–10084.

Bull, M.K., Zerdin, K., Howe, E., Goicoechea, D., Paramanandhan, P., Stockman, R., Sellahewa, J., Szabo, E.A., Johnson, R.L., Stewart, C.M. (2004). The effect of high pressure processing on the microbial, physical and chemical properties of Valencia and Navel orange juice. *Innovative Food Science and Emerging Technologies* 5(2): 135–149.

Burns, P., Patrignani, F., Serrazanetti, D., Vinderola, G.C., Reinheimer, J.A., Lanciotti, R., Guerzoni, M.E. (2008). Probiotic crescenza cheese containing *Lactobacillus casei* and *Lactobacillus acidophilus* manufactured with high-pressure homogenized milk. *Journal of Dairy Science* 91(2): 500–512.

Butz, P., Koller, W.D., Tauscher, B., Wolf, S. (1994). Ultra-high pressure processing of onions: Chemical and sensory changes. *LWT—Food Science and Technology* 27(5): 463–467.

Buzrul, S., Alpas, H., Largeteau, A., Demazeau, G. (2008). Inactivation of *Escherichia coli* and *Listeria innocua* in kiwifruit and pineapple juices by high hydrostatic pressure. *International Journal of Food Microbiology* 124(3): 275–278.

Calligaris, S., Foschia, M., Bartolomeoli, I., Maifreni, M., Manzocco, L. (2012). Study on the applicability of high-pressure homogenization for the production of banana juices. *LWT—Food Science and Technology* 45(1): 117–121.

Campos, F.P., Cristianini, M. (2007). Inactivation of *Saccharomyces cerevisiae* and *Lactobacillus plantarum* in orange juice using ultra high-pressure homogenisation. *Innovative Food Science and Emerging Technologies* 8(2): 226–229.

Cano, M.P., Hernandez, A., Ancos, B. (1997). High pressure and temperature effects on enzyme inactivation in strawberry and orange products. *Journal of Food Science* 62(1): 85–88.

Cao, X., Bi, X., Huang, W., Wu, J., Hu, X., Liao, X. (2012). Changes of quality of high hydrostatic pressure processed cloudy and clear strawberry juices during storage. *Innovative Food Science and Emerging Technologies* 16: 181–190.

Carle, R., Jauss, A., Fuesser, H. (1998). Cloud stability of pulp-containing tropical fruit nectars. *Fruit Processing* 8(7): 266–268, 270–272.

Carreño, J.M., Gurrea, M.C., Sampedro, F., Carbonell, J.V. (2011). Effect of high hydrostatic pressure and high-pressure homogenisation on *Lactobacillus plantarum* inactivation kinetics and quality parameters of mandarin juice. *European Food Research and Technology* 232(2): 265–274.

Castenmiller, J.J.M., West, C.E. (1998). Bioavailability and bioconversion of carotenoids. *Annual Review of Nutrition* 18: 19–38.

Castro, A., Bergenståhl, B., Tornberg, E. (2012). Parsnip (*Pastinaca sativa* L.): Dietary fibre composition and physicochemical characterization of its homogenized suspensions. *Food Research International* 48(2): 598–608.

Cerdán-Calero, M., Izquierdo, L., Sentandreu, E. (2013). Valencia late orange juice preserved by pulp reduction and high pressure homogenization: Sensory quality and gas chromatography–mass spectrometry analysis of volatiles. *LWT—Food Science and Technology* 51(2): 476–483.

Chaikham, P., Apichartsrangkoon, A., Jirarattanarangsri, W., Van de Wiele, T. (2012). Influence of encapsulated probiotics combined with pressurized longan juice on colon microflora and their metabolic activities on the exposure to simulated dynamic gastrointestinal tract. *Food Research International* 49(1): 133–142.

Charm, S.E., Longmaid, H.E., III, Carver, J. (1977). A simple system for extending refrigerated, nonfrozen preservation of biological material using pressure. *Cryobiology* 14: 625–636.

Cheftel, J.-C. (1991). Applications des hautes pressions en technologie alimentaire. *Industries alimentaires et agricoles* 108(3): 141–153.

Cheftel, J.-C. (1992). Effects of high hydrostatic pressure on food constituents: An overview. In: C. Balny, R. Hayashi, K. Heremans, P. Masson (eds.), *High Pressure and Biotechnology*, pp. 195–209. London: Colloque INSERM/John Libbey Euro-text.

Cheftel, J.-C. (1995). Hautes pressions, inactivation microbienne et conservation des aliments. *Comptes Rendus de l'Académie d'Agriculture de France* 81(1): 13–38.

Chicón, R., Belloque, J., Alonso, E., López-Fandiño, R. (2008). Immunoreactivity and digestibility of high-pressure-treated whey proteins. *International Dairy Journal* 18(4): 367–376.

Colle, I., Van Buggenhout, S., Van Loey, A., and Hendrickx, M. (2010). High pressure homogenization followed by thermal processing of tomato pulp: Influence on microstructure and lycopene *in vitro* bioaccessibility. *Food Research International* 43(8): 2193–2200.

Commission of the European Communities (2001). Commission Decision. 2001/424/EC, Authorising the placing on the market of pasteurised fruit-based preparations produced using high-pressure pasteurisation under regulation (EC) no 258/97 of the European Parliament and of the Council.

Cortés-Muñoz, M., Chevalier-Lucia, D., Dumay, E. (2009). Characteristics of submicron emulsions prepared by ultra-high pressure homogenisation: Effect of chilled or frozen storage. *Food Hydrocolloids* 23(3): 640–654.

Corwin, H., Shellhammer, T.H. (2002). Combined carbon dioxide and high pressure inactivation of pectin methylesterase, polyphenol oxidase, *Lactobacillus plantarum* and *Escherichia coli*. *Journal of Food Science* 67(2): 697–701.

Crandall, P.G., Davis, K.C. (1991). Viscosity reduction and reformation of structure in orange concentrate as affected by homogenization within commercial taste evaporators. *Journal of Food Science* 56(5): 1360–1364.

Crelier, S., Robert, M.C., Claude, J., Juillerat, M.A. (2001). Tomato (*Lycopersicon esculentum*) pectin methylesterase and polygalacturonase behaviors regarding heat- and pressure-induced inactivation. *Journal of Agricultural and Food Chemistry* 49(11): 5566–5575.

Curl, A.L. and Jansen, E.F. (1950). Effect of high pressures on trypsin and chymotrypsin. *Journal of Biological Chemistry* 184(1): 45–54.

da Cruz, A.G., Fonseca Faria, J.D.A., Isay Saad, S.M., André Bolini, H.M., Sant'Ana, A.S., and Cristianini, M. (2010). High pressure processing and pulsed electric fields: Potential use in probiotic dairy foods processing. *Trends in Food Science and Technology* 21(10): 483–493.

Daryaei, H. and Balasubramaniam, V.M. (2013). Kinetics of *Bacillus coagulans* spore inactivation in tomato juice by combined pressure–heat treatment. *Food Control* 30(1): 168–175.

Dede, S., Alpas, H., and Bayındırlı, A. (2007). High hydrostatic pressure treatment and storage of carrot and tomato juices: Antioxidant activity and microbial safety. *Journal of the Science of Food and Agriculture* 87(5): 773–782.

Diels, A.M.J., Michiels, C.W. (2006). High-pressure homogenization as a non-thermal technique for the inactivation of microorganisms. *Critical Reviews in Microbiology* 32(4): 201–216.

Dirix, C., Duvetter, T., Van Loey, A., Hendrickx, M., Heremans, K. (2005). The in situ observation of the temperature and pressure stability of recombinant *Aspergillus aculeatus* pectin methylesterase with Fourier transform IR spectroscopy reveals an unusual pressure stability of beta-helices. *The Biochemical Journal* 392(Pt 3): 565–571.

Donsì, F., Ferrari, G., Lenza, E., Maresca, P. (2009). Main factors regulating microbial inactivation by high-pressure homogenization: Operating parameters and scale of operation.
Chemical Engineering Science 64(3): 520–532.

Dumay, E., Chevalier-Lucia, D., López-Pedemonte, T. (2010). High pressure and food conservation. In: P. Sebert (ed.), *Comparative High Pressure Biology*, pp. 83–116. Enfield:
Science Publishers.

Dumay, E., Chevalier-Lucia, D., Picart-Palmade, L., Benzaria, A., Gràcia-Julià, A., Blayo,
C. (2013). Technological aspects and potential applications of (ultra) high-pressure
homogenisation. *Trends in Food Science and Technology* 31(1): 13–26.

Duvetter, T., Sila, D.N., Van Buggenhout, S., Jolie, R., Van Loey, A., Hendrickx, M. (2009).
Pectins in processed fruit and vegetables: Part I-stability and catalytic activity of pectinases. *Comprehensive Reviews in Food Science and Food Safety* 8(2): 75–85.

Ellis, P.R., Kendall, C.W., Ren, Y., Parker, C., Pacy, J.F., Waldron, K.W., Jenkins, D.J. (2004).
Role of cell walls in the bioaccessibility of lipids in almond seeds. *The American Journal
of Clinical Nutrition* 80(3): 604–613.

Erkmen, O. (2011). Effects of high hydrostatic pressure on *Salmonella typhimurium* and aerobic bacteria in milk and fruit juices. *Romanian Biotechnological Letters* 16: 5.

Eylen, D.V., Oey, I., Hendrickx, M., Van Loey, A. (2008). Effects of pressure/temperature treatments on stability and activity of endogenous broccoli (*Brassica oleracea* L. *cv. Italica*)
myrosinase and on cell permeability. *Journal of Food Engineering* 89(2): 178–186.

Fachin, D., Van Loey, A.M., Ly Nguyen, B., Verlent, I., Indrawati, I., Hendrickx, M.E. (2002).
Comparative study of the inactivation kinetics of pectin methylesterase in tomato juice
and purified form. *Biotechnology Progress* 18(4): 739–744.

Federighi, M., Vidon, M., Mescle, J.F., Pilet, M.F. (1995). Traitements hautes pressions et denrées
alimentaires: Revue bibliographique. *Microbiology, Foods and Nutrition* 13: 115–125.

Ferrari, G., Maresca, P., Ciccarone, R. (2010). The application of high hydrostatic pressure for
the stabilization of functional foods: Pomegranate juice. *Journal of Food Engineering*
100(2): 245–253.

Ferrua, M.J., Kong, F., Singh, R.P. (2011). Computational modeling of gastric digestion and
the role of food material properties. *Trends in Food Science and Technology* 22(9):
480–491.

Garau, M.C., Simal, S., Rosselló, C., Femenia, A. (2007). Effect of air-drying temperature on
physico-chemical properties of dietary fibre and antioxidant capacity of orange (*Citrus
aurantium v. Canoneta*) by-products. *Food Chemistry* 104(3): 1014–1024.

García-Graells, C., Hauben, K.J.A., Michiels, C.W. (1998). High-pressure inactivation and
sublethal injury of pressure-resistant *Escherichia coli* mutants in fruit juices. *Applied
and Environmental Microbiology* 64(4): 1566–1568.

Gassiot, M., Masoliver, P. (2010). Commercial high pressure processing of ham and other
sliced meat products at Esteban España, S.A. In: C.D. Doona, K. Kustin, F.E. Feeherry
(eds), *Case Studies in Novel Food Processing Technologies*, pp. 21–33. Cambridge:
Woodhead Publishing.

Gogate, P.R., Pandit, A.B. (2008). Application of cavitational reactors for cell disruption for
recovery of intracellular enzymes. *Journal of Chemical Technology and Biotechnology*
83(8): 1083–1093.

Gomes, M.R.A., Ledward, D.A. (1996). Effect of high-pressure treatment on the activity of
some polyphenoloxidases. *Food Chemistry* 56(1): 1–5.

Goodner, J.K., Braddock, R.J., Parish, M.E. (1998). Inactivation of pectinesterase in orange
and grapefruit juices by high pressure. *Journal of Agricultural and Food Chemistry*
46(5): 1997–2000.

Hauben, K.J.A., Wuytack, E.Y., Soontjens, C.C.F., Michiels, C.W. (1996). High-pressure transient sensitization of *Escherichia coli* to lysozyme and nisin by disruption of outer-
membrane permeability. *Journal of Food Protection* 59: 945–950.

Hayashi, R. (1989). Application of high pressure to food processing and preservation: Philosophy and development. *Engineering and Food* 2: 815–826.

Hayashi, R. (1990). *Pressure Processed Food: Research and Development*. Kyoto: San-Ei Publishing.

Heinisch, O., Kowalski, E., Goossens, K., Frank, J., Heremans, K., Ludwig, H., Tauscher, B. (1995). Pressure effects on the stability of lipoxygenase: Fourier transform-infrared spectroscopy (FT-IR) and enzyme activity studies. *Zeitschrift für Lebensmittel-Untersuchung und Forschung* 201(6): 562–565.

Hendrickx, M., Ludikhuyze, L., Van den Broeck, I., Weemaes, C. (1998). Effects of high pressure on enzymes related to food quality. *Trends in Food Science and Technology* 9(5): 197–203.

Heremans, K. (1982). High pressure effects on proteins and other biomolecules. *Annual Review of Biophysics and Bioengineering* 11: 1–21.

Heremans, K. (2005). Protein dynamics: Hydration and cavities. *Brazilian Journal of Medical and Biological Research* 38(8): 1157–1165.

Hite, B., Giddings, N.J., Weakly, C.E. (1914). The effect of pressure on certain microorganisms encountered in the preservation of fruits and vegetables. *West Virginia University. Agricultural Experiment Station Bulletin* 146: 1–67.

Holst, B., Williamson, G. (2008). Nutrients and phytochemicals: From bioavailability to bioefficacy beyond antioxidants. *Current Opinion in Biotechnology* 19(2): 73–82.

Hoover, D.G., Metrick, C., Papineau, A.M., Farkas, D.F., Knorr, D. (1989). Biological effects of high hydrostatic pressure on food microorganisms. *Food Science and Technology International* 3: 99–107.

Horie, Y., Kimura, K., Ida, M., Yosida, Y., Ohki, K. (1991). Jam preparation by pressurization. *Journal of the Japan Society for Bioscience Biotechnology and Agrochemistry* 65: 975–980.

Hu, W., Zhou, L., Xu, Z., Zhang, Y., Liao, X. (2013). Enzyme inactivation in food processing using high pressure carbon dioxide technology. *Critical Reviews in Food* 53(3): 5–6.

Huang, W., Bi, X., Zhang, X., Liao, X., Hu, X., Wu, J. (2013). Comparative study of enzymes, phenolics, carotenoids and color of apricot nectars treated by high hydrostatic pressure and high temperature short time. *Innovative Food Science and Emerging Technologies* 18: 74–82.

Izquierdo, L., Carbonell, J.V., Navarro, J.L., Sendra, J.M. (2007). Method of obtaining refrigerated pasteurized citrus juices. Patent WO/2007/042593. Consejo Superior de Investigaciones Científicas, Spain.

Jolibert, F., Tonello, C., Sagegh, P., Raymond, J. (1994). Les effets des hautes pressions sur la polyphénol oxydase des fruits. *Bios Boissons* 251: 27–35.

Kalchayanand, N., Sikes, A., Dunne, C.P., Ray, B. (1998). Interaction of hydrostatic pressure, time and temperature of pressurization and pediocin AcH on inactivation of foodborne bacteria. *Journal of Food Protection* 61(4): 425–431.

Kalchayanand, N., Sikes, T., Dunne, C.P., Ray, B. (1994). Hydrostatic pressure and electroporation have increased bactericidal efficiency in combination with bacteriocins. *Applied and Environmental Microbiology* 60(11): 4174–4177.

Kleinig, A.R., Middelberg, A.P.J. (1998). On the mechanism of microbial cell disruption in high-pressure homogenisation. *Chemical Engineering Science* 53(5): 891–898.

Knorr, D. (1999). Novel approaches in food-processing technology: New technologies for preserving foods and modifying function. *Current Opinion in Biotechnology* 10(5): 485–491.

Knorr, D., Heinz, V., Buckow, R. (2006). High pressure application for food biopolymers. *Biochimica et Biophysica Acta* 1764(3): 619–631.

Krebbers, B., Matser, A. (2003). Combined high-pressure and thermal treatments for processing of tomato puree: Evaluation of microbial inactivation and quality parameters. *Innovative Food Science and Emerging Technologies* 4: 377–385.

Kupper, P.L., Moore, K.L., Swaine, R.L. (1987). Fruit juice containing diet beverage. U.S. Patent 4690827.

Lacroix, N., Fliss, I., Makhlouf, J. (2005). Inactivation of pectin methylesterase and stabilization of opalescence in orange juice by dynamic high pressure. *Food Research International* 38(5): 569–576.

Lanciotti, R., Patrignani, F., Iucci, L., Saracino, P., Guerzoni, M.E. (2007). Potential of high pressure homogenization in the control and enhancement of proteolytic and fermentative activities of some *Lactobacillus* species. *Food Chemistry* 102(2): 542–550.

Lavinas, F.C., Miguel, M.A.L., Lopes, M.L.M., Valente Mesquita, V.L. (2008). Effect of high hydrostatic pressure on cashew apple (*Anacardium occidentale* L.) juice preservation. *Journal of Food Science* 73(6): M273–M277.

Lee, H.S., Coates, G.A. (2004). Pigment extraction system and method. U.S. Patent US20040258809-A1.

Lee, J., Durst, R.W., Wrolstad, R.E. (2002). Impact of juice processing on blueberry anthocyanins and polyphenolics: Comparison of two pretreatments. *Journal of Food Science* 67(5): 1660–1667.

Lemmens, L., Van Buggenhout, S., Oey, I., Van Loey, A., Hendrickx, M. (2009). Towards a better understanding of the relationship between the β-carotene in vitro bio-accessibility and pectin structural changes: A case study on carrots. *Food Research International* 42(9): 1323–1330.

Lortkipanidze, R.K., Anikeichik, N.M., Yakobashvili, R.A., Bolkovadze, M.K. (1972). Homogenizer in citrus juice production line. *Konservnaya i Ovoshchesushil'naya Promyshlennost* 7: 9–10.

Ly Nguyen, B., Van Loey, A., Fachin, D., Verlent, I., Indrawati, I., Hendrickx, M., Hendrickx, I.M. (2002). Purification, characterization, thermal, and high-pressure inactivation of pectin methylesterase from bananas (*cv. Cavendish*). *Biotechnology and Bioengineering* 78(6): 683–691.

Macheboeuf, M.A., Basset, J. (1934). Die Wirkung sehr hoher Drucke auf enzyme. *Ergebnisse der Enzymforschung* 3: 303–308.

Macpherson, A.J., Hunziker, L., McCoy, K., Lamarre, A. (2001). IgA responses in the intestinal mucosa against pathogenic and non-pathogenic microorganisms. *Microbes and Infection* 3: 1021–1035.

Maresca, P., Donsì, F., Ferrari, G. (2011). Application of a multi-pass high-pressure homogenization treatment for the pasteurization of fruit juices. *Journal of Food Engineering* 104(3): 364–372.

Masson, P., Tonello, C., Balny, C. (2001). High-pressure biotechnology in medicine and pharmaceutical science. *Journal of Biomedicine and Biotechnology* 1(2): 85–88.

McClements, D.J., Decker, E.A., Park, Y. (2009). Controlling lipid bioavailability through physicochemical and structural approaches. *Critical Reviews in Food Science and Nutrition* 49(1): 48–67.

McKay, A.M. (2009). Inactivation of fungal spores in apple juice by high pressure homogenization. *Journal of Food Protection* 72(12): 2561–2564.

McKay, A.M., Linton, M., Stirling, J., Mackle, A., Patterson, M.F. (2011). A comparative study of changes in the microbiota of apple juice treated by high hydrostatic pressure (HHP) or high pressure homogenisation (HPH). *Food Microbiology* 28(8): 1426–1431.

Middelberg, A.P.J. (1995). Process-scale disruption of microorganisms. *Biotechnology Advances* 13(3): 491–551.

Moore, E.K., Hoare, M., Dunnill, P. (1990). Disruption of baker's yeast in a high-pressure homogenizer: New evidence on mechanism. *Enzyme and Microbial Technology* 12(10): 764–770.

Morild, E. (1981). The theory of pressure effects on enzymes. *Advances in Protein Chemistry* 34: 93–166.

Nienaber, U., Shellhammer, T.H. (2001a). High-pressure processing of orange juice: Kinetics of pectin methylesterase inactivation. *Journal of Food Science* 66(2): 328–331.

Nienaber, U., Shellhammer, T.H. (2001b). High-pressure processing of orange juice: Combination treatments and a shelf life study. *Journal of Food Science* 66(2): 332–336.

Nindo, C.I., Tang, J., Powers, J.R., Singh, P. (2005). Viscosity of blueberry and raspberry juices for processing applications. *Journal of Food Engineering* 69(3): 343–350.

Norton, T., Sun, D. (2008). Recent advances in the use of high pressure as an effective processing technique in the food industry. *Food and Bioprocess Technology* 1(1): 2–34.

Oey, I., Lille, M., Van Loey, A., Hendrickx, M. (2008). Effect of high-pressure processing on colour, texture and flavour of fruit- and vegetable-based food products: A review. *Trends in Food Science and Technology* 19(6): 320–328.

Ogawa, H., Fukuhisa, K., Kubo, Y., Fukumoto, H. (1990) Pressure inactivation of yeasts, molds, and pectinesterase in satsumamandarin juice: Effects of juice concentration, pH, and organic acids, and comparison with heat sanitation. *Agricultural and Biological Chemistry* 54: 1219–1225.

Parada, J., Aguilera, J.M. (2007). Food microstructure affects the bioavailability of several nutrients. *Journal of Food Science* 72(2): R21–R32.

Park, S., Lee, J., Park, J. (2002). Effects of a combined process of high-pressure carbon dioxide and high hydrostatic pressure on the quality of carrot juice. *Journal of Food Science* 67(5): 1827–1834.

Pathanibul, P., Taylor, T.M., Davidson, P.M., Harte, F. (2009). Inactivation of *Escherichia coli* and *Listeria innocua* in apple and carrot juices using high pressure homogenization and nisin. *International Journal of Food Microbiology* 129(3): 316–320.

Patrignani, F., Tabanelli, G., Siroli, L., Gardini, F., Lanciotti, R. (2013). Combined effects of high pressure homogenization treatment and citral on microbiological quality of apricot juice. *International Journal of Food Microbiology* 160(3): 273 281.

Patrignani, F., Vannini, L., Kamdem, S.L.S., Lanciotti, R., Guerzoni, M.E. (2009). Effect of high pressure homogenization on *Saccharomyces cerevisiae* inactivation and physico-chemical features in apricot and carrot juices. *International Journal of Food Microbiology* 136(1): 26–31.

Patrignani, F., Vannini, L., Kamdem, S.L.S., Lanciotti, R., Guerzoni, M.E. (2010) Potentialities of high-pressure homogenization to inactivate *Zygosaccharomyces bailii* in fruit juices. *Journal of Food Science* 75(2): M116–M120.

Patterson, M.F. (2005). Microbiology of pressure-treated foods. *Journal of Applied Microbiology* 98(6): 1400–1409.

Patterson, M.F., McKay, A.M., Connolly, M., Linton, M. (2012). The effect of high hydrostatic pressure on the microbiological quality and safety of carrot juice during refrigerated storage. *Food Microbiology* 30(1): 205–212.

Picart, L., Thiebaud, M., René, M., Pierre Guiraud, J., Cheftel, J.C., Dumay, E. (2006). Effects of high pressure homogenisation of raw bovine milk on alkaline phosphatase and microbial inactivation. A comparison with continuous short-time thermal treatments. *Journal of Dairy Research* 73(04): 454.

Plaza, L., Colina, C., De Ancos, B., Sánchez-Moreno, C., Pilar Cano, M. (2012). Influence of ripening and astringency on carotenoid content of high-pressure treated persimmon fruit (*Diospyros kaki* L.). *Food Chemistry* 130(3): 591–597.

Polydera, A.C., Galanou, E., Stoforos, N.G., Taoukis, P.S. (2004). Inactivation kinetics of pectin methylesterase of Greek Navel orange juice as a function of high hydrostatic pressure and temperature process conditions. *Journal of Food Engineering* 62(3): 291–298.

Popper, L., Knorr, D. (1990). Applications of high pressure homogenization for food preservation. *Food Technology* 44: 84–89.

Rawson, A., Patras, A., Tiwari, B.K., Noci, F., Koutchma, T., Brunton, N. (2011). Effect of thermal and non thermal processing technologies on the bioactive content of exotic fruits and their products: Review of recent advances. *Food Research International* 44(7): 1875–1887.

Ritz, M., Tholozan, J.L., Federighi, M., Pilet, M.F. (2001). Morphological and physiological characterization of *Listeria monocytogenes* subjected to high hydrostatic pressure. *Applied and Environmental Microbiology* 67(5): 2240–2247.

Rivalain, N., Roquain, J., Demazeau, G. (2010). Development of high hydrostatic pressure in biosciences: Pressure effect on biological structures and potential applications in biotechnologies. *Biotechnology Advances* 28(6): 659–672.

Roger, H. (1895). Action des hautes pressions sur quelques bactéries. *Archives de Physiologie Normale et Pathologique* 7: 12–17.

Rossi, M., Giussani, E., Morelli, R., Lo Scalzo, R., Nani, R.C., Torreggiani, D. (2003). Effect of fruit blanching on phenolics and radical scavenging activity of highbush blueberry juice. *Food Research International* 36(9–10): 999–1005.

Rouse, A.H. and Atkins, C.D. (1955). Pectinesterase and pectin in commercial orange juice as determined by methods used at the citrus experiment station. *Florida Agricultural Experiment Station Bulletin* 570: 1–19.

Rovere, P., Carpi, G., Maggi, A., Gola, S., Dallaglio, G. (1994). Stabilization of apricot puree by means of high pressure treatments. *Prehrambeno-Tehnoloska I Biotehnoloska Revija* 32(4): 145–150.

Royer, C.A. (2005). Insights into the role of hydration in protein structure and stability obtained through hydrostatic pressure studies. *Brazilian Journal of Medical and Biological Research* 38(8): 1167–1173.

Sampedro, F., Fan, X., Rodrigo, D. (2010). *High Hydrostatic Pressure Processing of Fruit Juices and Smoothies: Research and Commercial Application*. Cambridge: Woodhead Publishing.

Seyderhelm, I., Boguslawski, S., Michaelis, G., Knorr, D. (1996). Pressure induced inactivation of selected food enzymes. *Journal of Food Science* 61(2): 308–310.

Siddiqi, S.F., Titchener-Hooker, N.J., Shamlou, P.A. (1997). High pressure disruption of yeast cells: The use of scale down operations for the prediction of protein release and cell debris size distribution. *Biotechnology and Bioengineering* 55(4): 642–649.

Silva, J.L., Foguel, D. (2009). Hydration, cavities and volume in protein folding, aggregation and amyloid assembly. *Physical Biology* 6(1): 015002.

Singh, S., Gamlath, S., Wakeling, L. (2007) Nutritional aspects of food extrusion: A review. *International Journal of Food Science and Technology* 42(8): 916–929.

Smeller, L. (2002). Pressure–temperature phase diagrams of biomolecules. *Biochimica Et Biophysica Acta (BBA)—Protein Structure and Molecular Enzymology* 1595(1–2): 11–29.

Smelt, J.P.P.M. (1998). Recent advances in the microbiology of high pressure processing. *Trends in Food Science and Technology* 9(4): 152–158.

Srivastava, A., Akoh, C.C., Yi, W., Fischer, J., Krewer, G. (2007). Effect of storage conditions on the biological activity of phenolic compounds of blueberry extract packed in glass bottles. *Journal of Agricultural and Food Chemistry* 55(7): 2705–2713.

Stang, M., Schuchmann, H., Schubert, H. (2001). Emulsification in high-pressure homogenizers. *Engineering in Life Sciences* 1(4): 151–157.

Suárez-Jacobo, Á., Rüfer, C.E., Gervilla, R., Guamis, B., Roig-Sagués, A.X., Saldo, J. (2011). Influence of ultra-high pressure homogenisation on antioxidant capacity, polyphenol and vitamin content of clear apple juice. *Food Chemistry* 127(2): 447–454.

Suárez-Jacobo, Á., Saldo, J., Rüfer, C.E., Guamis, B., Roig-Sagués, A.X., Gervilla, R. (2012). Aseptically packaged UHPH-treated apple juice: Safety and quality parameters during storage. *Journal of Food Engineering* 109(2): 291–300.

Suthanthangjai, W., Kajda, P., Zabetakis, I. (2005). The effect of high hydrostatic pressure on the anthocyanins of raspberry (*Rubus idaeus*). *Food Chemistry* 90: 193–197.

Svelander, C.A., Lopez-Sanchez, P., Pudney, P.D.A., Schumm, S., Alminger, M.A.G. (2011). High pressure homogenization increases the in vitro bioaccessibility of α- and β-carotene in carrot emulsions but not of lycopene in tomato emulsions. *Journal of Food Science* 76(9): H215–H225.

Tabanelli, G., Burns, P., Patrignani, F., Gardini, F., Lanciotti, R., Reinheimer, J., Vinderola, G. (2012). Effect of a non-lethal high pressure homogenization treatment on the *in vivo* response of probiotic lactobacilli. *Food Microbiology* 32(2): 302–307.

Tahiri, I., Makhlouf, J., Paquin, P., Fliss, I. (2006). Inactivation of food spoilage bacteria and *Escherichia coli* O157:H7 in phosphate buffer and orange juice using dynamic high pressure. *Food Research International* 39(1): 98–105.

Tanaka, T., Hatanaka, K. (1992) Application of hydrostatic pressure to yoghurt to prevent its after-acidification. *Journal of Japanese Society of Food Science and Technology* 39: 173–177.

Thiebaud, M., Dumay, E., Picart, L., Guiraud, J.P., Cheftel, J.C. (2003). High-pressure homogenisation of raw bovine milk. Effects on fat globule size distribution and microbial inactivation. *International Dairy Journal* 13(6): 427–439.

Timson, W.J., Short, A.J. (1965). Resistance of microorganisms to hydrostatic pressure. *Biotechnology and Bioengineering* 7: 139–159.

Tsou, C.L. (1986). Location of the active sites of some enzymes in limited and flexible molecular regions. *Trends in Biochemical Sciences* 11(10): 427–429.

Uckoo, R.M., Jayaprakasha, G.K., Somerville, J.A., Balasubramaniam, V.M., Pinarte, M., Patil, B.S. (2013). High pressure processing controls microbial growth and minimally alters the levels of health promoting compounds in grapefruit (*Citrus paradisi* Macfad) juice. *Innovative Food Science and Emerging Technologies* 18: 7–14.

Van den Broeck, I., Ludikhuyze, L.R., Van Locy, A.M., Hendrickx, M.E. (2000). Effect of temperature and/or pressure on tomato pectinesterase activity. *Journal of Agricultural and Food Chemistry* 48(2): 551–558.

Varela-Santos, E., Ochoa-Martinez, A., Tabilo-Munizaga, G., Reyes, J.E., Pérez-Won, M., Briones-Labarca, V., Morales-Castro, J. (2012). Effect of high hydrostatic pressure (HHP) processing on physicochemical properties, bioactive compounds and shelf-life of pomegranate juice. *Innovative Food Science and Emerging Technologies* 13: 13–22.

Velázquez-Estrada, R.M., Hernández-Herrero, M.M., Guamis-López, B., Roig-Sagués, A.X. (2012). Impact of ultra high pressure homogenization on pectin methylesterase activity and microbial characteristics of orange juice: A comparative study against conventional heat pasteurization. *Innovative Food Science Emerging Technologies* 13: 100–106.

Velázquez-Estrada, R.M., Hernández-Herrero, M.M., Rüfer, C.E., Guamis-López, B., Roig-Sagués, A.X. (2013). Influence of ultra high pressure homogenization processing on bioactive compounds and antioxidant activity of orange juice. *Innovative Food Science and Emerging Technologies* 18(0): 89–94.

Vervoort, L., Van der Plancken, I., Grauwet, T., Timmermans, R.A.H., Mastwijk, H.C., Matser, A.M., Hendrickx, M.E., Van Loey, A. (2011). Comparing equivalent thermal, high pressure and pulsed electric field processes for mild pasteurization of orange juice: Part II: Impact on specific chemical and biochemical quality parameters. *Innovative Food Science and Emerging Technologies* 12(4): 466–477.

Wilson, D.C. (1974). High pressure sterilization. Presented at 34th Annual Meeting of the Institute of Food Technologists. May 12–15, New Orleans, LA.

Winter, R., Dzwolak, W. (2005). Exploring the temperature–pressure configurational landscape of biomolecules: From lipid membranes to proteins. *Philosophical Transactions of the Royal Society A: Mathematical, Physical and Engineering Sciences* 363(1827): 537–563.

Wuytack, E.Y., Diels, A.M.J., Michiels, C.W. (2002). Bacterial inactivation by high-pressure homogenisation and high hydrostatic pressure. *International Journal of Food Microbiology* 77(3): 205–212.

Zabetakis, I., Leclerc, D., Kajda, P. (2000). The effect of high hydrostatic pressure on the strawberry anthocyanins. *Journal of Agricultural and Food Chemistry* 48(7): 2749–2754.

Zeece, M., Huppertz, T., Kelly, A. (2008). Effect of high-pressure treatment on *in-vitro* digestibility of β-lactoglobulin. *Innovative Food Science and Emerging Technologies* 9(1): 62–69.

Zhao, L., Wang, S., Liu, F., Dong, P., Huang, W., Xiong, L., Liao, X. (2013). Comparing the effects of high hydrostatic pressure and thermal pasteurization combined with nisin on the quality of cucumber juice drinks. *Innovative Food Science and Emerging Technologies* 17: 27–36.

13 Membrane Processes in Juice Production

María Isabel Iborra, María Isabel Alcaina, and Silvia Álvarez

CONTENTS

13.1 Fruit Juice Industry Background 265
13.2 Common Separations in the Juice Fruit Industry 266
13.3 Basic Concepts of Membrane Processes 268
    13.3.1 Membrane Definition 268
    13.3.2 Types of Membrane Processes 269
    13.3.3 Membrane Concepts, Terms, and Operations 269
    13.3.4 Concentration Polarization 270
    13.3.5 Membrane Fouling 272
    13.3.6 Membrane Structure 273
    13.3.7 Modules and Process Design 273
13.4 Membrane Processes 275
    13.4.1 Pressure-Driven Processes 275
    13.4.2 Electrodialysis 276
    13.4.3 Pervaporation 278
    13.4.4 Novel Membrane Processes 279
        13.4.4.1 Direct Osmosis Concentration 279
        13.4.4.2 Membrane Distillation 280
        13.4.4.3 Osmotic Distillation 280
13.5 Membrane Applications in the Fruit Juice Industry 281
    13.5.1 Clarification 281
    13.5.2 Concentration 287
    13.5.3 Deacidification 288
    13.5.4 Aroma Recovery 289
13.6 Integrated Membrane Processes 293
References 296

13.1 FRUIT JUICE INDUSTRY BACKGROUND

Nowadays the fruit juice industry needs a common basis for the assessment of quality, safety, and authenticity of fruit and vegetable juices that are produced in the single European market. In fruit juice processing, membrane technology is mainly used for several proposes: clarification of the juice by means of ultrafiltration (UF) and microfiltration (MF), deacidification by electrodialysis, recovery of aroma compounds by pervaporation and membrane distillation, and concentration or preconcentration of the juice by means of nanofiltration, reverse osmosis (RO), membrane distillation, or direct osmosis.

The high temperatures required during fruit juice production by means of traditional thermal evaporation processes produce a significant reduction of functional properties (vitamin content, flavors, and colors of the juices).

Membrane techniques are able to concentrate fruit juices up to 60°Brix–65°Brix (Jiao et al. 2004) or even higher, operating at or near room temperature, demonstrating their capacity to offer fruit juices of comparable quality to freshly squeezed fruit juices. These technologies offer a competitive and attractive alternative to the conventional separation techniques (filtration, evaporation, centrifugation, etc.), alone or in integrated hybrid membrane systems, which in most cases represent the best solution to a specific industrial separation problem, offering good-quality fruit juices for sale with reliable and stable properties.

Some of the advantages of membrane processes over conventional separation technologies are:

- Mild temperatures, which cause moderate changes in the product during processing
- High selectivity of the separation mechanisms (sieving, solution-diffusion or ion-exchange mechanisms)
- Compact and modular design, ease of installation, operation, and modification
- Low energy consumption compared with the evaporative process
- Clean technology, because no additional chemicals are required

However, the main disadvantage of membrane processes is the fouling of the membrane, which causes a decline in the flux and, therefore, a loss of productivity. This effect can be minimized by means of regular cleaning steps; it is common in this type of industry to clean equipment at least every 24 h. Other options to minimize fouling are directly related to the design and operation of the plant, membrane selection parameters (e.g., hydrophilic membranes result in a low level of fouling), and the choice of membrane modules with the appropriate dimensions and configuration (Malik et al. 2013; Susanto et al. 2007).

The lifetime of the membrane is crucial for the implementation of these processes at the industrial scale, as they usually require pressures and temperatures that may negatively affect the durability of the membrane materials over time.

Both the requirement of periodic replacement of the membranes and the fact that they are easy to damage will ultimately affect the economics of the process, which may become too expensive.

13.2   COMMON SEPARATIONS IN THE JUICE FRUIT INDUSTRY

Nowadays, most fruit juices are concentrated up to 60°Brix–75°Brix in order to reduce storage, packaging, handling, and shipping costs. Concentration has also solved the problem of the seasonal nature of crops and allowed the economic utilization of perishable products.

Juice characteristics may vary according to the type of fruit juice considered and the market region. For example, grape and apple juices are normally commercialized only after a clarification process, and orange juice is preferentially consumed at a lower level of clarity.

The conventional method for fruit juice concentration is evaporation. It is performed in multiple-effect evaporators at temperatures between 45°C and 90°C. It is common practice to recover and concentrate the volatile aroma compounds from the vapor by means of distillation. Therefore, an aroma concentrate and a concentrated dearomatized juice are obtained. This conventional process has a number of drawbacks, such as important losses of volatile aroma compounds, heat degradation of valuable compounds, color changes, development of a "cooked" aftertaste, and high energy consumption. Membrane concentration processes, such as RO, nanofiltration, membrane distillation, direct osmosis, and osmotic distillation can overcome most of these problems. In addition, certain membrane processes (pervaporation, membrane distillation) can also be used to obtain fruit juice aroma concentrates (Cassano and Drioli 2007).

In pulpy juices, the raw juice obtained after pressing is very turbid, viscous, and of a dark color, and contains a lot of colloidal compounds that are stabilized in suspension by polysaccharides such as pectin, starch, cellulose, and gums. Therefore, many juices are clarified prior to their concentration. Clarification is performed to remove the juice components that cause cloudiness, mainly pectin.

In conventional processes, juice clarification begins with depectinization by the addition of proteolytic enzymes. The enzymes are able to hydrolyze pectin molecules and cause pectin–protein complexes to flocculate. The viscosity of the juice is reduced, so that it is much easier to filter. Amylases are usually added as well to break down the starch molecules, which can cause cloudiness during storage. Afterward, fining agents are added to enhance the settling of the formed flocs, gelatin being the most common agent. Other suitable fining agents are bentonite, tannic acid, and silica sol. Settled solids and suspended matter are then removed by conventional filtration. Filter aids such as diatomaceous earth (kieselguhr) are used to facilitate the filtration step. These processes are labor-intensive, time-consuming, and discontinuously operated. The utilization of additives (fining agents and filter aids) may leave a slight aftertaste in the juice. Moreover, the solids removed after filtration, which contain enzymes, fining agents, and filter aids, cannot be reused and cause pollution problems (Alvarez et al. 2000).

Dark colors in fruit juices are caused by browning reactions. The browning of fruit and fruit products is a major problem in the fruit industry and one of the main causes of loss of quality during processing. It has not only a negative impact on color, but also on other sensory properties, including aroma and texture. The process that makes fruit and fruit products turn brown can be enzymatic or nonenzymatic. Enzymatic browning starts with the oxidation of phenols to quinones by the enzyme polyphenol oxidase in the presence of oxygen. Nonenzymatic browning is mainly due to the Maillard reaction between amino groups and reducing sugars. This reaction takes place during the thermal treatment of fruit products (Echavarría et al. 2011). Therefore, operation at low temperatures is of interest.

MF and UF are very promising alternatives to conventional clarification processes. Membranes can be continuously operated, they require less labor and processing time, and work at mild temperatures. Moreover, MF and UF membranes are able to retain microorganisms, avoiding the need for thermal pasteurization processes, and UF is able to remove polyphenol oxidases, which is effective in stabilizing the colors of fruit juices.

Finally, the high acidity of some juices, especially tropical fruit juices, limits their use. Some conventional processes that have been tested to deacidify fruit juices include calcium salt precipitation, which involves the addition of chemicals, and ion exchange, which strongly modifies the aroma profile and provides effluents during the regeneration process. The membrane process of electrodialysis can overcome most of these drawbacks (Vera et al. 2003).

13.3 BASIC CONCEPTS OF MEMBRANE PROCESSES

13.3.1 Membrane Definition

The membrane is a semipermeable barrier that separates two phases and limits the transport of several species, soluble or not, in a specific way. It is permeable to some and impermeable to others (Figure 13.1). The feed composition changes in the membrane, creating two separate streams: *permeate* and *retentate* or concentrate stream. Such membranes are termed *semipermeable* and are usually in the form of thin sheets of synthetic material in different configurations. Depending on the material used for membrane preparation, synthetic membranes can be organic (polymeric or liquid) or inorganic (ceramic, glass, or metal) membranes.

Since the amount of a species transported across a membrane is inversely proportional to the thickness of the membrane, it is advantageous to have the thinnest membrane possible. In practice, considerations such as mechanical strength usually determine the lower limit of membrane thickness. In many cases, synthetic polymers are used, and many have been developed especially to provide the required

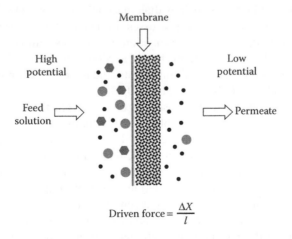

FIGURE 13.1 Transport of components from membrane.

semipermeable characteristics. The particle or molecule is transported across the membrane because of the action of a driving force. The extent of this is determined by the gradient in the driving force across the membrane (i.e., the difference in potential across the membrane divided by the membrane thickness).

The main applications in the food industry are: concentration, sterilization, and fractionation of products; solute removal from solutions (e.g., desalination and demineralization); purification; and clarification. Some of the factors that are utilized in membrane-based separation are: solute size, solute shape, electrostatic charge, and diffusivity.

13.3.2 TYPES OF MEMBRANE PROCESSES

Depending on the process, the driving force may be mechanical (pressure), chemical (concentration), thermal (temperature), or electric potential (voltage). In the majority of industrial applications, this membrane is a thin solid barrier, although the active component of a membrane may also be a liquid, gas, or vapor.

In Table 13.1, the main membrane processes are classified according to the driving forces.

13.3.3 MEMBRANE CONCEPTS, TERMS, AND OPERATIONS

The performance or efficiency of a membrane can be defined in terms of several parameters:

- *Permeation flux* is defined as the volume flowing through the membrane per unit area and time. The SI units used are meters cubed per meter squared per second ($m^3 \cdot m^{-2} \cdot s^{-1}$) although other units are often used as well.

TABLE 13.1

Driving Forces in Membrane Processes

Driving Force	Membrane Processes	Permeate Compounds	Retentate Compounds
Pressure gradient	Reverse Osmosis	Solvents	Solutes
	Nanofiltration	Small molecules	Large molecules
	Ultrafiltration		
	Microfiltration		
Partial pressure gradient	Pervaporation	Volatile compounds	Nonvolatile solutes
	Gas separation	Gas molecules	Larger gas molecules
Electric potential gradient	Electrodialysis	Ionic solutes	Solvents
	Membrane electrolysis		Nonionic solutes
			Larger solutes
Concentration gradient	Dialysis	Solvents	Solutes
		Small molecules	Larger solutes
Temperature gradient	Membrane distillation	Solvents	Ionic solutes
		Volatile compounds	Nonvolatile solutes
			Larger molecules

- *Selectivity* indicates the ability of a membrane to discriminate between species in the original solution. The selectivity of a membrane can be expressed in two ways depending on the membrane process being considered.

The retention coefficient R is generally used in membrane systems that use pressure as the driving force. A definition of the retention coefficient is shown in Equation 13.1:

$$R = \frac{c_{R,m} - c_P}{c_{R,m}} \tag{13.1}$$

where $c_{R,m}$ is the concentration of species at the membrane surface on the retentate side and c_p is the concentration in the permeate.

- *Separation factor* (α): Selectivity is normally expressed in terms of a separation factor for mixtures containing two components i and j. For these cases, and with i as the most mobile component, the separation factor (α_{ij}) is expressed as:

$$\alpha_{ij} = \frac{c_{i,P}/c_{j,P}}{c_{i,R}/c_{j,R}} \tag{13.2}$$

where $c_{i,P}$, $c_{i,R}$ and $c_{j,P}$, $c_{j,R}$ are the concentrations in the permeate and retentate at the membrane interfaces for components i and j, respectively.

13.3.4 CONCENTRATION POLARIZATION

In membrane separation processes, the fluid flow through the membrane convectively transports the solute molecules to the membrane surface. At the beginning of the process (the nonsteady state), the amount of solute that is transported toward the membrane is much larger than the amount of solute that turns back to the bulk solution by diffusion. Therefore, solute accumulation occurs at the membrane surface until the equilibrium between convective and diffusive fluxes is reached (Miranda and Campos 2001). This phenomenon is called concentration polarization and is illustrated in Figure 13.2.

Due to the increase of solute concentration at the membrane surface, concentration polarization causes a decrease of solvent flux across the membrane. Moreover, at a certain concentration of solutes, the mixture of solutes and solvent can form a gel on the membrane surface.

The ratio of feed solution concentration at the membrane surface (c_m) to the bulk solution concentration (c_b) is known as the *concentration polarization modulus* (γ_{CP}), and is a useful measure of the extent of concentration polarization. This modulus can be larger or smaller than 1.0, depending on the separation process considered:

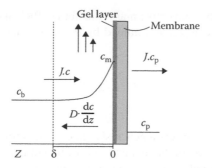

FIGURE 13.2 Concentration polarization: concentration profile under steady-state conditions.

$$\gamma_{CP} = \frac{c_m}{c_p} \tag{13.3}$$

The *membrane concentration factor* (η) is defined as the ratio of the retentate concentration (c_R) with respect to the bulk solution concentration (c_b) as:

$$\eta = \frac{c_R}{c_b} \tag{13.4}$$

Once a gel layer is formed, the permeate flux decreases significantly. At the steady state, the local concentration does not change with time; hence, the two effects (solute transport toward the membranes and back diffusion) must be in equilibrium. Assuming Fick's law for back diffusion, the steady state condition can be written as follows:

$$J \cdot c - D \cdot \frac{dc}{dz} = J \cdot c_p \quad \Rightarrow \quad \int_0^\delta J \cdot (c - c_p) \cdot dz = \int_{c_m}^{c_b} D \cdot dc \tag{13.5}$$

where:
c is the concentration of the solute (c_m at the membrane interface, c_b in the bulk) (kg·m^3)
J is the solvent flux (m^3·m^{-2}·s^{-1})
D is the diffusivity of the solute in the solvent (m^2·s^{-1})
z is the distance from the membrane (m)
δ is the thickness of the boundary layer for diffusion (m)
The integration of Equation 13.5 gives

$$J = \frac{D}{\delta} \cdot \ln \frac{c_m - c_p}{c_b - c_p} \tag{13.6}$$

where (D/δ) is called the convective mass transfer coefficient in liquid phase (k).

When the solute is completely retained by the membrane $(c_p=0)$, Equation 13.6 becomes

$$J = k \cdot \ln \frac{c_m}{c_b} \tag{13.7}$$

The gel polarized layer offers a new resistance to mass transfer. The formation of a gel layer is very common in the membrane filtration of macromolecules in specific proteins, and is considered a type of membrane fouling.

13.3.5 MEMBRANE FOULING

One of the main drawbacks of membrane technology is the fouling of the membrane, which is caused by the accumulation of solute molecules on the membrane surface or inside the pores. Membrane fouling causes a reduction of the permeate flux and also causes changes in selectivity and decreases the overall process productivity. The permeate flux can be restored by means of cleaning procedures, but the process must be stopped and large amounts of chemicals, energy, water, and time are consumed. Moreover, successive membrane cleaning operations can reduce the life of the membrane.

In porous membranes, fouling is mainly caused by two phenomena: the formation of a gel or cake layer on the membrane surface and the obstruction of the membrane pores. The obstruction of the pores may be complete when particles are larger than the pore size or partial when the particles are small enough to enter a pore. In this case, the particles enter the pores and are deposited or adsorbed, reducing the pore volume. The different modes of membrane fouling are shown in Figure 13.3. Different physical or chemical phenomena may take place and contribute to membrane fouling, such as physical adsorption, deposition of molecules on the membrane surface, interactions between different solutes in the feed stream, formation of complexed species, and so on (Martí-Calatayud et al. 2010).

Membrane fouling is a complex phenomenon that is greatly affected by the operating conditions, membrane properties, and feed characteristics, and also by the complex

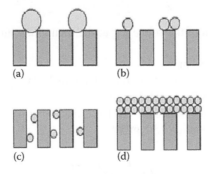

FIGURE 13.3 Illustration of membrane fouling mechanisms. (a) Complete pore blocking. (b) Partial pore blocking. (c) Internal pore blocking. (d) Cake layer formation.

interactions among all these factors. Therefore, the right choice of operating conditions (temperature, pressure, cross-flow velocity, and volume concentration ratio) and membrane characteristics (membrane material, dimensions, and configuration) can significantly reduce the effect of fouling on the performance of the process. Mathematical models can predict the permeate flux decline with time due to fouling and can identify the type of fouling that takes place. Some of the models can describe the effect of the operating parameters on fouling, which is useful when optimizing the process.

13.3.6 MEMBRANE STRUCTURE

The separation ability of a synthetic material depends on its physical and chemical properties (pore size, structure, design, chemical characteristics, and electrical charge).

Allowing for the structure, membranes can be divided into two main groups: *porous* and *nonporous*. Porous membranes achieve separation due to the size, shape, and charge of the species, while nonporous membranes achieve separation due to the selective adsorption and diffusion of the species.

Again, two types of membranes may be distinguished depending on the morphology of the cross-section structure: symmetric (when it is uniform) or asymmetric membranes (when it is not uniform).

We can observe in Figure 13.4 that both structures are asymmetric. In these kinds of membranes, selectivity and resistance to mass transfer are both determined largely or completely by the thin top layer.

13.3.7 MODULES AND PROCESS DESIGN

Membrane plants often require large membrane areas to carry out a given separation; therefore, for good development of technology on an industrial scale, it becomes necessary to employ smaller units into which the membrane area is packed, offering a higher area/volume ratio of membrane. The smallest unit into which the membrane area is packed is called a module.

The membranes can be cast in two types of configuration: flat sheets and tubular. To accommodate such types, a number of module designs are possible. Plate-and-frame

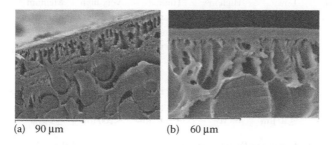

(a) 90 μm   (b) 60 μm

FIGURE 13.4 Cross-section of asymmetric membranes. (a) Porous ultrafiltration membrane. (b) Nonporous reverse-osmosis membrane.

and spiral-wound modules involve flat membrane configurations, whereas tubular, capillary, and hollow-fiber modules are based on tubular membrane configurations. The difference between the latter types of module arises mainly from the dimensions of the diameter of the tubes employed, as shown in Figure 13.5.

Table 13.2 shows a summary of the characteristics of these membrane elements.

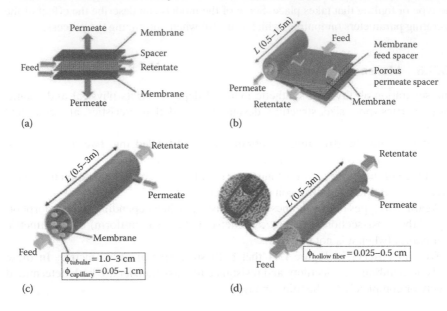

FIGURE 13.5   Schematic module designs. (a) Plate and frame. (b) Spiral wound. (c) Tubular and capillary. (d) Hollow fiber.

TABLE 13.2

Characteristics of Membrane Elements

Element Type	Spiral Wound	Tubular	Plate and Frame	Capillary	Hollow Fiber	Ceramic
Membrane area density (m² m⁻³)	High	Low	Average	Average	Very high	Low
Investment costs	Low	High/low	High	Very high	Medium	Very high
Fouling capacity	Average	Low	Average	Low	Very high	Medium
Easy to clean	Good	Good	Good	Poor	Impossible	Very good
Variable costs	Low	High/low	Average	Average	Low	High
Membrane replacement	No	Yes/no	Yes	No	No	Yes
Feed flow demand	Medium	High/ medium	Medium	High	Low	Very high
Prefilter grade	≤50 μm	Sieve	≤100 μm	≤100 μm	≤5 μm	Sieve

Source: Wagner, J., *Membrane Filtration Handbook: Practical Tips and Hints*, 2nd edn, Minnetonka, Osmonics, MN: 2001.

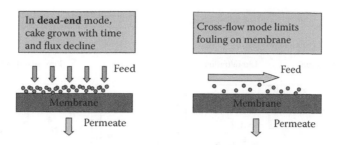

FIGURE 13.6 Operation modes: dead-end and cross-flow modes.

Membranes can be operated in two different ways, as depicted in Figure 13.6. The simplest operating mode is the dead-end operation; in this case, all feed is forced through the membrane, resulting in a buildup of fouling, which results in a loss of performance. In dead-end membrane filtration, frequent cleaning is a necessity. For the more industrial applications, the cross-flow mode is preferred, because membrane fouling is lower. In the cross-flow mode the feed flows parallel to the membrane surface.

13.4 MEMBRANE PROCESSES

13.4.1 PRESSURE-DRIVEN PROCESSES

Pressure-driven processes are most often used. The driving force or transmembrane pressure, which is necessary for these filtration processes, has to overcome the resistance of the feed solution to filtration. This resistance is due to the addition of the resistance of the membrane, the resistance by adsorption, and the clogging of the pores of the membrane, the covering layer at feed side (osmotic pressure) and concentration polarization.

The classification of pressure-driven processes is carried out according to the range of pressures applied to them. Table 13.3 and Figure 13.7 provide an overview of the pressure-driven membrane process, with possible applications.

There are essentially two mechanisms responsible for the mass transfer in these processes: *transfer by pores* and *transfer due to diffusion*. In MF and UF the separation is by transfer through the pores. All the particles that are larger than the membrane pores

TABLE 13.3

Pressure-Driven Membrane Processes

Membrane Processes	Size of Particles Separated	Transmembrane Pressure (MPa)
Microfiltration	Solids >0.1 μm	0.01–0.3
Ultrafiltration	20,000–200,000 Da	0.01–0.5
Nanofiltration	200–20,000 Da	0.3–2.0
Reverse osmosis	<200 Da	0.5–7.0

Note: Da, Dalton: numerically equivalent to molecular weight (g mol⁻¹).

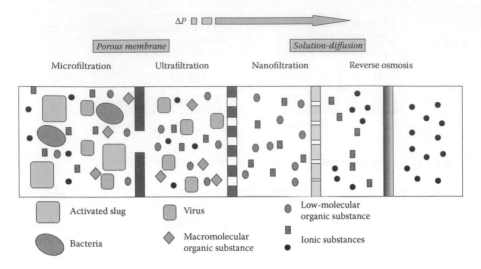

FIGURE 13.7 Applications of characteristics of pressure-driven membrane process.

are retained completely while the smaller ones cross the membrane. Nevertheless, the particles retained on the membrane surface can develop a covering layer that could retain small particles which, without this layer, would pass through the membrane.

Nanofiltration (NF) is a pressure-driven membrane process where the operational pressure and separation size are categorized between those of RO and UF. By means of NF membranes, the retention rate for particles with a molecular mass greater than 200 Da is high. Typical of NF membranes is their ion selectivity. The retention of a dissolved salt is determined by the valence of the anion. Therefore, most of the anions (e.g., Cl^-) can pass through the membrane, while multivalent anions (e.g., SO_4^{2-}) are retained by the membranes.

Finally, RO membranes are nonporous membranes that can retain completely dissolved matter with a molecular weight of less than 200 Da.

The solution-diffusion model is the generally accepted mechanism for describing permeation through RO membranes:

$$J = A \cdot (\Delta P - \Delta \pi) \tag{13.8}$$

where:
J is the permeate flux
A is the water permeability of the membrane
ΔP is the transmembrane pressure
$\Delta \pi$ is the osmotic pressure difference between both sides of the membrane

13.4.2 ELECTRODIALYSIS

Electrodialysis (ED) is a membrane process in which an electrical potential difference acts as a driving force. The charged ions or molecules are transported through permselective membranes under the effect of an electrical field, whereas uncharged molecules are not affected, and hence electrically charged components can be separated from their uncharged counterparts (Mulder, 2000; Baker, 1999).

ED membranes are sheets of ion-exchange materials. Two types of membranes may be distinguished:

- Cation-exchange membranes, which allow the passage of positively charged cations
- Anion-exchange membranes, which allow the passage of negatively charged anions

In the ED process, only ions are transferred through the membranes, while the diluate and concentrate streams are pumped at the same pressure. One of the first uses of ED was the desalination of brackish water. The principal applications of ED in food processing are desalting, demineralization, deacidification, and acidification of liquid foods.

The principle of the ED process is depicted in Figure 13.8. The electrically charged membranes are assembled in an alternating pattern between a cathode and an anode to remove ions from aqueous solutions.

The discrimination between ions of the same charge depends on the pore size of the membrane. Electrodes (an anode and a cathode) are placed between the stack compartments, and when the voltage source is connected, the migration of ions occurs. Cations tend to move toward the negative electrode (cathode) and are stopped by anion-exchange membranes, while anions move toward the anode and are stopped by cation-exchange membranes.

The purpose of the ED system shown is to deplete the product stream (diluate) from its ions by transporting them to the carrier stream (concentrate). For commercial applications, several hundreds of cell pairs are assembled in a stack.

Conventional ED can be combined with so-called bipolar membranes constituting a bipolar membrane electrodialysis (BME) stack. Bipolar membranes are composed of a cation-exchange membrane, an anion-exchange membrane, and a hydrophilic interface at their junction. When a direct current is applied in an aqueous media, the

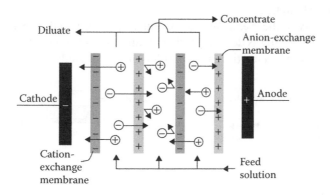

FIGURE 13.8 Scheme of electrodialysis principle.

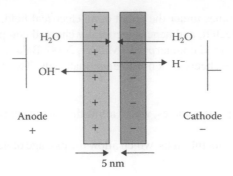

FIGURE 13.9   Scheme of bipolar membrane electrodialysis.

water molecules migrate into the hydrophilic layer where they are dissociated, generating hydroxyl ions (OH−) and protons (H+) that move to the opposite electrodes (Figure 13.9). The H+ and OH− ions can react with anions (organic or inorganic) or cations to obtain acids and alkalis simultaneously with high energy efficiency (Riera and Alvarez 2012).

13.4.3   PERVAPORATION

Pervaporation is a relatively new membrane separation process based on the selective vaporization of some components through the membranes due to their higher affinity with and quicker diffusivity in the membrane (Neel 1991) by the action of the driving force.

In pervaporation, the liquid mixture to be separated (feed) is placed in contact with one side of a membrane and the permeated product is removed as a low-pressure vapor from the other side (Figure 13.10). The permeate vapor can be condensed and collected or released as desired. The chemical potential gradient across the membrane is the driving force for mass transport. The driving force can be created by applying either a vacuum pump or an inert purge (normally air or steam) on the permeate side to maintain the permeate vapor pressure lower than the partial pressure of the feed liquid.

The selectivity of the membrane may be quantified by two dimensionless ratios, the *separation factor* (α) as defined previously, and the *enrichment factor* (β), which is most often used when multicomponent solutions are treated:

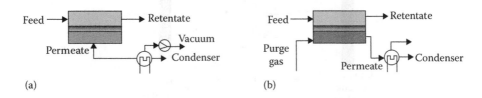

FIGURE 13.10   Schematic diagram of the pervaporation separation. (a) Vacuum pervaporation. (b) Purge gas pervaporation.

$$\beta_i = \frac{x_{P,i}}{x_{F,i}} \tag{13.9}$$

where:

x is the mole fraction

i and j are the fastest and the slowest permeants, respectively

F and P refer to the feed and permeate streams, respectively

Vacuum pervaporation is the most standard operation mode, while inert purge pervaporation is normally of interest if the permeate can be discharged without condensation. Besides these two modes of operation, there are several other variants, including thermal pervaporation, osmotic distillation, and saturated vapor permeation (Franken et al. 1990).

Pervaporation involves simultaneous mass and heat transfer, but the principle of separation is different from that of distillation, since it does not depend on vapor–liquid equilibrium; rather, it is dependent on the solubilities and diffusivities of the components of the mixture in the membrane material.

Most of the industrial applications are focused on the recovery of highly diluted compounds from the feed liquid mixture.

13.4.4 Novel Membrane Processes

The main disadvantage of RO is its inability to reach concentrations similar to those obtained by evaporation techniques, due to osmotic pressure limitations. Novel techniques such as direct osmosis concentration (DOC), membrane distillation (MD), and osmotic distillation (OD) can achieve improvements in this area.

13.4.4.1 Direct Osmosis Concentration

Direct osmosis concentration (DOC) is a membrane process that is capable of concentrating streams at low pressures and temperatures, thereby maintaining the original flavor and color characteristics.

An osmotic agent (OA) solution is used to establish an osmotic pressure gradient across a semipermeable membrane and thus remove water from the feed.

An OA is generally a solid that is highly soluble in water, hygroscopic, inert as regards the flavor, odor, and color, and nontoxic (sodium chloride, glucose, glycerol, etc.). The OA solution should have an osmotic pressure higher than the concentrated stream.

Unlike RO, pressure differences across the membrane are negligible and flux depends on the gradient in the osmotic potential. The only hydraulic pressure necessary is to pump the feed solution and the OA over the membrane surface (Figure 13.11).

The DOC process utilizes a new generation of thin film composite (TFC) RO membranes with a molecular weight cutoff (MWCO) lower than 100 Da. The solute retention is higher than 99% and the permeate flux is relatively low (5–6 L m^{-2} h^{-1}), and is necessary to evaluate the duration of the membrane.

This process is a novel technology that requires evaluation on an industrial scale.

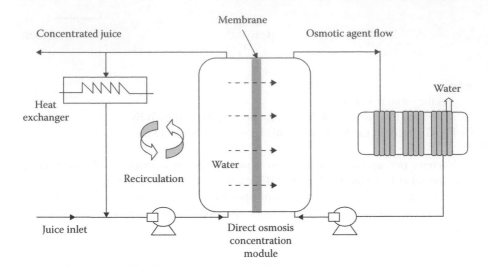

FIGURE 13.11 Concentration process by direct osmosis. (From Jiao, B., Cassano, A., and Drioli, E., *Journal of Food Engineering*, 63, 303–624, 2004.)

13.4.4.2 Membrane Distillation

Membrane distillation (MD) is a relatively new process in which two aqueous solutions at different temperatures are separated by a microporous hydrophobic membrane.

Under these conditions, a net flow of water from the warm side to the cold side occurs. This process occurs at atmospheric pressure and the temperatures may be much lower than the boiling points of the solutions. The driving force, in this case, is the vapor pressure difference between the two interfaces (solution–membrane) due to the temperature gradient.

This phenomenon consists of three steps:

1. Formation of a vapor gap at the warm side of the solution–membrane interface
2. Transport of the vapor phase through the microporous membrane
3. Condensation on the cold side of the membrane–solution interface

The MD process can be used to concentrate solutes that are sensitive to high temperatures, also at high osmotic pressure (e.g., fruit juice). The membranes usually employed are laminated hydrophobic microporous membranes, typical UF membranes, with pore sizes between 0.2 and 0.4 µm.

13.4.4.3 Osmotic Distillation

This is a relatively recent membrane process (Lefebvre 1988), also known as "osmotic evaporation," "membrane evaporation," "isothermal membrane distillation," or "gas membrane extraction," which has been successfully applied to the concentration of liquid foods such as milk, fruit and vegetable juices, instant coffee and tea, and various nonfood aqueous solutions. This technique can be used to selectively extract the water from aqueous solutions under atmospheric pressure and at room temperature, thus avoiding thermal degradation of the solutions. A microporous hydrophobic membrane separates two circulating aqueous solutions at different solute concentrations.

While the operating pressure is kept below the capillary penetration pressure of the liquid into the pores, the membrane cannot be wetted by the solutions. The difference in the solute concentrations of both solutions generates a vapor pressure difference, causing a vapor transfer from the dilute solution toward the stripping solution in the vapor–liquid interface.

The water transport through the membrane can be summarized in three steps:

1. Evaporation of water at the dilute vapor–liquid interface
2. Diffusion or convective transport of vapor through the membrane pore
3. Condensation of water vapor at the membrane–brine interface

The osmotic distillation (OD) process involves the use of concentrated brines on the downstream side of the membrane as stripping solutions. Those most often employed are $MgSO_4$, $CaCl_2$, and K_2HPO_4. The solution's most commonly used module is the Hoeschst-Celanese Liqui-Cel, containing microporous hollow-fiber membranes of polypropylene (PP) with a mean pore diameter of about 30 nm and porosity of about 40%.

13.5 MEMBRANE APPLICATIONS IN THE FRUIT JUICE INDUSTRY

13.5.1 CLARIFICATION

In the field of fruit juices, the main application of membrane technology concerns clarification by MF or UF. As indicated in Section 13.2, both membrane processes can be continuously operated, they work at mild temperatures, and they are able to retain microorganisms, and, in the case of UF, polyphenol oxidases are removed as well. The main drawback of MF and UF is the rapid permeate flux decline due to fouling or concentration polarization. In fruit juice clarification, fouling is mainly caused by pectin, tannins, proteins, starch, hemicelluloses, and cellulose (Santón et al. 2008). To enhance filtration performance, fruit juices are usually treated before filtration with enzyme preparations able to hydrolyze the main polysaccharides responsible for the high viscosity of the juice. Echavarría et al. (2011) reviewed the different types of enzymes used in fruit juice processing and their effects on the properties of juice.

Several industrial plants have already incorporated membranes to perform fruit juice clarification. They operate with an average permeate flux around $100 \, L \, m^{-2} \, h^{-1}$, depectinization with enzymes previously carried out at 50°C, transmembrane pressures of 0.5–5 bar, and cross-flow velocities of 3–7 m s⁻¹, depending on the characteristics of the membrane (Daufin et al. 2001).

Tables 13.4 and 13.5 show a summary of the optimal operating conditions reported by several authors to perform fruit juice clarification. In all these works, the resulting juices after membrane filtration showed very low turbidity, a significant reduction in color intensity, and the complete removal of suspended solids without significant loss of the other physicochemical characteristics of the original juice. Several authors investigated the clarification of the juice obtained just after pressing without any further pretreatment (Table 13.4). Severe membrane fouling was observed in all the studies due to cake layer formation or internal pore blockage. Nevertheless, in all cases the membranes were easily cleaned by means of simple alkaline methods.

Taking into account the low values of the permeate flux obtained when the raw juice was directly treated by MF or UF, most of the works considered an enzymatic treatment of the juice with pectinases or amylases prior to the filtration process (Table 13.5). Alvarez et al. (1998) investigated the UF of apple juice when it had been pretreated by different amounts of pectinases. A commercial zirconium oxide UF membrane (MWCO, 15 kDa) was used. A threefold increase in the permeate flux (from 50 to 150 L m^{-2} h^{-1} at 50°C, 400 kPa, and 3.7 m s^{-1}) was observed when the optimum enzyme amount was used in comparison with the UF of raw juice. Nandi et al. (2009) also observed a large increase in the permeate flux when mosambi juice was pretreated by pectinase prior to being microfiltered with a ceramic membrane of 0.285 μm pore size. Some authors compared the effects of various pretreatments on the MF and UF of different fruit juices. Youn et al. (2004) reported that the best pretreatment for apple juice MF and UF was the utilization of filter aids, especially bentonite. When mosambi juice was ultrafiltered with a 50 kDa membrane, Rai et al. (2007) obtained the maximum permeate flux when an enzymatic treatment with pectinases was followed by adsorption using bentonite.

Some works investigated the effect of the operating conditions and MWCO on the permeate flux and juice properties. The flux was observed to increase with temperature and feed flow rate, while it reached a maximum at certain transmembrane pressures due to concentration polarization. Most of the authors obtained the best results in terms of the permeate flux and juice quality with UF membranes of MWCO up to 50 kDa (Youn et al. 2004; Rai et al. 2007; Vladisavljevic et al. 2003). However, in the clarification of enzyme-treated pineapple juice, MF membranes produced higher permeate flux and better recovery of valuable compounds (vitamin C, total phenolic content, and antioxidant capacity) than UF membranes (De Carvalho et al. 2008; Laorko et al. 2010). Due to severe fouling, membrane clarification of fruit juices with a very high pulp content, such as mango, is complicated. Vaillant et al. (2001b) reported that MF of this type of juice with a 0.2 μm pore size tubular ceramic membrane would only be economically viable if a fully continuous process was carried out, with constant feeding and removal of retentate.

The preservation of clarified juice properties during storage was also investigated. De Bruijn et al. (2003) reported that apple juice ultrafiltered with 15 and 50 kDa ceramic membranes had a shelf life of at least 5 months when stored in glass containers at 16°C in the dark. Nandi et al. (2009) microfiltered mosambi juice with a ceramic membrane of 0.285 μm pore size and stored it in refrigerated conditions for more than 30 days without significant changes in juice quality.

TABLE 13.4

Operating Conditions during Membrane Clarification of Nonpretreated Fruit Juices

Type of Juice	Membrane	Operating Conditions	Flux (L m^{-2} h^{-1})	Rejection	References
Pineapple	Alumina monolith, 19 chan., MWCO 50 kDa (NGK Filtech, Japan)	25°C, 300 kPa, 2.0 m s^{-1}	15.8	Macromolecules: 91% Sugars: 10.5%	Jiraratananon et al. (1997)
Pineapple	Alumina monolith, 19 chan., 0.1 µm pore size (NGK Filtech, Japan)	25°C, 300 kPa, 2.0 m s^{-1}	6	Macromolecules: 84%–87% Sugars: 6%	Jiraratananon et al. (1997)
Apple	ZrO$_2$ tubular, MWCO 15 kDa (Orelis, France)	50°C, 400 kPa, 3.7 m s^{-1}, VRF 1	50		Alvarez et al. (1998)
Blood orange	PVDF tubular, MWCO 15 kDa (Koch Glitsch Italia S.r.l., Italy)	25°C, 85 kPa, 300 L h^{-1}, VRF 6	15	Total rejection of insoluble solids; 8.4% loss of ascorbic acid; 1%–5% loss of TAA. No other changes in composition	Cassano et al. (2007)
Pomegranate	PVDF flat sheet, 0.22 µm (Millipore, USA)	50 kPa	3	Reduction of turbidity: 99.3% Reduction of color intensity: 62% Reduction of acidity: 1% Reduction of viscosity: 15%	Mirsaeedghazi et al. (2010)
Pomegranate	PVDF flat sheet, 0.45 µm (Millipore, USA)	50 kPa	6	Reduction of turbidity: 97% Reduction of color intensity: 74% Reduction of acidity: 10% Reduction of viscosity: 3%	Mirsaeedghazi et al. (2010)

Notes: VRF, volume reduction factor; TAA, total antioxidant activity.

TABLE 13.5

Operating Conditions during Membrane Clarification of Pretreated Fruit Juices

Type of Juice	Pretreat	Membrane	Operating Conditions	Flux (L m^{-2} h^{-1})	Rejection	References
Apple	Pectinases	ZrO$_2$ tubular, MWCO 15 kDa (Orelis, France)	50°C, 400 kPa, 3.7 m s^{-1}	150		Alvarez et al. (1998)
Apple	Pectinases and amylases	ZrO$_2$ tubular, MWCO 15 kDa (Orelis, France)	50°C–55°C, 400 kPa, 7 m s^{-1} 50°C–55°C, 400 kPa, 2 m s^{-1}	157.4 102.4	Reduction of color intensity: 67.4% Reduction of TSS: 7.9% Reduction of turbidity: 93.2% Reduction of acidity: 9.1% Rejection of proteins: 92%; ashes: 88%; fiber: 78%; phenols: 50%	De Bruijn et al. (2003)
Apple	Pectinases and amylases	ZrO$_2$ tubular, MWCO 50 kDa (Orelis, France)	50°C–55°C, 400 kPa, 7 m s^{-1} 50°C–55°C, 400 kPa, 2 m s^{-1}	150.7 96.2	Reduction of color intensity: 56.5% Reduction of TSS: 7.1% Reduction of turbidity: 94.1% Reduction of acidity: 9.1%	De Bruijn et al., 2003
Apple	Pectinases	ZrO$_2$ tubular, MWCO 30 kDa (Orelis, France)	55°C, 200 kPa, 800 mL min^{-1}	30	Total solids: 4.7%; sugars: 1%; malic acid: 2.2%; total phenolics: 27.8%; pectin: 100%	Vladisavljevic et al. (2003)
Tangerine Pineapple Naranjilla Passion Blackberry Mango	Pectinases	Ceramic tubular, 0.2 μm pore size (SCT-USF-France)	150 kPa, 7 m s^{-1}, VRF 3.5 150 kPa, 7 m s^{-1}, VRF 3.2 150 kPa, 7 m s^{-1}, VRF 3.0 150 kPa, 7 m s^{-1}, VRF 3.0 150 kPa, 7 m s^{-1}, VRF 1.3	50 ± 2 70 ± 5 65 ± 5 40 ± 2 70 ± 8 60 ± 5		Vaillant et al. (2001b)

Fruit	Enzyme	Membrane	Operating conditions	Flux	Results	Reference
Kiwifruit	Pectinases	PVDF tubular, MWCO 15 kDa (Koch Glitsch Italia, Italy)	25°C, 90 kPa, 700 mL min⁻¹, VRF 3.75	7.5	Reduction of turbidity: 100% Reduction of TSS: 11.1% Reduction of ascorbic acid: 16% Reduction of TAA: 7.8%	Cassano et al. (2007)
Kiwifruit	Pectinases	Homemade modified PEEKWC hollow fiber	25°C, 75 kPa, 40 L h⁻¹, VRF 2	25	Reduction of color intensity: 97.1% Reduction of TSS: 16.7% Reduction of suspended solids: 100% Reduction of acidity: 0.9%	Tasselli et al. (2007)
Clementine mandarin	Pectinases	Homemade modified PEEKWC hollow fiber	25°C, 30 kPa, 90 L h⁻¹, VRF 2	38	Reduction of color intensity: 97.3% Reduction of TSS: 5.4% Reduction of suspended solids: 100% Reduction of acidity: 0.0% Reduction of total phenolics: 16.4% Reduction of TAA: 32%	Cassano et al. (2009)
Pineapple	Pectinases	Al_2O_3/ZrO_2 tubular, 0.1 μm pore size	50°C, 200 kPa, 4.17 m s⁻¹, VRF 1.8	124	Recovery of reduced sugars: >100% Recovery of ascorbic acid: >100% Recovery of total solids: 83.1% Removal of pulp: 100% Removal of turbidity: 100%	De Barros et al. (2003)
Pineapple	Pectinases	Polysulfone hollow fiber, MWCO 100 kDa	40°C, 30 kPa, 1.19 m s⁻¹, VR 2.8	46	Recovery of reduced sugars: >100% Recovery of ascorbic acid: >100% Recovery of total solids: 95.6% Removal of pulp: 100% Removal of turbidity: 99.9%	De Barros et al. (2003)
Pineapple	Pectinases and cellulases	Polysulfone flat sheet, MWCO 50 kDa Polyethersulfone tubular, 0.3 μm pore size	25°C, 700 kPa 25°C, 150 kPa	16.0 57.5	Total sugars recovery: 90.79% Total sugars recovery: 80.0%	De Carvalho et al. (2008)

(continued)

TABLE 13.5 (Continued)

Operating Conditions during Membrane Clarification of Pretreated Fruit Juices

Type of Juice	Pretreat	Membrane	Operating Conditions	Flux (L m^{-2} h^{-1})	Rejection	References
Pineapple	Pectinases	Polysulfone hollow fiber, 0.2 μm pore size (Amersham Biosciences, UK)	20°C, 70 kPa, 3.4 m s^{-1}, batch concentration mode	37	Recovery of phytochemical compounds: 94.3% Recovery of total phenolics: 93.4% Recovery of antioxidant capacity: 99.6% Total variable cells, mold, yeast, and coliforms were completely removed	Laorko et al. (2010)
Passion fruit	Centrifugation and depectinization	Al$_2$O$_3$/ZrO$_2$ tubular, 0.3 μm pore size	25°C, 50 kPa, 500 L h^{-1}	42.4	Color: 97% Turbidity: 100% Soluble solids: 14% Total sugar: 49% Reducing sugar: 15% Vitamin C: 26% The microbiological analysis of the permeate complied with the Brazilian legislation	De Oliveira et al. (2012)
Passion fruit	Centrifugation and depectinization	Polyamide hollow fiber, 0.3 μm pore size	25°C, 100 kPa, 325 L h^{-1}	18.7	Color: 97.6% Turbidity: 100% Soluble solids: 15.1% Total sugar: 62% Reducing sugar: 16.2% Vitamin C: 13.0% The microbiological analysis of the permeate complied with the Brazilian legislation	De Oliveira et al. (2012)

Notes: TSS, total soluble solids; VRF, volume reduction factor; TAA, total antioxidant activity.

Several studies focused on modeling the flux decline during membrane filtration of fruit juices (Mondor et al. 2000; De Barros et al. 2003; Yazdanshenas et al. 2010; De Oliveira et al. 2012). The dominant fouling mechanisms were cake formation and pore blocking, depending on the MWCO of the membrane, while different mathematical models (model of Metha [1973]; model of Field et al. [1995]; concentration polarization model; model of Cheryan and Han [1995]; etc.) were proposed to predict permeate flux reduction with time.

A few researchers investigated the immobilization of the enzymes on the membranes or the utilization of enzymatic membrane reactors (EMR) to perform the clarification of fruit juices. However, the permeate fluxes obtained were not high (Carrín et al. 2001).

Finally, several authors proposed the utilization of turbulence promoters and electric fields to increase the permeate flux (Pal et al. 2008; Sarkar et al. 2008a,b,c).

13.5.2 CONCENTRATION

Membrane technology can also be used to concentrate fruit juices. For this purpose, the membrane processes of NF, RO, DOC, MD, and OD may be considered. Nowadays, the utilization of membranes for juice concentration may be more expensive than evaporation. However, product quality can be significantly improved. Moreover, these processes are easy to scale up and they require less energy consumption. One of the main aims of the process of concentration by membrane technology is to determine how membrane separation affects juice quality. Some papers compared the total antioxidant activity (TAA) of juices concentrated by evaporation and by membrane separation. The TAA of the juice concentrated by membrane processes was higher than that of the juice concentrated by evaporation; however, of the various membrane separation techniques tested, RO caused a slight decrease in TAA (Jiao et al. 2004).

Replacing RO by NF can improve the efficiency of the process, first, because the high pressure required in RO may damage the juice (Warczok et al. 2004) and, second, because the cost of RO is higher. However, aroma losses may be greater.

The value of the permeate flux obtained decreases as the osmotic pressure of the feed solution increases during the concentration process. Therefore, it is not possible to concentrate fruit juices by RO over 30°Brix–35°Brix due to the high osmotic pressure of concentrated juices. A subsequent process (conventional evaporation or a novel membrane process, such as OE, DO, or MD) is required to reach a final concentration of 60°Brix–72°Brix.

Polyamide membranes were reported to have greater retention of aroma and other constituents and higher permeation fluxes than cellulose acetate membranes (Jiao et al. 2004). The effect of operation parameters on the permeate flux was investigated by several authors. The permeate flux was observed to increase with pressure temperature and flow rate, pressure being the most important parameter. On the other hand, it was reported that aroma rejection increased with transmembrane pressure and feed flow rate and decreased with temperature and concentration. Alvarez et al. (2002) studied the rejection of aroma compounds and the permeate flux during the RO concentration of apple juice at laboratory and pilot-plant scales using RO spiral-wound aromatic polyamide membranes (MSCB2521 R99 and MSCE 4040 R99, respectively [Separem SpA, Biella, Italy]).

Experiments were performed at different transmembrane pressures (1.5–7.0 MPa), feed flows (200–600 L h^{-1} at laboratory scale and 4200 L h^{-1} at pilot-plant scale), temperatures (20°C–30°C), and concentrations (10.0°Brix–22.7°Brix). When working at 7.0 MPa transmembrane pressure, 4200 L h^{-1} feed flow, and 25°C temperature, concentrations higher than 22°Brix can be reached with high permeate fluxes (higher than 25 L m^{-2} h^{-1}) and high aroma retention (higher than 80% for most of the compounds).

By means of DOC, OE, and MD, very high concentrations (above 60°Brix) can be achieved, since the driving force is not a hydraulic pressure difference (Jiao et al. 2004). Moreover, they require much less energy consumption than RO and, in the case of MD and OD, capital investment is also lower than that required for RO. The application of these processes to concentrate fruit juices has been studied at laboratory and pilot-plant scales (Laganà et al. 2000; Rodrigues et al. 2004; Vaillant et al. 2001a). They have been applied alone or integrated with other processes such as UF and RO (Bailey et al. 2000; Calabró et al. 1994; Cassano et al. 2002). However, as they are relatively new, there is a lack of a systematic comparison of these processes, not only regarding the water flux obtained, but also concerning the retention of aroma compounds. In fact, some studies on the transport of volatile compounds have been made, but only for the OE process (Ali et al. 2002).

The main drawback of these processes is the low permeation fluxes obtained (operating at mild temperatures) when compared to RO. Therefore, they seem economically uncompetitive. However, when the product to be concentrated is a solution containing compounds that are sensitive to shear degradation, RO could cause significant product deterioration. For these applications, OD may be applied with important advantages (Jiao et al. 2004).

13.5.3 DEACIDIFICATION

The membrane process of ED is a very promising technique for the deacidification of very acid fruit juices. The main acids present in fruit juices are citric and malic acids. Therefore, the deacidification consists of the partial removal of citrate and malate ions and the partial neutralization of protons by hydroxyl ions. Vera et al. (2003, 2007a,b, 2009a,b) investigated the utilization of ED with homopolar (three compartments) and bipolar (two compartments) membranes to perform the clarification of several tropical fruit juices (passion fruit, castilla mulberry, naranjilla, and araza) at laboratory and preindustrial scales. The final pH value was limited to 4.0 or 4.5 in order to avoid microorganism growth and spoilage. The sensory characteristics of the juices were preserved, although a slight decrease in odor and slight changes of color were detected. In terms of juice characteristics, small differences were found whatever the ED configurations (conventional or bipolar ED) and operating conditions used.

Membrane fouling is the main limitation of the process, but it can be reduced by selecting the appropriate current density and flow rate specifically for each juice. The worst ED performance was observed for fruit juices with high malic acid content (araza juice). Conventional ED gave a better performance than bipolar ED, but the latter allowed the production of a solution of citric or malic acid, and avoided the NaOH consumption required in the conventional ED process.

Regarding the effect of the operating conditions on the ED performances, these were improved by increases in temperature and current densities. However, temperatures that are too high could affect the sensory properties of juices and the occurrence of fouling limits the increase in the current density. The flow rate does not have a substantial influence on the transport of ions, but high values of this parameter can significantly reduce membrane fouling.

Finally, several pretreatments were tested in the deacidification of passion fruit by ED with bipolar membranes. At the preindustrial scale, the deacidification of the juice at the initial pulpy state was possible, but better ED performances were found when the juice was microfiltered or centrifuged before the deacidification process.

13.5.4 AROMA RECOVERY

Traditional concentration techniques, based on evaporation processes such as distillation or partial condensation, may cause an appreciable decrease in the functional and organoleptic properties of fruit juice processing, due to a significant loss in the volatile aroma fraction. In other cases, such as vine and cider dealcoholization (Alcaina 1991; Iborra 2001), it is possible that these compounds, which are important for the sensorial quality of juices, can be recovered and added back to the dearomatized juice. Currently, because these compounds are at very low concentrations, the conventional techniques may be complex and expensive. However, the pervaporation technique constitutes a satisfactory substitute for or supplement to evaporative techniques (Pereira et al. 2005). In recent years, the literature on the application of this technology for recovering aroma compounds is extensive; as well as evaluating both experimental studies and modeling, they also consider membrane materials, equipment, operating parameters, and their effects.

The aromatic fraction of fruit juices is made up of a wide variety of different organic compounds (of the order of hundreds) that are present at very low concentrations (of the order of parts per million or less). However, these compounds are of great importance and in most cases they may determine the acceptability of products.

Membrane processes such as pervaporation offer great advantages, namely, high selectivity and the possibility of operation at moderate temperatures, allowing the preservation of functional properties and organoleptic characteristics.

Compared to other membrane processes such as UF and RO, pervaporation exhibits a very low flux (<10 kg m^{-2} h^{-1}) and is considered a process under development, although it has already been adopted on an industrial scale for some application solvents, with more than 100 industrial units installed worldwide (Anglerot 1994). However, it exhibits high selectivities and is therefore particularly suitable for the recovery of highly diluted species.

Hydrophilic membranes are the most commonly used on an industrial scale and the process is especially directed toward the separation of close-boiling components or azeotropic-like dehydration, esterification, acetalization, or etherification, where it is considered that pervaporation is more advantageous than distillation from both the technical and economic points of view.

Table 13.6 shows a summary of the experimental studies on aroma recovery of fruit juice by pervaporation reported in the literature using several polymeric

TABLE 13.6
Summary of Experimental Studies on Natural Aroma Juice Recovery by Pervaporation

System	Membrane	Module	Operating Range	References
Industrial condensate from apple juice concentration	MTR-100 and MTR-200[a]	SW	$c = 1.0$ wt% $T = 40°C$ $P_p = 20$ mmHg	Kaschemekat et al. (1989)
Natural apple essence	PDMS[b]	PF	$T = 22°C$ $P_p = 2.2$ mmHg	Zhang and Matsuura (1991)
Industrial condensate from apple juice concentration	PDMS[d]	PF	$5°C \leq T \leq 20°C$ $P_p = 4.5$ mmHg	Bengtsson et al. (1992)
Commercial grape essence	PDMS-b-PC[c]	PF	$11 \leq c \leq 200$ ppm $33°C \leq T \leq 50°C$ $1 < P_p \leq 20$ mmHg	Rajagopalan and Cheryan (1995)
Binary, ternary, and multicomponent solutions industrial condensate from orange juice concentration	PDMS-1060[d]	PF	$0.002 \leq c \leq 13.65\%b$ $5°C \leq T \leq 45°C$ $P_p < 10$ mmHg	Adão (1998)
Clarified and depectinized apple juice multicomponent solution	PDMS[d], PDMS-PT[d], POMS-PEI[d], POMS-VDF[e], PEBA[e]	PF	$0.002 \leq c \leq 13.65\%b$ $5°C \leq T \leq 45°C$ $P_p < 10$ mmHg	Alvarez et al. (1998)
Cocoa aroma extract	PDMS (ns)	HF	$T = 55°C$ $P_p = 7$ mmHg	Kattenberg and Willemsen (2002)
Pineapple juice–passion fruit juice binary solutions	PDMS-1060[d], PDMS-1070[d], PDMS[f], EVA, EDPM[g]	PF, HF	$T = 25°C$ $P_p < 10$ mmHg	Pereira et al. (2002)
Binary solution (EtBu) industrial condensate from orange juice concentration	PDMS[h]	HF	$25 \leq T \leq 45°C$ $P_p < 10$ mmHg	Shepherd et al. (2002)

| Binary and multicomponent solutions hot-water tea extract | PDMS[g], POMS-PEI[e] | PF | $25 \leq T \leq 45°C$ $P_P < 10$ mmHg | Kanani et al. (2003) |
| Binary and multicomponent solutions hot-water tea extract | PDMS-1070[d], EVA, EPDM[g] | HF | $100 \leq c \leq 900$ ppm $T = 25°C$ $P_P < 2.2$ mmHg | Pereira et al. (2005) |

Source: Pereira, C.C., Rufino, J.R.M., Habert, A.C., Nobrega, R., Cabral, L.M.C., and Borges, C.P., *Journal of food engineering*, 66, 77–87, 2005.

Notes: Module configuration: capillary (CAP), hollow fiber (HF), plate and frame (PF), and spiral wound (SW); supplier: (ns) not specified.

[a] Membrane Technology and Research, Inc.
[b] General Electric Co.
[c] Membrane Products Co.
[d] Sulzer Chemtech Membranetechnik GA.
[e] GKSS Forschungzentrum.
[f] Sigma Products.
[g] Tailor-made.
[h] LPI France.

membrane materials (Pereira et al. 2006): polyethylene-propylene-diene (EPDM); polyethylene-vinyl acetate (EVA); polydimethylsiloxane (PDMS); polyether-polyamide block (PEBA); polyoctylmethylsiloxane (POMS); and polyetherimide (PEI).

Due to the intrinsic complexity of fruit juice aromas containing hundreds of different organic compounds, some of which are in very low concentrations, many authors have opted for working with model solutions, usually binary ones.

The potential of pervaporation for recovering aroma compounds has been clearly demonstrated in the literature by a considerable amount of experimental work at laboratory scale. Almost 70 different components have already been tested and were recovered with high selectivity with the aid of this membrane technique.

PDMS is by far the most tested membrane material, providing selectivity for the aroma compounds investigated and also a somewhat high water flux, which implies a high cost for condensing the permeate. Consequently, alternative materials are still sought. Whenever a new material is developed and tested for aroma recovery by pervaporation, its performance, assessed in terms of flux and selectivity, should always be compared with that of PDMS.

Aroma recovery by pervaporation has not yet been achieved at the industrial scale. Further studies on the subject should contribute to overcome this limitation, despite the favorable results obtained at the laboratory scale. In particular, experimental data on the pilot-scale processing of real juices and industrial streams (such as condensate from juice evaporators) with an assessment of the sensory quality of the final product, as well as comprehensive models for process design and simulation, are highly desirable (Pereira et al. 2005).

Aroujalian and Raisi (2007) have studied the effects of key parameters such as feed temperature (25°C, 40°C, and 50°C), permeate pressure (1, 20, and 40 mmHg), and feed flow rate (from 500 to 2500 Re) on the pervaporative recovery of volatile aroma compounds from real orange juice using a commercial PDMS membrane. They concluded that pervaporation is an attractive technique for the recovery of orange aroma compounds. As the feed flow rate increased, the flux and enrichment factor exhibited no significant changes, but the feed temperature was a key parameter. As the feed temperature rose, the flux increased linearly and followed an Arrhenius-type relation. The activation energy for various aroma compounds (ethyl acetate, ethyl butyrate, hexanal, linalool, terpineol, water, and the overall value) was calculated from Arrhenius plots. The enrichment factor also increased in line with the feed temperature.

Permeate pressure is another important parameter that affects pervaporation performance. Its effect on pervaporation performance has been investigated by only a few researchers. The results showed that the permeation flux dropped as the permeate pressure rose. However, the enrichment factor of ethyl acetate, ethyl butyrate, and hexanal increased, but limonene, linalool, and terpineol exhibited a different behavior when the permeate pressure increased. Ethyl acetate had the highest enrichment factor; however, its concentration was lower than that of other components detected in orange juice, and α-terpineol had the lowest enrichment factor. On the other hand, the increase in the Reynolds number from 500 to 2500 had no significant effect on aroma recovery.

13.6 INTEGRATED MEMBRANE PROCESSES

A very attractive alternative for the industrial production of concentrated or clarified fruit juices is the utilization of integrated membrane processes. The main advantages are a high-quality product and lower energy consumption when compared with conventional processes. Jiao et al. (2004) reviewed different processes for the production of fruit juice concentrates.

Alvarez et al. (2000) proposed an integrated membrane process for the production of apple juice and aroma concentrates. The process involves the following operations: a membrane reactor to clarify the raw juice, an RO process to preconcentrate the juice up to 25°Brix, pervaporation to recover and concentrate aroma compounds, and finally evaporation to concentrate the apple juice up to 72°Brix. These operations were tested at laboratory and pilot-plant scales. The resulting products proved to be clearer and more brilliant than apple juice produced by conventional methods. The organoleptic evaluation of the clarified and preconcentrated apple juices was excellent in terms of odor and flavor. An economic evaluation of the proposed and conventional processes was performed: The authors reported that the integrated membrane process showed comparable or slightly higher profitability than the conventional process.

Some juices, such as orange and kiwifruit, are usually produced with a lower level of clarity. However, they have high solid and pectin content. Therefore, they represent a very viscous stream when directly submitted to concentration by RO or OD, and low permeate fluxes are obtained. If only RO is used, concentrations higher than 25°Brix 30°Brix cannot be achieved due to osmotic pressure limitations (Rao et al. 1987). MF or UF can be combined with RO to separate suspended solids and pectin, thus reducing the viscosity and increasing the permeate flux. Lawhon and Lusas (1987) proposed the separation of the pulp and the serum of fruit juices by UF. The serum was concentrated by RO to levels above 42°Brix, and was observed to contain almost all the flavor and aroma components. The UF concentrate, which contained the suspended solids, pectins, and microorganisms, was heated and added to the RO concentrate. The reconstituted juice had a quality similar to that of fresh juice, as claimed in a commercial patent (Lawhon and Lusas 1987).

A new patent developed by Walker (1990) has proposed a combined membrane process, which is called the *FreshNote system*, to concentrate pulpy juices up to 50°Brix while almost retaining the flavors of fresh juice (Figure 13.12). The method consists of MF or UF followed by a two-stage RO process. The first stage of the RO process involves three high-rejection membrane units in series, with 98.5% salt rejection, and the second stage uses two low-rejection RO units in series, the first membrane having a 93% and the second a 97% salt rejection. The reconstituted juice showed better flavor characteristics than thermally concentrated products, and was very similar to freeze-concentrated juice and the feed juice itself. Production costs are greater than those of the conventional concentration process, but they are significantly lower than those of the freeze concentration process (Cross, 1989).

Nabetani (1996) developed an integrated RO–NF membrane process to produce highly concentrated fruit juices. The feed juice is first concentrated to 30°Brix by RO and afterward to above 45°Brix by means of NF. The NF permeate is then

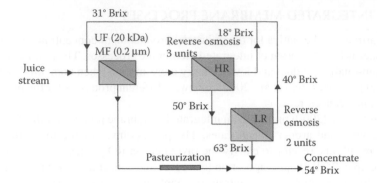

FIGURE 13.12 Diagram of the combined UF/RO process for juice concentration. (Adapted from Walker, J.B., *Proceedings of the 1990 International Congress on Membrane and Membrane Processes*, Chicago, North American Membrane Society, 1990.)

recycled back into the RO unit. The process was reported to retain the fresh juice flavor and to reduce energy consumption when compared with evaporation and freeze concentration.

Membrane retention is a very important variable. The use of low-retention membranes allows higher retentate concentrations to be achieved, because, as part of the solute crosses the membrane, the effective osmotic pressure difference is reduced. However, part of the solute is lost in the permeate stream. Therefore, in order to improve solute recovery, the permeate stream can be recycled to a high retention module. Hollow fibers have been reported to show better performance for this process than spiral-wound modules, as they have lower concentration polarization effects and a larger packing density, which compensates for the lower permeation fluxes (Walker 1990; Gostoli et al. 1995).

A complex processing scheme was proposed by Watanabe et al. (1990) to produce highly concentrated juices. The juice was separated into pulpy suspended solids (retentate) and clarified juice (permeate) by UF. Then, the clarified juice was concentrated by conventional evaporation using a thermally accelerated short-time evaporator (TASTE) evaporator. The pulpy retentate from the UF system was pasteurized by a heat exchanger. The clear juice concentrate obtained from the combined membrane–evaporation system can reach a higher concentration (>80°Brix) than the conventional concentrate produced in a TASTE evaporator under similar conditions (Hernandez et al. 1995). Thus, significant energy savings during storage and distribution can be achieved (Crandall and Graumlich 1982; Chen 1998). The storage stability of orange juice concentrated by this process was evaluated. The major changes during storage were reported to be due to chemical reactions rather than microbial deterioration (Johnson et al. 1995). Lee and Chen (1998) studied the vitamin C loss and discoloration in the clear orange juice concentrate (80.2°Brix) produced by this technique during 19 weeks of storage. They indicated that vitamin C degradation occurred slowly during storage at 4°C.

Karode et al. (2000) proposed a coupling of RO and OD processes to concentrate sucrose solutions. The process was theoretically and experimentally tested.

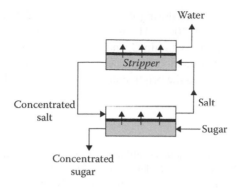

FIGURE 13.13   Osmotic dehydration coupled reverse-osmosis concentration process for concentrating fruit juice enriched stripper configuration. (Adapted from Karode, S.K., Kulkarni, S.S., and Ghorapade, M.S., *Journal of Membrane Science*, 164(1–2), 277–288, 2000.)

The flowchart of the process is shown in Figure 13.13. This configuration is able to concentrate a sucrose solution from 5% to 60% using a natural source of brine (seawater: 3.5% salt). The maximum operating pressure is 54.4 bar (800 psi). The integrated system could also be used to concentrate fruit juices.

The coupling of UF and MD has been investigated for the concentration of kiwifruit and orange juices (Cassano et al., 2003). The process is depicted in Figure 13.14. Firstly, the fruit juices are separated into serum and pulp by UF. Then, RO is used to preconcentrate the juices up to 20°Brix–25°Brix. Finally, the RO retentates are concentrated to above 60°Brix by OD (using microporous PP hollow fibers). The proposed process considers continuous countercurrent recycling and evaporative reconcentration of the brine strip. The UF retentate is pasteurized and then added to the final OD

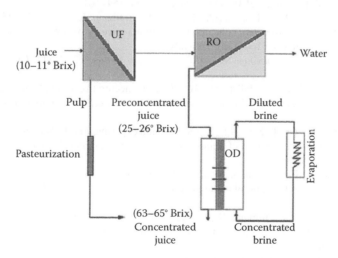

FIGURE 13.14   Integrated membrane process for the production of concentrated orange juices. (Adapted from Cassano, A., Drioli, E., Galaverna, G., Marchelli, R., Di Silvestro, G., and Cagnasso, P., *Journal of Food Engineering*, 57, 153–163, 2003. With permission.)

concentrate. The TAA stability during the concentration of blood orange juice was investigated (Galaverna et al. 2008). The results showed that the content of ascorbic acid, phenolics, anthocyanins, vitamin C, and TAA remained almost unchanged during the proposed integrated membrane process. Moreover, the juice concentrated by means of this process retained the bright color and flavor of fresh juice.

REFERENCES

Adäo, L.G. (1998). Treatment of aqueous effluent for orange juice concentration with aroma recovery. MSc. Thesis, COPPE/Federal University of Rio de Janeiro, Brazil.

Alcaina, M.I. (1991). Optimización del Proceso de Desalcoholización de Vinos por Pervaporación: Caracterización y Selección de Membranas Compuestas. MSc. Thesis, Universitat Politècnica de Valencia, Spain.

Ali, F., Dornier, M., Duquenoy, A., Reynes, M. (2002). Transfer of volatiles through FE membrane during osmotic distillation. *Proceedings of the 2002 International Congress on Membrane and Membrane Processes*, Toulouse, France, European Membrane Society.

Alvarez, S., Alvarez, R., Riera, F.A., Coca, J. (1998). Influence of depectinization on apple juice ultrafiltration. *Colloids and Surfaces A: Physicochemical and Engineering Aspects* 138: 377–382.

Alvarez, S., Riera, F.A., Alvarez, R., Coca, J. (2002). Concentration of apple juice by reverse osmosis at laboratory and pilot-plant scales. *Industrial and Engineering Chemistry Research* 41: 6156–6164.

Alvarez, S., Riera, F.A., Alvarez, R., Coca, J., Cuperus, F.P., Bouwer, S., Boswinkel, G., et al. (2000). A new integrated membrane process for producing clarified apple juice and apple juice aroma concentrate. *Journal of Food Engineering* 46(2): 109–125.

Anglerot, D. (1994). Process of making alcohol-free beer and beer aroma concentrates. U.S. Patent 5,308,631 A.

Aroujalian, A., Raisi, A. (2007). Recovery of volatile aroma components from orange juice by pervaporation. *Journal of Membrane Science* 303: 154–161.

Bailey, A.F.G., Barbe, A.M., Hogan, P.A., Johnson, R.A., Sheng, J. (2000). The effect of ultrafiltration on the subsequent concentration of grape juice by osmotic distillation. *Journal of Membrane Science* 164(1–2): 195–204.

Baker, R.W. (1991). *Membrane Technology and Applications*, 2nd edn. Chichester, UK: Wiley.

Bengtsson, E., Trägårdh, G., Hallströom, B. (1992). Concentration of apple juice aroma from evaporator condensate using pervaporation. *LWT—Food Science and Technology* 25: 29–34.

Calabró, V., Jiao, B., Drioli, E. (1994). Theoretical and experimental study on membrane distillation in the concentration of orange juice. *Industrial Engineering Chemistry Research* 33(7): 1803–1808.

Carrín, M.E., Ceci, L.N., Lozano, J. (2001). Effects of co-immobilization of pectinase and amylase on ultrafiltration of apple juice simulate. *Journal of Food Process Engineering* 24: 423–435.

Cassano, A., Conidi, C., Timpone, R., D'Avella, M., Drioli, E. (2007a). A membrane-based process for the clarification and the concentration of the cactus pear juice. *Journal of Food Engineering* 80: 914–921.

Cassano, A., Donato, L., Drioli, E. (2007b). Ultrafiltration of kiwifruit juice: Operating parameters, juice quality and membrane fouling. *Journal of Food Engineering* 79: 613–621.

Cassano, A., Drioli, E. (2007). Concentration of clarified kiwifruit juice by osmotic distillation. *Journal of Food Engineering* 79(4): 1397–1404.

Cassano, A., Drioli, E., Galaverna, G., Marchelli, R., Di Silvestro, G., Cagnasso, P. (2003). Clarification and concentration of citrus and carrot juice by integrated membrane process. *Journal of Food Engineering* 57: 153–163.

Cassano, A., Jiao, B., Drioli, E. (2002). Integrated membrane process for production of concentrated kiwifruit juice. *Proceedings of 1st Workshop Italy–China on State of Research and Applications of Membrane Operations for a Sustainable Growth.* Cetraro (CS), Italy, s.n.

Cassano, A., Tasselli, F., Conidi, C., Drioli, E. (2009). Ultrafiltration of clementine mandarin juice by hollow fibre membranes. *Desalination* 241: 302–308.

Chen, C.S. (1998). Methods for producing ready to pour frozen concentrated clarified fruit juice, fruit juice produced therefrom, and high solids fruit product. US Patent 5,756,141, May 26.

Cheryan, M., Han, I.S. (1995). Nanofiltration of model acetate solutions. *Journal of Membrane Science* 107: 107–113.

Crandall, P.G., Graumlich, T.R. (1982). Storage stability and quality of high Brix orange concentrate. *Proceedings of Florida State Horticultural Society* 95: 198–210.

Cross, S. (1989). Membrane concentration of orange juice. *Proceedings of Florida State Horticultural Society* 102: 146–152.

Daufin, G., Escudier, J.P., Carrère, H., Bérot, S., Fillaudeau, L., Decloux, M. (2001). Recent and emerging applications of membrane processes in the food and dairy industry. *Transactions of the Institution of Chemical Engineers, Part C* 79: 89–102.

De Barros, S.T.D., Andrade, C.M.G., Mendesa, E.S., Peres, L. (2003). Study of fouling mechanism in pineapple juice clarification by ultrafiltration. *Journal of Membrane Science* 215: 213–224.

De Bruijn, J.P.F., Venegas, A., Martínez, J.A., Bórquez, R. (2003). Ultrafiltration performance of Carbosep membranes for the clarification of apple juice. *Lebensmittel-Wissenschaft und -Technologie* 36: 397–406.

De Curvalho, L.M., Miranda, I., Bento da Silva, C.A. (2008). A study of retention of sugars in the process of clarification of pineapple juice (*Ananas comosus, L. Merril*) by micro- and ultrafiltration. *Journal of Food Engineering* 87: 447–454.

De Oliveira, R.C., Caleffi, R., Davantel, S.T. (2012). Clarification of passion fruit juice by microfiltration: Analyses of operating parameters, study of membrane fouling and juice quality. *Journal of Food Engineering* 111(2): 432–439.

Echavarría, A.P., Torras, C., Pagán, J., Ibarz, A. (2011). Fruit juice processing and membrane technology application. *Food Engineering Reviews* 3: 136–158.

Field, R.W., Wu, D., Howell, J.A., Gupta B.B. (1995). Critical flux concept for microfiltration fouling. *Journal of Membrane Science* 100(3): 259–272.

Franken, A.C.M., Mulder, M.H.V., Smolders, C.A. (1990). Pervaporation process using a thermal gradient as the driving force. *Journal of Membrane Science* 53(1–2): 127–141.

Galaverna, G., Di Silvestro, G., Cassano, A., Sforza, S., Dossena, A., Drioli, E., Marchelli, R. (2008). A new integrated membrane process for the production of concentrated blood orange juice: Effect on bioactive compounds and antioxidant activity. *Fruit Chemistry* 106: 1021–1030.

Gostoli, C., Bandini, S., Di Franscesca, R., Zardi, G. (1995). Concentrating fruit juices by reverse osmosis. The low retention-high retention method. *Fruit Processing* 6: 417–421.

Hernandez, E., Chen, C.S., Johnson, J., Carter, R.D. (1995). Viscosity changes in orange juice after ultrafiltration and evaporation. *Journal of Food Engineering* 25(3): 387–396.

Iborra, A. (2001). Bebidas de bajo contenido alcohólico a partir de sidra. Estudio del comportamiento de la fracción aromática en el proceso de desalcoholización por pervaporación. MSc. Thesis, Universitat Politècnica de Valencia, Spain.

Jiao, B., Cassano, A., Drioli, E. (2004). Recent advances on membrane processes for concentration of fruit juices: A review. *Journal of Food Engineering* 63: 303–624.

Jiraratananon, R., Uttapap, D., Tangamornsuksun, C. (1997). Self-forming dynamic membrane for ultrafiltration of pineapple. *Journal of Membrane Science* 129: 135–143.

Johnson, J.R., Braddock, R.J., Chen, C.S. (1995). Kinetics of ascorbic acid loss and nonenzymatic browning in orange juice serum: Experimental rate constants. *Journal of Food Science* 60(3): 502–505.

Kanani, D.M., Nikhade, B.P., Balakrishnan, P., Singh, G., Pangarkar, V.G. (2003). Recovery of valuable tea aroma components by pervaporation. *Industrial and Engineering Chemistry Research* 42: 6924–6932.

Karode, S.K., Kulkarni, S.S., Ghorapade, M.S. (2000). Osmotic dehydration coupled reverse osmosis concentration: Steady-state model and assessment. *Journal of Membrane Science* 164(1–2): 277–288.

Kaschemekat, J., Wijmans, J.G., Baker, R.W. (1989). Removal of organic solvent contaminants from industrial effluent streams by pervaporation. In: Bakish, R. (ed.), *Proceedings of the Fourth International Conference on Pervaporation Process in the Chemical Industry*, pp. 321–331. Englewood, NJ: Bakish Materials Corporation.

Kattenberg, H.R., Willemsen, J.H.A. (2002). Aroma extracts from cocoa. *Manufacturing Confectioner* 82: 73.

Laganà, F., Barbieri, G., Drioli, E. (2000). Direct contact membrane distillation: Modelling and concentration experiments. *Journal of Membrane Science* 166(1): 1–11.

Laorko, A., Li, Z., Tongchitpakdee, S., Chantachum, S., Youravong, W. (2010). Effect of membrane property and operating conditions on phytochemical properties and permeate flux during clarification of pineapple juice. *Journal of Food Engineering* 100: 514–521.

Lawhon, J.T., Lusas, E.W. (1987). Method of producing sterile and concentrated juices with improved flavor and reduced acid. US Patent 4,643,902, February 17.

Lee, H.S., Chen, C.S. (1998). Rates of vitamin C loss and discoloration in clear orange juice concentrate during storage at temperatures of 4–24°C. *Journal of Agricultural and Food Chemistry* 46(11): 4723–4727.

Lefebvre, M.S.M. (1988). Method of performing osmotic distillation. US Patent 4,781,837, November 1.

Malik, A.A., Kour, H., Bhat, A., Kaul, R.K., Khan, S., Khan, S.U. (2013). Commercial utilization of membranes in food industry. *International Journal of Food Nutrition and Safety* 3(3): 147–170.

Martí-Calatayud, M.C., Vincent-Vela, M.C., Álvarez-Blanco, S., Lora-García, J., Bergantiños-Rodríguez, E. (2010). Analysis and optimization of the influence of operating conditions in the ultrafiltration of macromolecules using a response surface methodological approach. *Chemical Engineering Journal* 156: 337–346.

Mehta, B. (1973). Processing of model compositional whey solutions with pressure driven membranes. PhD thesis, Ohio State University.

Miranda, J.M., Campos, J.B.L.M. (2001). An improved numerical scheme to study mass transfer over a separation membrane. *Journal of Membrane Science* 188: 49–59.

Mirsaeedghazi, H., Emam-Djomeh, E., Mohammad, S., Aroujalian, A., Mahdi, N. (2010). Clarification of pomegranate juice by microfiltration with PVDF membranes. *Desalination* 264: 243–248.

Mondor, M., Girard, B., Moresoli, C. (2000). Modeling flux behavior for membrane filtration of apple juice. *Food Research International* 33: 539–548.

Mulder, M. (2000). *Basic Principles of Membrane Technology*, 2nd edn. Dordrecht: Kluwer Academic Publishers.

Nabetani, H. (1996). Development of a membrane system for highly concentrated fruit juice. *Journal of Membrane (Japanese)* 21(2): 102–108.

Nandi, B.K., Das, B., Uppaluri, R., Purkait, M.K. (2009). Microfiltration of mosambi juice using low cost ceramic membrane. *Journal of Food Engineering* 95: 597–605.

Neel, J. (1991). Introduction to pervaporation. In: Huang, R.Y.M. (ed.), *Pervaporation Membrane Separation Processes*, vol. 1, pp. 1–109. Amsterdam: Elsevier.

Pal, S., Ambastha, S., Ghosh, T.B., De, S., DasGupta, S. (2008). Optical evaluation of deposition thickness and measurement of permeate flux enhancement of simulated fruit juice in presence of turbulence promoters. *Journal of Membrane Science* 315: 58–66.

Pereira, C.C., Ribeiro, C.P., Nobrega, R., Cristiano, P.B. (2006). Pervaporative recovery of volatile aroma compounds from fruit juices. *Journal of Membrane Science* 274: 1–23.

Pereira, C.C., Rufino, J.R.M., Habert, A.C., Nobrega, R., Cabral, L.M.C., Borges, C.P. (2002). Membrane for processing tropical fruit juice. *Desalination* 148: 57.

Pereira, C.C., Rufino, J.R.M., Habert, A.C., Nobrega, R., Cabral, L.M.C., Borges, C.P. (2005). Aroma compounds recovery of tropical fruit juice by pervaporation: Membrane material selection and process evaluation. *Journal of Food Engineering* 66: 77–87.

Rajagopalan, N., Cheryan, M. (1995). Pervaporation of grape juice aroma. *Journal of Membrane Science* 104: 243–250.

Rai, P., Majumdar, G.C., Das Gupta, S., De, S. (2007). Effect of various pretreatment methods on permeate flux and quality during ultrafiltration of mosambi juice. *Journal of Food Engineering* 78: 561–568.

Rao, M.A., Acree, T.E., Cooley, H.J., Ennis, R.W. (1987). Clarification of apple juice by hollow fiber ultrafiltration: Fluxes and the odor-active volatiles. *Journal of Food Science* 52(2): 375–378.

Riera, F., Alvarez, S. (2012). Purification of lactic acid obtained by fermentative processes by means of membrane techniques and ion exchange. In: Jiménez-Migallón, A., Ruseckaite, R.A. (eds), *Lactic Acid: Production, Properties and Health Effects*, pp. 1–46. New York: Nova Science Publishers.

Rodrigues, R.B., Menezes, H.C., Cabral, L.M.C., Dornier, M., Rios, G.M., Reynes, M. (2004). Evaluation of reverse osmosis and osmotic evaporation to concentrate camu-camu juice (*Myrciaria dubia*). *Journal of Food Engineering* 63(1): 97–102.

Santón, M., Treiche, H., Valduga, E., Cabra, L., Di Luccio, M. (2008). Evaluation of enzymatic treatment of peach juice using response surface methodology. *Journal of the Science of Food and Agriculture* 88: 507–512.

Sarkar, B., DasGupta, S., De, S. (2008a). Effect of electric field during gel-layer controlled ultrafiltration of synthetic and fruit juice. *Journal of Membrane Science* 307: 268–276.

Sarkar, B., De, S., DasGupta, S. (2008b). Pulsed electric field enhanced ultrafiltration of synthetic and fruit juice. *Separation and Purification Technology* 63: 582–591.

Sarkar, B., Pal, S., Ghosh, T.B., De, S., DasGupta, S. (2008c). A study of electric field enhanced ultrafiltration of synthetic fruit juice and optical quantification of gel deposition. *Journal of Membrane Science* 311: 112–120.

Shepherd, A.G., Habert, A.C., Borges, C.P. (2002). Hollow fibre modules for orange juice aroma recovery using pervaporation. *Desalination* 148: 111–114.

Susanto, H., Franzkab, S., Ulbrichta, M. (2007). Dextran fouling of polyethersulfone ultrafiltration membranes: Causes, extent and consequences. *Journal of Membrane Science* 296: 147–155.

Tasselli, F., Cassano, A., Drioli, E. (2007). Ultrafiltration of kiwifruit juice using modified poly(ether ether ketone) hollow fibre membranes. *Separation and Purification Technology* 57: 94–102.

Vaillant, F., Jeanton, E., Dornier, M., O'Brien, G.M., Reynes, M., Decloux, M. (2001a). Concentration of passion fruit juice on an industrial pilot scale using osmotic evaporation. *Journal of Food Engineering* 47(3): 195–202.

Vaillant, F., Millan, A., Dornier, M., Decloux, M., Reynes, M. (2001b). Strategy for economical optimisation of the clarification of pulpy fruit juices using cross-flow microfiltration. *Journal of Food Engineering* 48: 83–90.

Vera, E., Ruales, J., Dornier, M., Sandeaux, J., Persin, F., Pourcelly, G., Vaillant, F., Reynes, M. (2003). Comparison of different methods for deacidification of clarified passion fruit juice. *Journal of Food Engineering* 59: 361–367.

Vera, E., Sandeaux, J., Persin, F., Pourcelly, G., Dornier, M., Ruales, J. (2007a). Deacidification of clarified tropical fruit juices by electrodialysis. Part I. Influence of operating conditions on the process performances. *Journal of Food Engineering* 78: 1427–1438.

Vera, E., Sandeaux, J., Persin, F., Pourcelly, G., Dornier, M., Piombo, G., Ruales, J. (2007b). Deacidification of clarified tropical fruit juices by electrodialysis. Part II. Characteristics of the deacidified juices. *Journal of Food Engineering* 78: 1439–1445.

Vera, E., Sandeaux, J., Persin, F., Pourcelly, G., Dornier, M., Ruales, J. (2009a). Deacidification of passion fruit juice by electrodialysis with bipolar membrane after different pretreatments. *Journal of Food Engineering* 90: 67–73.

Vera, E., Sandeaux, J., Persin, F., Pourcelly, G., Dornier, M., Ruales, J. (2009b). Modeling of clarified tropical fruit juice deacidification by electrodialysis. *Journal of Membrane Science* 326: 472–483.

Vladisavljevic, G.T., Vukosavljevic, P., Bukvic, B. (2003). Permeate flux and fouling resistance in ultrafiltration of depectinized apple juice using ceramic membranes. *Journal of Food Engineering* 60: 241–247.

Wagner, J. (2001). *Membrane Filtration Handbook: Practical Tips and Hints*. 2nd edn. Minnetonka, MN: Osmonics.

Walker, J.B. (1990). Membrane process for the production of superior quality fruit juice concentrate. In: *Proceedings of the 1990 International Congress on Membrane and Membrane Processes*, Chicago: North American Membrane Society.

Warczok, J., Ferrando, M., López, F., Güell, C. (2004). Concentration of apple and pear juices by nanofiltration at low pressures. *Journal of Food Engineering* 63(1): 63–70.

Watanabe, A., Nabetani, H., Nakajima, M. (1990). Development of multi-stage RO combined system for high concentration of apple juice. In: *Proceedings of the 1990 International Congress on Membrane and Membrane Processes*, Chicago: North American Membrane Society.

Yazdanshenas, M., Tabatabaee-Nezhad, S.A.R., Soltanieh, M., Roostaazad, R., Khoshfetrat, A.B. (2010). Contribution of fouling and gel polarization during ultrafiltration of raw apple juice at industrial scale. *Desalination* 258: 194–200.

Youn, K.S., Hong, J.H., Bae, D.H., Kim, S.J., Kim, S.D. (2004). Effective clarifying process of reconstituted apple juice using membrane filtration with filter-aid pretreatment. *Journal of Membrane Science* 228: 179–186.

Zhang, S.Q., Matsuura, T. (1991). Recovery and concentration of flavour compounds in apple essence by pervaporation. *Journal of Food Process Engineering* 14: 291–296.

14 Juice Packaging

Maribel Cornejo-Mazón, Darío Iker
Téllez-Medina, Liliana Alamilla-Beltrán,
and Gustavo Fidel Gutiérrez-López

CONTENTS

14.1 Introduction 301
14.2 Primary and Secondary Containers 302
    14.2.1 Hermetic Containers 302
14.3 Materials Commonly Used for Primary Containers 303
    14.3.1 Glass 303
    14.3.2 Metal 303
    14.3.3 Laminates 304
    14.3.4 Polyethylene Terephthalate: Rugged, Reasonably Inert, Visible 304
14.4 Packaging Techniques 304
    14.4.1 Sterile Filtration 305
    14.4.2 Canning 305
    14.4.3 Hot Fill 305
    14.4.4 Aseptic Processing 306
    14.4.5 Novel Techniques for Juice Preservation 306
        14.4.5.1 High Pressures 306
        14.4.5.2 Pulsed Electric Fields 306
        14.4.5.3 Irradiation 307
14.5 Preservation of Nutrients by Packaging 307
14.6 Final Remarks 308
References 309

14.1 INTRODUCTION

The consumption and commercialization of semisolid and liquid foodstuffs need appropriate storage and distribution systems. This need has been recognized since ancient times when consumers and producers first had to store and transport food supplies, and rudimentary containers were developed from leaves; fruit shells; tree barks; and animal skins, entrails, and horns. Later, pottery containers made from wood, glass, and metal were used to reduce leakage during storage and transportation, reduce incidences of contamination, and improve the shelf life of the product. It was also discovered that, by dividing batches of semisolid/liquid foodstuffs into several containers, transportation and storage became easier to achieve for the consumption of individual rations (Brody, 1999).

As a result of the continuous search for new methods to protect and transport food-stuffs, functional packaging and a number of engineered methods for product protection using environmentally friendly materials have been developed. Also, packing materials and products have been used as effective media to label the different characteristics of the content (and packaging material) and have become important tools in advertising and marketing practices. Nowadays, packaging is manufactured from different sources including plants (Brody, 1999; Taylor, 2005), and barcodes and quick response (QR) codes are included on labels, providing information about the contents, their durability, and use of the product.

The purpose of this chapter is to summarize the materials, techniques, and technologies that are currently used in the packaging of fruit juices, emphasizing the role of packaging in the preservation of both the sensory and quality characteristics and the safety and nutritional values of the product, as well as the novel methods that focus on increasing the shelf life of the product and reducing the environmental impact of manufacturing materials.

14.2   PRIMARY AND SECONDARY CONTAINERS

The term *primary container* refers to the material that is in direct contact with the product, while the *secondary container* is in direct contact with the primary container but not with the product. The secondary container (outer box, wrap, or drum) holds the units together and gives gross protection (Dauthy, 1995).

Commonly, fruit concentrates are packed into primary containers such as plastic linings that are then packaged within suitable secondary containers, which minimize the requirements that must be met by the primary container. As primary containers are in direct contact with the food, this chapter refers to them more than to secondary ones. The following are among the main general requirements that primary containers must meet (Dauthy, 1995; Baroni and Torri, 2012):

- Must be nontoxic and compatible with food
- Must be sanitary, look good, and be printable
- Must protect against gases, moisture, light, and odors
- Must be robust and resistant to impact
- Must have features that ensure absence of adulteration (e.g., different types of sealing)
- Must be easy to open, pour, and reseal
- Must be easy to dispose of and be environmentally friendly
- Must have low cost

14.2.1   HERMETIC CONTAINERS

Hermetic means impermeable to something and refers mainly to gases and vapors. A hermetic container has this characteristic and includes adequate closure features. Thus, as long as it remains intact, a hermetic container is impermeable to microorganisms and solid particles. However, a container that prevents the entry of microorganisms might be nonhermetic (Baroni and Torri, 2012).

Hermetic containers are essential for vacuum and pressure packaging techniques, in addition to protecting the product from moisture gain or loss and from oxygen. Depending on their flexibility and resistance to fracture, containers may exhibit hermetic or nonhermetic properties. The hermetic characteristic of the container might be lost through failures or faulty closures or because of minimal pinholes in the container's wall, even though the transfer rates of gas and water vapor may be considerably low. Also, containers are considered hermetic provided their lids or closure features are tight. For many vacuum-packed containers, the tightness of the lid or cover will be increased by the differential of atmospheric pressure pushing down the cover. Regarding nonhermetic properties, glass bottles fail more often than cans (Dauthy, 1995; Bates et al., 2001).

14.3 MATERIALS COMMONLY USED FOR PRIMARY CONTAINERS

14.3.1 GLASS

Originally, glass packaging was used for storing all kinds of solids and liquids, protecting them from light, heat, and moisture. The technique of glassblowing appeared centuries later and enabled the production of glass containers of different shapes and sizes and for different applications. The large-scale production of glass began in the nineteenth century, which considerably reduced the importance of the glassblowing method and initiated the mass production of glass packaging. The first automatic machines to produce glass bottles were developed at the beginning of the twentieth century and were used for liquids.

The glass used for containers in juice packaging is a controlled blend of sand, limestone, and other materials, and it is made by heating these materials to 1500°C. Glass containers have several advantages: they do not react with food; they are transparent, colored, or opaque according to different needs; they can be manufactured in various shapes; and they use low-cost, recyclable materials. Their main disadvantages are their substantial weight and brittleness with respect to metal cans of the same capacity, as well as their low thermal conductance and low resistance to thermal shocks (Dauthy, 1995; Baroni and Torri, 2012).

Another important aspect of glass containers is the lid, cover, or system that closes the container, which must ensure a hermetic seal. This commonly consists of metallic, glass, or plastic caps and specific materials for tightness. Currently, there are two closure methods for glass containers: mechanical and pneumatic closure (Baroni and Torri, 2012).

14.3.2 METAL

The use of metal packaging is relatively new. The development of metal manufacturing industries and the invention of preservation at the beginning of the nineteenth century triggered the use of metal cans. Shortly thereafter, aluminum was used for the first time in the production of food containers (Baroni and Torri, 2012).

The cans that are used nowadays are made of tinplate. Tinplate consists of a thin sheet of low-carbon steel that is coated with a layer of tin on both sides (commonly by electrodeposition). In most cases, the plate is differentially coated, that is, the tin layer on one plate's surface is thicker than the the tin layer on the other surface. Tin is not completely resistant to corrosion, but its rate of reaction with many food materials is considerably slower than that of steel; furthermore, the effectiveness of a tin coating depends on its thickness, which may range from 1.0 to 2.0 µm. However, when tin reacts unfavorably with a particular juice product, the tin may be coated with enamel, which consists of a resinous base coat and a vinyl top coat; this is particularly common for red fruit juices (Dauthy, 1995).

14.3.3 Laminates

In order to protect fruit juices from microorganisms, water vapor, oxygen, and light, a frequently used alternative is laminates, which can have as many as eight layers of flexible materials such as paper sheets, plastic films, and metal foils. Among the advantages offered by laminates are their aseptic and inert characteristics in addition to their low weight and cost; however, the preference for this type of packaging is due to the ease with which it can be sealed and resealed.

Laminates are manufactured using different processes, for instance, wet or dry bonding of the layers with a thermoplastic adhesive or hot-melt laminating and extrusion techniques (Baroni and Torri, 2012). These plastic layers can be bonded to paper or metal sheets to produce thicker structures with more and improved functions.

For laminate production, paper and reprocessed wastepaper are whitened and coated with resins, plastics, and aluminum layers to improve the laminate's impermeability to water vapor and other gases, as well as its sealability and appearance (Dauthy, 1995).

14.3.4 Polyethylene Terephthalate: Rugged, Reasonably Inert, Visible

Currently, plastic is the most commonly used packaging material due to its wide range of applications and valuable qualities. The manufacture of polyethylene terephthalate (PET) bottles dates back to the late 1980s (Baroni and Torri, 2012).

The physical appearance of PET is very similar to glass. The low cost of raw materials and their mechanical resistance to bulk storage and transportation have driven the increased use of primary containers made from PET. Since the end of the twentieth century, new PET bottles also incorporate recycled PET (Bates et al., 2001). Other advantages of PET containers for fruit juice packaging are their reasonably inert nature with respect to juice components and the possibility of using nonthermal sterilization methods without modifying their physical and chemical safety.

Originally conceived as a textile fiber, since its first use as a material to produce containers for food packaging, PET is the polymer that most international automation engineering companies have focused their efforts on (Bates et al., 2001).

14.4 PACKAGING TECHNIQUES

Advances in packaging technology have been achieved in parallel with the development of processing systems not only for juice packaging but also for other applications.

Traditional tin cans and glass containers may be replaced in some applications by aluminum cans, lightweight shock-resistant glass, plastic, and laminated materials. All these facilitate high production efficiencies resulting in improved product protection and lower associated costs.

14.4.1 Sterile Filtration

All microorganisms and viruses may be removed by filtration through membranes with pore sizes of less than 200 nm. Filtered juices may have long storage periods assuming that fruit enzymes are not active and a reasonably low-temperature storage is maintained. Juices in which turbidity is normally present or those with precipitates cannot be treated this way (Bates et al., 2001). However, some experimental systems that separate the juice into a turbid portion for pasteurization and a clear fluid portion for sterile filtration, followed by homogenizing and combining the sterile streams, have been developed (Dauthy, 1995). For juices containing considerable amounts of pulp, the sterilization strategy is to separate the pulp from the fluid juice and to rapidly process the juice in a heat exchanger, whereas the pulp is treated using slower heating methods, such as using batch stirring tanks and large-diameter holding tubes. The two streams are then combined by homogenization to stabilize the blend and the juice is then packaged under aseptic conditions (Bates et al., 2001).

14.4.2 Canning

Canning is an effective method for processing fresh juices and initially involves heating clean, whole fruit for up to 1 min at 80°C. By doing this, contamination is considerably reduced without affecting either the pericarp or the pulp that, which give fresh juice its sensory qualities. Currently, several research works are in progress with the aim of combining surface heat with other decontamination practices (Bates et al., 2001).

Cans are filled with hot juice and are sealed and processed at 105°C for 10 min and then cooled (Bates et al., 2001). The juice is agitated inside the can due to the movement of bubbles caused by the continuous rotation of the can, which results from rapid heating and cooling; this prevents lower-quality juice that would be obtained by slow heating and cooling.

14.4.3 Hot Fill

A process called flash pasteurization can be used to obtain good quality, safely packaged juices. Hot fill is the process of rapidly heating the juice (up to 90°C), and then filling the containers with the hot juice. After sealing, the filled containers are cooled by spinning for short time periods (Dauthy, 1995; Bates et al., 2001).

Juice may be heated be means of a coil that is submerged in boiling water with the juice flow adjusted to the desired pasteurization temperature. However, for turbid juices or juices with a large amount of pulp, a swept surface unit can continuously heat the juice stream. Some systems use the hot juice stream for preheating the cool juice at the entrance to the heat exchanger; this increases energy efficiency, although the hot juice stream needs to be quickly filled and sealed in an aseptic environment (Bates et al., 2001).

14.4.4   ASEPTIC PROCESSING

The systems used for juice packaging should perform all the processing steps in sterile surroundings and conditions; that is, the system should quickly heat, pasteurize, and cool the juice as well as fill the sterile containers with the sterile juice. As mentioned above, the rapid heating and cooling of the product increase the quality and shelf life of the juice due to microbial and enzyme destruction. A system that works in this way is called an aseptic processing system and, of course, it requires sophisticated control and maintenance (Bates et al., 2001; Baroni and Torri, 2012).

Certainly, in order to allow for an aseptic processing system to work adequately, the selection of the material for the primary container is critical. The container should be capable of resisting the rapid heat changes required for container sterilization and for juice pasteurization. Laminates are regularly used because of their versatility to produce containers of different capacities.

14.4.5   NOVEL TECHNIQUES FOR JUICE PRESERVATION

This section introduces the most recent techniques being researched that aim to increase the shelf life not only of juices but also of food products in general. Although these techniques are not described in depth, the reader may find the references cited for each topic useful.

14.4.5.1   High Pressures

High-pressure processing of fruit juices, at several hundred megapascals, causes cell destruction as well as a significant decrease in the microbial population. Higher pressures than these are even capable of producing spore and enzyme inactivation, once the exposure times are sufficient and the pressuring system is stable.

Of course, the equipment required to generate high pressures in a short time is very expensive. Nonetheless, many studies on the effect of high pressures on the properties of foodstuffs have been carried out and are currently in progress, including the application of high pressures to semisolid and liquid products (Bates et al., 2001).

14.4.5.2   Pulsed Electric Fields

This nonthermal method uses short pulses of electricity to inactivate microorganisms. It has the important advantage of having almost no effect on food quality; thus, pulsed electric fields (PEFs) minimize harmful changes in the sensory and physical properties of foods (Mohamed and Eissa, 2006). This technology helps to preserve the original physical form and characteristics (such as color, flavor, and texture) of foods, in addition to preserving the nutrients contained in the food products. By applying high-voltage pulses to liquid or semisolid foods placed between two

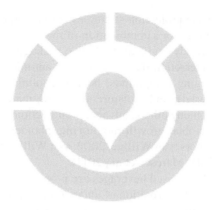

FIGURE 14.1 "Radura" international symbol required on the label of food products treated with ionizing radiation.

electrodes, it is possible to pasteurize fruit juices at slightly increased temperatures. However, a different method is required to achieve the inactivation of enzymes.

14.4.5.3   Irradiation

By applying ionizing radiation, the shelf life of fruit juices may be increased. This physical agent can be applied to fruit before the juice is extracted or it can be applied directly to the juice. A reduction in the microbial population is achieved with radiation doses close to 400 Gy (Bates et al., 2001; Niemira and Fan, 2006), although enzymes require more energy per unit mass to be inactivated. This technique is safe and effective to preserve the freshness of the fruit juice and to increase its shelf life, assuming appropriate storage conditions.

Current regulations include the requirement to display the "Radura" on the product's label, which is the international symbol for products treated with ionizing radiation (see Figure 14.1). Ionizing radiation, unlike the general assumption, is a safe aid to packaging and preserving by thermal methods as well as an extraordinary technique for insect disinfestation (Niemira and Fan, 2006).

14.5   PRESERVATION OF NUTRIENTS BY PACKAGING

One of the main purposes of the packaging of juice and juice-like products is to preserve the quality of the packed product. Many efforts have been made not only to produce adequate packaging to physically protect the product, but also to develop active packaging to aid in the preservation of the contents. Even though juices can be treated by any of the above-mentioned packaging methods to reduce and eliminate microorganisms, decomposition may occur mainly due to the juice constituents or the environment. Alterations to juices that might be attributed to the environment, such as the Maillard reaction (sugar-amine browning), can be reduced by active packaging (Bates et al., 2001; Kerry and Butler, 2008). Many efforts have been made not only to produce adequate packaging to physically protect the product, but also to develop active packaging to aid in the preservation of the contents (Labuza and Breene, 1989).

One of the most frequent protection strategies is to incorporate antioxidant, chelating, or antimicrobial agents or a combination of these into the packaging material (Vermeiren et al., 1999; Brody et al., 2001). Active packaging implies a level of container–food–consumer interaction that may include antimicrobial agents; ethylene, oxygen, and CO_2-scavenging compounds; heating/cooling aids; odor- and flavor-absorbing/releasing materials; and moisture-absorbing materials; while intelligent packaging may include, among others, advanced interactions such as time–temperature history records, microbial growth monitoring, photochromic light protection, and physical shock indicators (van Willige, 2002; van Willige et al., 2002; Kerry and Butler, 2008; Bolouri, 2011; Maresca et al., 2011).

Most components of fruit-based beverages are prone to oxidation with the consequent loss of vitamins and the formation of undesirable sensorial attributes. A number of studies discuss the nutritional implications of storage and types of packaging. Vermeiren et al. (1999) reported developments in the active packaging of foods and focused on O_2-scavenging and ethylene-scavenging technology and moisture regulators (including sachets), emphasizing antimicrobial films whose main applications are claimed to include meat, fish, poultry, bread, cheese, fruits, vegetables, and so forth. Suppakul et al. (2003) mentioned the different categories of active packaging concepts with particular emphasis on the activity of antimicrobial packaging and its effects on food products and proposed that future research on antimicrobial active packaging should focus on a combination of naturally derived agents, biopreservatives, and biodegradable packaging and consider aspects such as food safety, shelf life, and environmental friendliness. The effect of an Ag-containing nanocomposite active packaging system on the survival of *Alicyclobacillus acidoterrestris* was studied by del Nobile et al. (2004), who observed that an active film successfully inhibited the growth of the microorganism in two different media.

Ayhan et al. (2001) studied the effects of nonthermal processing on the flavor, color, and vitamin C retention of PEF-processed orange juice in different packaging materials, while a comprehensive review of antimicrobial food packaging was published by Appendini and Hotchkiss (2002). Özkan et al. (2004) investigated the influence of H_2O_2 on low-pH juices and found that the degradation of vitamin C fitted a zero-order model. Rate constants increased slightly in the presence of 0.5 ppm H_2O_2, but increasing the H_2O_2 concentration from 0.5 to 5 ppm enhanced the decomposition rates of ascorbic acid.

14.6   FINAL REMARKS

Packaging constitutes a major issue in the preservation of fruit and vegetable juices and has greatly evolved over the last two decades. The practice involves traditional, new, and emerging technologies and technical knowledge such as hardware development; the evaluation of stored and packed products based on high levels of detection and fine measurements; methodologies involving molecular biology and microbiology, advanced physics and chemistry, and micro- and nanotechnologies; the design of novel equipment incorporating robotics; the development of new materials, updating processing control schemes, and modern process design and synthesis; and all of this within a sustainable and environmentally friendly philosophy.

REFERENCES

Appendini, P., Hotchkiss, J. H. (2002). Review of antimicrobial food packaging. *Innovative Food Science and Emerging Technologies* 3: 113–126.

Ayhan, Z., Yeom, H. W., Zhang, Q. H., Min, D. B. (2001). Flavor, color, and vitamin C retention of pulsed electric field processed orange juice in different packaging materials. *Journal of Agricultural and Food Chemistry* 49: 669–674.

Baroni, M. R., Torri, L. (2012). *Packages and Foods*. Artek, Italy.

Bates, R. P., Morris, J. R., Crandall, P. G. (2001). *Principles and Practices of Small- and Medium-Scale Fruit Juice Processing*. Food and Agriculture Organization of the United Nations, Rome.

Bolouri, B. (2011). Predicted versus steady state aroma transfer through packaging films. In: P. S. Taoukis, N. G. Stoforos, V. T. Karathanos, G. D. Saravacos (eds), *ICEF 11th Congress Proceedings*, volume I, pp. 999–1000. May 22–26, NTUA, School of Chemical Engineering, Athens, Greece.

Brody, A. L. (1999). Development of packaging for food products. In: A. L. Brody, J. B. Lord (eds), *Developing New Food Products for a Changing Marketplace*, pp. 313–351. CRC Press, Boca Raton, FL.

Brody, A. L., Strapinsky, E. R., Kline, L. R. (2001). Antimicrobial packaging. In: *Active Packaging for Food Applications*, pp. 131–196. CRC Press, Boca Raton, FL.

Dauthy, M. E. (1995). *Fruit and Vegetable Processing*. FAO Agricultural Services Bulletin No. 119. Food and Agriculture Organization of the United Nations, Rome.

del Nobile, M. A., Cannarsi, M., Altieri, C., Sinigaglia, M., Favia, P., Iacoviello, G., D'Agostino, R. (2004). Effect of Ag-containing nano-composite active packaging system on survival of *Alicyclobacillus acidoterrestris*. *Journal of Food Science* 69(8): 379–383.

Kerry, J., Butler, P. (2008). *Smart Packaging Technologies for Fast Moving Consumer Goods*. Wiley, Chichester.

Labuza, T. P., Breene, W. M. (1989). Applications of "active packaging" for improvement of shelf-life and nutritional quality of fresh and extended shelf-life foods. *Journal of Food Processing and Preservation* 13(1): 1–69.

Maresca, P., Donsì, F., Ferrari, G. (2011) Application of a multi-pass high-pressure homogenization treatment for the pasteurization of fruit juices. *Journal of Food Engineering* 104: 364 372.

Mohamed, M. E. A., Eissa, A. H. A. (2006). Pulsed electric fields for food processing technology, structure and function of food engineering. In: A. H. A. Eissa (ed.), *Food Irradiation Research and Technology*, pp. 177–184. Blackwell Publishing, Oxford.

Niemira, B. A., Fan, X. (2006). Low-dose irradiation of fresh and fresh-cut produce: Safety, sensory, and shelf life. In: C. H. Sommers, X. Fan (eds) *Food Irradiation Research and Technology*, pp. 169–184. Blackwell, Ames, IA.

Özkan, M., Kirca, A., Cemeroğlu, B. (2004). Effects of hydrogen peroxide on the stability of ascorbic acid during storage in various fruit juices. *Food Chemistry* 88: 591–597.

Suppakul, P., Miltz, J., Sonneveld, K., Bigger, S. W. (2003). Active packaging technologies with an emphasis on antimicrobial packaging and its applications. *Journal of Food Science* 68(2): 408–420.

Taylor, B. (2005). Fruit and juice processing. In: P. R. Ashurst (ed.), *Chemistry and Technology of Soft Drinks and Fruit Juices*, 2nd edn., pp. 35–66. Wiley-Blackwell, New York.

van Willige, R. W. G. (2002). Effects of flavour absorption on foods and their packaging materials. PhD thesis, Wageningen Universiteit.

van Willige, R. W. G., Linssen, J. P., Meinders, M. B., van der Stege, H. J., Voragen, A. G. (2002). Influence of flavour absorption on oxygen permeation through LDPE, PP, PC and PET plastics food packaging. *Food Additives and Contaminants* 19(3): 303–313.

Vermeiren, L., Devlieghere, F., van Beest, M., de Kruijf, N., Debevere, J. (1999). Developments in the active packaging of foods. *Trends in Food Science & Technology* 10: 77–86.

15 Spoiling Microorganisms in Fruit Juices

Antonio J. Ramos and Sonia Marín

CONTENTS

15.1 Introduction 311
15.2 Fruit Juices as a Suitable Medium for Growth of Microorganisms 311
15.3 Sources of Fruit Juice Contamination 312
15.4 Microorganisms Involved in Fruit Juice Spoilage 313
    15.4.1 Yeasts 313
    15.4.2 Bacteria 314
        15.4.2.1 *Alicyclobacillus* spp. 317
    15.4.3 Molds 321
15.5 Methods for Detection of Spoilage Microorganisms in Fruit Juice 322
    15.5.1 Yeast Enumeration and Identification 322
    15.5.2 *Alicyclobacillus* spp. Analysis 323
References 325

15.1 INTRODUCTION

According to EU Directive 2001/112/EC of December 20, 2001, relating to fruit juices and certain similar products intended for human consumption, a fruit juice is a fermentable but unfermented product having the characteristics of the fruit from which it comes. This definition emphasizes one of the main aspects of concern from the microbiological point of view: fruit juices are a suitable substrate for the growth of microorganisms, such as fermenting yeasts. However, not only yeasts are responsible for fruit juice spoilage. A wide variety of microorganisms can cause alterations in fruit juices, including aciduric bacteria, xerophilic yeasts, and molds. This chapter will review the main microorganisms involved in fruit juice spoilage, including data on the effect that fruit juice treatments can have on them and the analytical methods most commonly used to detect them. Aspects related to the presence of pathogenic microorganisms in fruit beverages are described in the following chapter.

15.2 FRUIT JUICES AS A SUITABLE MEDIUM FOR GROWTH OF MICROORGANISMS

Fruit juices and fruit beverages contain water, a high carbohydrate concentration (sugars and polymers such as pectin, hemicellulose, or cellulose), organic acids (mainly citric, tartaric, malic, lactic, acetic, and ascorbic acid), minerals (such as calcium, magnesium, phosphorus, and sodium), vitamins, soluble and insoluble fibers, and other growth-promoting factors, and enough nutrients to make fruit juices an adequate medium for the growth of most microorganisms, were it not for their low pH values. Fruit juices typically have low pH values, which inhibit most bacteria but leave a wide variety of yeasts unaffected. The pH value of fruit usually ranges between 2.5 and 4.5, although limes may have a lower pH value (1.8–2.0) and melons a considerably higher range (6.3–6.7). A low pH makes fruit juices susceptible to the growth of yeasts, filamentous fungi, and lactic acid bacteria (LAB), due to their growth pH range (with relatively low optimum values) and ability to grow in high-acid environments. Some thermoacidophilic bacteria belonging to the genus *Alicyclobacillus* have also demonstrated the ability to grow in this acid substrate.

On the other hand, the redox potential (Eh) is a physicochemical parameter that determines the oxidizing or reducing properties of the medium, and depends on the composition of the food (thiol-containing amino acids, peptides, proteins, and reducing sugars), pH, and temperature, and, to a greater extent, on the concentration of dissolved oxygen. This parameter plays an important role in the cellular physiology of microorganisms such as their growth capacity, enzyme expression, and thermal resistance (Alwazeer et al. 2003). The Eh of fruit juices tends to range from +300 to +400 mV, which enables spoilage of these products by aerobic bacteria and molds.

After water, which represents 70%–95% of the edible part of a fruit, carbohydrates are the main component of fruits, and represent more than 90% of their dry matter. Carbohydrates include sugars and other carbon sources that act as sources of energy for microorganisms, whereas the nitrogen requirement for microbial growth is provided by proteolysis of proteins present in fruits and the use of amino acids, nucleotides, and certain polysaccharides and fats.

Due to their nutritional value, natural juices, even when kept under refrigeration, have a short shelf life. Several factors ultimately encourage, prevent, or limit the growth of microorganisms in commercialized juices; the most important are pH value, water activity (a_w), quality of raw material, hygiene practice, processing method, presence of preservatives, packaging material, and storage conditions.

Processed fruit products, such as fruit concentrates, jellies, syrups, or similar products have reduced water activity due to the added sugar and water reduction. This, together with the usual heat treatments applied to these products, causes highly osmophilic yeasts and certain spore-forming *Clostridium* or *Bacillus* species to occur within the usual spoiling microbiota. In pasteurized fruit juices and nectars, as thermal treatments kill most vegetative bacteria, yeasts, and molds, the main microbiota are heat-resistant ascospores or sclerotia from *Paecilomyces* spp., *Aspergillus* spp., or *Penicillium* spp., or endospore-forming bacteria such as *Alicyclobacillus acidoterrestris* (Kalia and Gupta 2006).

15.3 SOURCES OF FRUIT JUICE CONTAMINATION

With regard to the origin of contamination, fruit juices may ultimately be contaminated with microorganisms from soil-contaminated or insect-damaged fruits; visibly spoiled fruits and fallen fruits must be avoided where possible. Fruits can be also contaminated by the air, dust, handling, and creatures such as birds. Soil is the main source of spoilage microorganisms such as *Alicyclobacillus* spp. and heat-resistant molds. Environmental fomites may also make the fruits unsafe and could contribute to the spread of pathogenic or spoilage microorganisms.

Water, flavorings, and other chemicals added to juices are all potential sources of microbial contamination. Water used in fruit juice preparation can be a major source of microorganisms such as coliforms, fecal coliforms, fecal streptococci, *Escherichia coli*, *Salmonella*, *Shigella*, *Vibrio cholerae*, and protozoa such as *Cryptosporidium* spp. Sugars and sugar concentrates are commonly contaminated with osmophilic yeasts such as *Zygosaccharomyces rouxii*.

On the other hand, machinery and filling lines are particularly problematic, and strict hygiene measures are essential (Wareing and Davenport 2004). Contamination can take place in inadequately cleaned presses, mills, extractors, pipelines, and filling machines, and in contaminated packaging materials. Improper sanitation procedures will result in juice recontamination after pasteurization and the possibility of microorganisms establishing themselves inside the plant (Tribst et al. 2009). In fact, it has been suggested that poor factory hygiene accounts for 95% of yeast infections; improvements in factory hygiene may dramatically reduce spoilage.

Bearing in mind that the fruits themselves may be the most important source of juice contamination, the step of washing the fruits with sanitizers is of obvious importance. However, as commonly used sanitizers have limited effectiveness, depending on the microorganism considered, selection of raw material and discarding visibly altered fruits is a key process.

15.4 MICROORGANISMS INVOLVED IN FRUIT JUICE SPOILAGE

15.4.1 YEASTS

Many microorganisms are frequently found in fruits and fruit juices, but relatively few can ultimately grow in this acidic environment. Bacterial growth is controlled to a large extent by acidity; bacterial spores will not germinate on foods with a pH of less than 4.5, and vegetative cells of pathogenic bacteria will not usually grow at a pH lower than 4.0 (Smelt et al. 1982), a low temperature, or a high osmotic strength (generally caused by a high sugar concentration) (Stratford 2006). In the absence of competing bacteria, yeasts are the main group associated with fruit juice spoilage.

To compose an exhaustive list of all yeasts that have, on occasion, been isolated from any kind of fruit juice would be an endless task. In fact, it has been estimated that nearly 120 yeast species, belonging to 30 genera, could be associated with foods (Barnett et al., 1983), although Pitt and Hocking (1985) stated that most of these 120 species grow poorly in properly formulated foods, where low water activity, heat treatment, or the addition of preservatives could inhibit the growth of many of them. Stratford (2006), when considering only spoilage of fruit juices and soft drinks, gave as the most significant spoilage yeasts a reduced list that includes (using current names): *Dekkera anomala*, *D. bruxellensis*, *D. naardenensis*, *Hanseniaspora uvarum*, *Saccharomyces bayanus*, *S. cerevisiae*, *S. exiguus*, *Schizosaccharomyces pombe*, *Torulaspora delbrueckii*, *Zygosaccharomyces bailii*, *Z. bisporus*, *Z. microellipsoides*, and *Z. rouxii*. On the other hand, other authors added to this list species of the genera *Candida, Hansenula, Pichia, Rhodotorula*, and *Trichosporon* (Tribst et al. 2009). Recently, Hutzler et al. (2012) have published a complete review of spoilage yeasts relevant to the beverage industry, where information about important beverage yeast species can be found. In this review, yeasts found in fruit juices comprise the following genera/species: *Brettanomyces/Dekkera* spp., *Candida* sp., *Debaryomyces hansenii, H. uvarum, Issatchenkia orientalis, Kazachstania exigua, Pichia fermentans, P. guilliermondii, P. membranefaciens, Saccharomyces sensu stricto* sp., *Schizosaccharomyces pombe, Torulaspora delbrueckii, Wickerhamomyces anomalus, Z. bailii, Z. rouxii*, and *Zygotorulaspora florentinus*.

The most frequent alterations produced by yeasts in fruit juices are gas and alcohol production, cloudiness, phase separation, sediment or pellicle formation, off-flavors dominated by a slight fermentation smell, and off-tastes (Loureiro and Querol 1999).

Most spoilage yeasts are highly fermentative; fermentation can cause cans and cartons to split and glass or plastic packages to explode. The yeast species that are capable of forming sufficient gas pressure to cause bottles to explode include *Z. bailii, S. cerevisiae, D. bruxellensis*, and *S. ludwigii*; species such as *Candida parapsilosis* or *C. pseudointermedia* can also produce CO_2 but to a lesser extent: not enough to cause breakage of bottles but enough to cause complaints from consumers due to organoleptic changes (Stratford 2006). However, many yeast species do not ferment, and these are termed respiring species.

A second sign of yeast spoilage is related to the visible observation of macroscopic symptoms of yeast growth (presence of hazes, clouds, flocks, particulates, surface films or colonies, and sediments in undisturbed bottles).

Off-tastes and off-odors are other frequent symptoms of yeast spoilage and, in some cases, obvious enough to be detected by consumers. The production of volatile metabolites such as alcohol, acetaldehyde, acetic acid, ethyl acetate, diacetyl, acetoin, and other volatile acids can influence the flavor and smell of juices, contributing to the undesired formation of unexpected and surprising flavors.

Due to the widespread use of preservatives in fruit juice products, preservative-resistant yeasts are a matter of concern in these kinds of products. The main species in this group are *Z. bailii, Z. rouxii, S. pombe, C. krusei, Z. bisporus*, and *P. membranaefaciens* (Tribst et al. 2009). Most of these yeasts are not only able to grow in the presence of preservatives, such as sorbic or benzoic acid, but also in beverages with low water activity, such as syrups. For these reasons, these yeast strains are a major problem for the soft drink industry, as the stability of these products frequently depends on the pasteurization of the sugar syrup before it is mixed with the beverage base (fruit juice, preservatives, flavorings, sweeteners, etc.) and carbonated (Tribst et al. 2009).

15.4.2 BACTERIA

The bacteria that are able to proliferate in fruit juices are restricted to a few acid-tolerant groups (main genera in parentheses): LAB (*Lactobacillus* and *Leuconostoc*), acetic bacteria (*Acetobacter* and *Gluconobacter*), spore-forming bacteria (mainly *Bacillus* and *Clostridium*), ethanol-producing bacteria (*Zymomonas, Zymobacter*, and *Saccharobacter*), and acidothermophilic sporulated bacteria (*Alicyclobacillus*)

(Vasavada 2003). In the last 30 years, *Alicyclobacillus* spp., mainly *A. acidoterrestris*, has emerged as one of the main spoilage bacteria in pasteurized fruit juices, thereby causing a serious concern for the industry. Therefore, it will be described in detail in the following section.

LAB are microaerophilic, Gram-positive bacilli or cocci. They can grow in substrates with low oxygen content, fermenting sugars predominantly to produce lactic acid. Some strains produce diacetyl (causing a buttermilk off-flavor), and can produce extracellular fructose or glucose polymers from sucrose (generating a gummy slime or an appearance of "ropiness"). Also, LAB spoilage of fruit juices is often associated with the production of acids such as acetic, formic, and succinic, and with the generation of a sour or off-taste, a buttermilk off-flavor, cloudiness and turbidity formation, and gas (CO_2) and ethanol production. Common species are *Lactobacillus paracasei* and *Leuconostoc mesenteroides*, although other species such as *Lactobacillus brevis*, *L. buchneri*, *L. plantarum*, *L. perolens*, *L. collinoides*, *L. mali*, and *Weissella confusa* are also commonly found (Dicks and Endo 2009; Juvonen et al. 2011). LAB are not heat-resistant bacteria; therefore, fruit juice pasteurization is expected to control this type of microorganism efficiently. Although the presence of LAB is more commonly reported in unpasteurized juices, recontamination after thermal treatment plays an important role (Tribst et al. 2009). Frequently, spoilage episodes are the result of failures in cleaning and sanitation programs, especially of the equipment used after the thermal treatment. To control LAB in fruit juices, attention must be paid to three important points: washing of fruit, proper pasteurization, and improved sanitation of equipment.

Acetic acid bacteria (AAB) consist of strictly aerobic species of the acid-tolerant Gram-negative genera *Acetobacter* (such as *A. aceti* and *A. pasteurianus*) and *Gluconobacter* (such as *G. oxydans*), which are responsible for such undesirable effects as browning of juices, production of acetic acid in the presence of ethanol, and production of buttermilk- and sauerkraut-like flavors. In addition, *Gluconacetobacter* and *Asaia* spp. have been associated with the spoilage of soft drinks. AAB acquire energy from the oxidation of sugars, organic acids, sugar alcohols, and alcohols that produce acetic, gluconic, lactic, and succinic acids, and acetaldehyde and ketone compounds (Juvonen et al. 2011). As with LAB, AAB are easily controlled by heat treatments, thus they are more frequently found in fresh juices. Control measures in the industry are the same as described for LAB.

Besides *Alicyclobacillus*, other spore-forming bacteria have been found in fruit juices, mainly represented by the *Bacillus* and *Clostridium* species. Thus, some *Bacillus* spp., such as *B. coagulans*, *B. macerans*, *B. polymyxa*, *B. licheniformis*, and *B. subtilis*, have been connected with flat-sour spoilage (due to the production of lactic acid without gas formation) of tomato juice, soft drinks, and canned fruits (Lucas et al. 2006; Vasavada 2003). *B. megaterium* and *B. coagulans* have also been connected with spoilage in mango and orange juices, as well as in tomato paste (Silva and Gibbs, 2004).

On the other hand, some species of *Clostridium* have been isolated from spoiled fruit juices, such as *C. pasteurianum* and *C. butyricum*, which produce an increase in acidity and gas, and a strong butyric odor (Vasavada, 2003). *C. pasteurianum* is an anaerobic, saccharolytic, spore-forming microorganism that produces hydrogen and carbon dioxide gas as a by-product of its growth, which results in swollen packages of spoiled foods. It produces butyric acid, which gives an off-odor and off-flavor that are easily detected and produce results that are unacceptable to consumers. Spores of *C. pasteurianum* are widely distributed in soil and, as a result, fruits coming into direct contact with soil may become contaminated with the spores, and consequent spoilage of processed food products becomes possible given anaerobic conditions, adequate pH conditions, or inadequate thermal processing. *C. pasteurianum* is an important spoilage organism in acid foods since it can tolerate high concentrations of sugar at low pH levels. The spoilage of apple juice by *C. pasteurianum* was identified from multiple large spoilage outbreaks of shelf-stable juice that exhibited severely swollen containers and turbid juices with a strong butyric acid odor (Feng et al. 2010). *C. pasteurianum* spores were found to be able to germinate at a pH as low as 4.3 in pH-adjusted apple juice at low contamination levels. Maintaining the finished juice at a pH below 4.0 in combination with mild heating was proposed to prevent potential *C. pasteurianum* spoilage of shelf-stable apple juices (Fweng et al. 2010). Spoilage by *C. butyricum* is less frequent, but it seems that this microorganism could be relevant in juice-based beverages, such as soy and milk beverages, containing fruits and vegetables that have been in close contact with soil (such as carrots or beetroots) (Tribst et al. 2009).

Other relevant spore-forming species include *Streptomyces griseus* and *Sporolactobacillus inulinus*. *S. griseus* is a rod-shaped, aerobic, Gram-positive actinomycete that forms branched filaments and spores resistant to high temperatures, and that produce musty, moldy, or earthy off-flavors in pasteurized apple juices (Siegmund and Pöllinger-Zierler 2007). Growth is possible with a limited oxygen supply even at 4°C, and the spores of thermophilic actinomycetes can be highly resistant to high temperatures, surviving in a sucrose solution up to 100°C for 10 min–4 h (Fergus, 1967). On the other hand, *Sporolactobacillus* is a genus of the anaerobic endospore-forming, Gram-positive, motile, rod-shaped LAB. *S. inulinus*, the type species of the genus, is a mesophilic, homofermentative lactic acid bacterium that is capable of efficient lactic acid production from glucose, which produces spores that are moderately heat resistant. Although it has been found in thick juices with a high sugar content (Justé et al. 2008), due to its close association with soil it is very likely to occur in fruits, and it may have been misidentified as a *Bacillus* or *Clostridium* species in the past (Tribst et al. 2009).

With regard to ethanol-producing bacteria, *Zymomonas mobilis* is a Gram-negative facultative anaerobe that has been linked to apple-cider spoilage (cider sickness), which is most often observed in sweet ciders containing residual sugars with a pH higher than 3.7 (Coton and Coton 2003). The pH value is known to be a key factor in its development, as bacteria are typically sensitive to low pH values (less than 3.5) (Drilleau 1977). This bacterium produces ethanol five to six times faster than yeasts, using only glucose, fructose, and sucrose as carbon sources. Cider sickness is characterized by an off-flavor and off-aroma, due at least in part to the production of acetaldehyde, described as "rotten lemon skin" or "grassy," by an almost explosive production of gas, a decrease in density, and sometimes by a marked turbidity of the product. Cider is in a risk zone for *Z. mobilis* contamination as this bacterium is able to grow at temperatures as low as 4°C, in the pH range from 3.5 to 6.0, in 0–8 mL ethanol/100 mL, at 200 mg/L SO$_2$, and in the presence of a cider polyphenol extract up to 3 g/L (Coton et al. 2006). *Z. mobilis* has also been shown to be a spoilage microorganism in beer and pear-cider beverages (perries).

Finally, another spoilage bacterium that has been occasionally found in fruit juices is *Propionibacterium cyclohexanicum*, a Gram-positive, acid-tolerant, aerotolerant, and catalase-negative bacterium, which has been isolated from fruit juice. *P. cyclohexanicum* is heat resistant but it is non-spore-forming, and grows at temperatures of 20°C–40°C with a reported optimum temperature of 35°C and a pH range of 3.2–7.5. Although *P. cyclohexanicum* does not produce spores, it has been isolated from pasteurized orange juice (Kusano et al. 1997), and previous studies have demonstrated that it is able to survive a heat treatment of 95°C for 10 min (Walker and Phillips 2007). Sodium benzoate (0.5 and 1.0 mg/mL) and potassium sorbate (1.0 mg/mL), both alone and in combination with 2.5, 5, or 10 IU/mL of nisin, inhibit the growth of *P. cyclohexanicum* in orange juice at 30°C for 29 days; however, nisin alone, at concentrations up to 1000 IU/mL, was not effective in inhibiting the multiplication of *P. cyclohexanicum*, suggesting that this microorganism may be resistant to nisin (Walker and Phillips 2008).

15.4.2.1 *Alicyclobacillus* spp.

Alicyclobacillus spp. spoilage is becoming an important issue in heat-treated fruit juices, as these microorganisms produce endospores that are sufficiently heat resistant to enable them to survive the hot-fill–hold pasteurization process to which fruit juice and similar products are exposed in order to render them commercially sterile.

Alicyclobacillus species are nonpathogenic, rod-shaped, thermophilic, and acidophilic spore-forming bacteria. All species are Gram-positive, with the exception of *A. sendaiensis*, which is Gram-negative. Likewise, all species are obligate aerobic, and *A. pohliae* is sometimes facultatively anaerobic. *Alicyclobacillus* grows generally over a pH range of 2.0 to 6.5 (optimum values 3.0–5.5) (Smit et al. 2011), although some species can grow at pH levels below 1.5. The temperature growth range for the juice-associated species is 20°C–70°C (Juvonen et al. 2011), with optimum temperatures for growth between 35°C and 65°C. Growth requires a water activity of more than 0.90 a_w, and some species grow in fruit juices up to 18.2°Brix, but growth inhibition has been seen at 21.6°Brix (Splittstoesser et al. 1994).

The genus *Alicyclobacillus* was proposed in 1992 (Wisotzkey et al. 1992) in order to reclassify thermoacidophilic isolates obtained from hot springs and terrestrial acid thermal environments that were previously classified as *Bacillus* spp. (*B. acidocaldarius*, *B. acidoterrestris*, or *B. cycloheptanicus* and some isolates of *B. coagulans*) (Smit et al. 2011). The comparative sequence analyses carried out on the 16S ribosomal RNA (rRNA) genes of these isolates showed that these strains were different from any other *Bacillus* species. In the same way, isolates previously classified in the genus *Sulfobacillus* were also reclassified into the genus *Alicyclobacillus* (Karavaiko et al. 2005).

To date, 20 species, 2 subspecies, and 2 genomic species belonging to the genus *Alicyclobacillus* have been identified (Smit et al. 2011; Steyn et al. 2011): *A. acidiphilus*, *A. acidocaldarius*, *A. acidocaldarius* subsp. *acidocaldarius*, *A. acidocaldarius* subsp. *rittmannii*, *A. acidoterrestris*, *A. aeris*, *A. contaminans*, *A. cycloheptanicus*, *A. disulfidooxidans*, *A. fastidiosus*, *A. ferrooxydans*, *A. herbarius*, *A. hesperidum*, *A. kakegawensis*, *A. macrosporangiidus*, *A. pohliae*, *A. pomorum*, *A. sacchari*, *A. sendaiensis*, *A. shizuokensis*, *A. tolerans*, *A. vulcanalis*, *Alicyclobacillus* genomic species 1 (*A. mali*), and *Alicyclobacillus* genomic species 2.

Although not all *Alicyclobacillus* species are characterized as spoilage microorganisms, *A. acidoterrestris*, *A. acidocaldarius*, *A. herbarius*, *A. hesperidum*, *A. cycloheptanicus*, *A. acidiphilus*, *A. fastidiosus*, and *A. pomorum* have frequently been implicated in spoilage incidents in high-acid fruit and vegetable products (McKnight et al. 2010; Steyn et al. 2011), *A. acidoterrestris* being recognized as the most important species.

The name *Alicyclobacillus* refers to the presence of unusual ω-alicyclic fatty acids in the membranes of these species. These fatty acids provide the exceptional heat and acid resistance of *Alicyclobacillus* spp., as it has been demonstrated that lipids containing ω-cyclohexane fatty acids pack densely, resulting in low diffusion at high temperatures, which generates an advantage when these microorganisms are grown at high temperatures or low pHs. Lipids containing fatty acids with a cyclohexane ring may stabilize the membrane structure and help to maintain the barrier functions of prokaryotic membranes at high temperatures. These fatty acids contribute to the heat resistance of *Alicyclobacillus* by forming a protective coating with strong hydrophobic bonds that stabilize and reduce the membrane's permeability. Thus, ω-cyclohexane fatty acids may be important in the thermoacidophilic adaptation of bacterial membranes (Merle and Montville 2012). However, it should be noted that *A. pomorum* does not contain ω-alicyclic fatty acids in its membrane (Goto et al. 2003).

Alicyclobacillus spp. have been isolated from hot springs, fruit and acidic fruit juices, concentrates, and beverages. Many acidic juices and concentrates, predominantly apple and orange products, but also including cranberry, white grape, cherry, grapefruit, pear, mango, and pineapple derivatives, have been found to be contaminated with *Alicyclobacillus* (Durak et al. 2010). Tea and other herbal drinks have also been spoiled by this genus (Goto et al. 2002). It has also been detected in fruit juice blends, carbonated fruit juice drinks, fruit pulps, lemonade, and isotonic water, and even in canned diced tomatoes (Smit et al. 2011). As the fruit juice industry is now aware of the problem originated by *Alicyclobacillus* in fruit juices, there is now a challenge to prevent spoilage of newer products that combine fruit juices with vegetable juices. Vegetable root crops such as carrots and beets can also be easily contaminated with soil-based *Alicyclobacillus* spores and, therefore, can be problematic if added to fruit juices (Mermelstein 2012).

Spoilage by *Alicyclobacillus*, which can occur from inoculum levels as low as one spore per 10 mL, can be difficult to detect, as it typically only involves off-flavor development and lacks the typical gas production, turbidity, and heavy sediment associated with other microbial spoilage. Spoilage incidents occur mainly in spring or summer, and spoilage is mainly apparent as an off-flavor or off-odor, with or without sediment, and in some products discoloration or cloudiness occur. Manufacturers often only became aware of the problem because of consumer complaints, since the absence of gas production made spoilage difficult to detect.

The origin of the off-flavor and off-odor caused by *Alicyclobacillus* has been correlated not only with the production of guaiacol (2-methoxyphenol), but also with the halophenols 2,6-dichlorophenol (2,6-DCP) and 2,6-dibromophenol (2,6-DBP). The off-odor is described as medicinal, disinfectant-like, antiseptic, phenolic, smoky, and hammy. These compounds are detectable by the senses when *A. acidoterrestris* reaches 10^5–10^6 CFU/mL. Taste thresholds for guaiacol in orange and noncarbonated fruit juice were reported to be as low as $2\,\mu g/L$ (ppb) (Pettipher et al. 1997) and 2.33 ppb in apple juice, while the concentrations of 2,6-DCP and 2,6-DBP in spoiled mixed fruit drinks were reported to be 16–20 ng/L (ppt) and 2–4 ppt, respectively (Jensen and Whitfield 2003). However, the guaiacol content in fruit juices does not always correlate with the number of *Alicyclobacillus* cells in the juices, and sometimes the off-odor is detected prior to the visual detection limit for bacterial growth in juices or beverages (Pettipher et al. 1997).

Soil is considered to be the primary environment and the main source of contamination of fresh fruits during harvesting, as *Alicyclobacillus* spp. are soil-borne microorganisms. Soil can cling to the fruits that have fallen on the ground and can also be carried into processing facilities by employees. It is therefore highly recommended not to use fruit that has been collected directly from the ground, as well as to perform a fruit-sorting procedure, and to clean and disinfect the surface of the fruit before processing.

Process water has also been identified as an important source of contamination; therefore particular attention must be paid to the quality of flume (transportation) and condensate (recovered) water. Flume water is used to unload and transport the fruits to the processing line and, if the quality of water is appropriate, it is beneficial to clean the fruit and to remove the soil and other particles from the fruits' surfaces. Obviously, the frequency with which this water is renewed and the disinfectant treatment applied to the water can influence the level of *Alicyclobacillus* contamination (Steyn et al. 2011). On the other hand, condensate water from evaporators is a by-product of the juice concentration process that is reused for fruit-cleaning purposes. As this water is warm and has a low pH, it is a suitable substrate for *Alicyclobacillus* development and may therefore contain high counts of *Alicyclobacillus* endospores, increasing the contamination of fruits cleaned with this water unless controlled.

A very useful guideline to avoid problems derived from *Alicyclobacillus* contamination in the fruit industry is the "*Alicyclobacillus* Best Practice Guideline" by the European Fruit Juice Association (AIJN) for the reduction and control of *Alicyclobacillus* in the production, packaging, and distribution of fruit juices, juice concentrates, purees, and nectars (AIJN 2008).

Due to the heat-resistant properties of the *Alicyclobacillus* endospores, the fruit juice industry has focused its efforts on increasing the intensity of the pasteurization step, and it has been suggested that *A. acidoterrestris* must be designated as the target microbe in the design of pasteurization processes for acidic foods and beverages. In fact, *A. acidoterrestris* spores are highly heat resistant, with a $D_{90^\circ C}$ value ranging between 5.95 and 23 min and a $D_{95^\circ C}$ value between 0.06 and 8.55 min, depending on the soluble solids (SS) concentration and the pH of the juice (Tribst et al. 2009). A standard procedure that involves heating at 90°C–95°C for 15–20 s, followed by package filling while the product cools to 82°C–84°C (in 2 min) before chilling (Solberg et al. 1990), may not be enough to control this microorganism. According to Vieira et al. (2002), thermal treatment at 115°C/8 s guarantees juice stability, with a 5-log reduction of *A. acidoterrestris*.

The main factors that determine the heat resistance of *Alicyclobacillus* endospores are temperature, pH, SS content, water activity, species/strain, divalent cations, and sporulation temperature.

Temperature has the greatest influence on D-values, greater than that of the pH level; slight changes in temperature may have a considerable effect. An increase in the total SS content leads to an increase in D-values and a higher heat resistance, which explains the greater difficulty of destroying the *Alicyclobacillus* endospores in fruit juice concentrates than in a single-strength juice.

The different species/strains of *Alicyclobacillus* also differ in their heat resistance, which can be explained by the fact that, depending on the species, the ω-cyclohexane fatty acids of the cell membranes can vary from 15% to 91% of the total fatty acid content (Hippchen et al. 1981) and, as previously explained, these fatty acids play an important role in thermal resistance, although differences in the sporulation temperature, the pH value, the nutrient composition of the heating medium, and water activity can also influence the resistance of spores.

Other factors that have been associated with the heat resistance of *Alicyclobacillus* endospores include the presence of heat-stable proteins and enzymes, and the mineralization by divalent cations with dipicolinic acid (DPA), especially the calcium dipicolinate (Ca-DPA) complex. The structural integrity of *A. acidoterrestris* endospores under low pH conditions was shown to be affected by divalent cations as their heat resistance was associated with strong binding characteristics to calcium (Ca) and manganese (Mn) (Steyn et al. 2011).

To control *Alicyclobacillus* in the fruit juice industry, as previously commented, fallen fruits must be discarded, and control of water quality is a key point; for water treatment, AIJN suggests the use of ozone, hydrogen peroxide, chlorine dioxide, hypochlorite, peracetic acid, ultraviolet (UV) radiation, filtration, or heat treatment to control *Alicyclobacillus* (AIJN 2008). Fruit cleaning and sorting must remove rotten fruits, and for the surface disinfection of fruits, aqueous, chlorine-based disinfectants could be used, as well as the application of 2% H_2O_2 (Orr and Beuchat 2000). Disinfectants can lose their effectiveness in fruits with a waxy surface, and the use of a vigorous wash or a detergent or food-grade surfactant could enhance the effect of disinfectants (Orr and Beuchat 2000).

The control of *Alicyclobacillus* in processed fruit juice is still subject to an exhaustive study. Effective control can be achieved by the use of potassium sorbate or sodium benzoate, the removal of oxygen, the addition of ascorbic acid, or the use of an appropriate pasteurization regime (Wareing and Davenport 2004). Rapid chilling of juice below 20°C after pasteurization, and transportation and storage of fruit juice under refrigerated conditions, are other options (Steyn et al. 2011).

There is increasing interest in the use of bacteriocins, such as nisin, which are not considered to be chemical preservatives. The presence of nisin during heating increases the inactivation of *A. acidoterrestris* spores (Komitopoulou et al. 1999; Peña et al. 2009). However, while nisin inhibits spore germination in orange juice, it does not do so in clear apple juice, most likely due to the competitive effect of phenols (Yamazaki et al. 2000).

The use of essential oils has been also attempted. It has been found that cinnamaldehyde and eugenol can inhibit *A. acidoterrestris* endospores (Bevilacqua et al. 2008a).

Different nonthermal processes such as the use of high electric field alternating current (Uemura et al. 2009), ohmic heating (Baysal and Icier 2010), high hydrostatic pressures (Vercammen et al. 2012), and high-pressure homogenization (Bevilacqua et al. 2012) have been attempted with promising results. A very interesting review on these new nonthermal methods for *A. acidoterrestris* control is the work by Bevilacqua et al. (2008b).

15.4.3 MOLDS

Molds are acid-tolerant aerobic microorganisms that, in many cases, can grow in foods with a high sugar content, which accounts for their occasional occurrence as spoilage microorganisms in fruit juices. Filamentous fungi can cause gas, off-odors and off-flavors (described as "stale" or "old"), tainting, discoloration, formation of mycelial mats on the juice's surface, and reduction of sugar content. Despite their oxygen requirement, some species can grow under anaerobic conditions with fermentation metabolism or, more frequently, at low oxygen concentrations (Juvonen et al. 2011).

Molds usually produce extracellular degradative enzymes that contribute to fruit juice spoilage, such as pectinases, proteases, carbohydrases, and lipases, as well as some allergens and toxins. Also, mycotoxigenic fungi growing on fruits can produce mycotoxins, such as patulin or ochratoxins (see Chapter 16), which can persist in the pasteurized fruit juices due to their high thermal resistance.

Molds encountered in the juice industry come not only from spoiled fruits, air, dust, or soil containing spores but also from mycelium fragments, soil being the main source of heat-resistant molds related to fruit juice contamination (Tribst et al. 2009).

According to their heat resistance, mold problems are generally caused by two types of fungi: heat-sensitive and heat-resistant molds. In the first case, the presence of molds usually indicates poor hygiene within the factory or field environment, the use of highly spoiled fruits, postpasteurization contamination, or improper manufacturing practices. Heavy fungal infection of raw material may lead to the production of gushing inducers, such as hydrophobins; a problem that has been described in beers, but also in some apple- and grape-based products (Khalesi et al. 2012). Gushing inducers could produce an extensive overfoaming in ciders and sparkling wines due to heavy fungal contamination with *Penicillium* or other molds (Juvonen et al. 2011).

Heat-resistant fungi encompass representatives from a considerable list of fungal genera, including *Byssochlamys*, *Neosartorya*, *Paecilomyces*, *Talaromyces*, *Eupenicillium*, *Phialophora*, and *Thermoascus*, although fungi of the genera *Monascus*, *Aureobasidium*, *Cladosporium*, *Penicillium*, and *Aspergillus* have also been found (Wareing and Davenport 2004). Fungal heat-resistant structures include ascospores, chlamydospores, aleurospores, and sclerotia. It is important to note that the thermal tolerance of the heat-resistant structures of molds such as ascospores varies among different species and strains, and due to factors such as the age of the organism, heating media, pH values, the presence of sugars, fats, and acids in the heating media, and growth conditions (Tournas 1994).

Byssochlamys and *Neosartorya* are the heat-resistant genera most often implicated in the spoilage of fruit juices, with species such as *B. nivea*, *B. fulva*, and *N. fischeri* (anamorph *Aspergillus fischerianus*) frequently found in fruit juices (Vasavada 2003). *Byssochlamys* species produce heat-resistant ascospores and survive for considerable periods of time above 85°C. In addition to their heat resistance, *Byssochlamys* species can grow under very low oxygen tensions and can produce pectinolytic enzymes. The combination of these three physiological characteristics causes *Byssochlamys* species to be very significant spoilage fungi in pasteurized fruit juices, such as strawberry, pineapple, passion fruit, mango, grape, and citrus fruit juices, as well as other acidic beverages and dairy products (Hosoya et al. 2012). *Byssochlamys* has a *Paecilomyces* anamorph and only six accepted species: *B. nivea*, *B. fulva*, *B. spectabilis*, *B. lagunculariae*, *B. zollerniae*, and *B. verrucosa*, with similar anamorphs. With regard to food safety, it should be noted that both *B. lagunculariae* and *B. nivea* are able to produce the mycotoxin patulin (Hosoya et al. 2012), and that certain strains of *N. fischeri* are able to produce gliotoxin, verruculogen, and fumitremorgins A, B, and C (Tournas 1994; Yaguchi et al. 2012).

Other fungi such as *Paecilomyces variotii* (the anamorph of *B. spectabilis*), *Eupenicillium brefeldianum* (syn. *Penicillium dodgei*), *Phialophora mustea*, *Thermoascus aurantiacus*, *Monascus purpureus*, *Talaromyces flavus*, *T. macrosporus*, and *T. trachyspermus* have been described in fruit juices such as apple, grape, and pineapple juice (Vasavada 2003).

15.5 METHODS FOR DETECTION OF SPOILAGE MICROORGANISMS IN FRUIT JUICE

Generally, the routine microbiological analysis of fruit juices is carried out through the classical microbiological counting techniques, using general or specific culture media. Thus, to quantify the global contamination of a fruit juice, use of plate count agar (PCA) medium is frequent in order to perform an aerobic enumeration of viable microorganisms. In the same way, for a total estimation of fungal contamination, acidified potato dextrose agar, Sabouraud agar media, or dichloran-glycerol agar (for xerotolerant molds) are frequently used media (among others); whereas for BAL enumeration the Man–Rogosa–Sharpe medium is usually employed. An analysis of pathogenic bacteria often requires sample preenrichment steps and more specific media. Due to the importance of yeast contamination and the occurrence of *Alicyclobacillus* spp. in fruit juices, both traditional and new methods for the detection of these two groups of microorganisms are explained below.

15.5.1 Yeast Enumeration and Identification

As a rule, the general isolation and enumeration media for food-borne spoilage yeasts are the same as those used for food-borne molds (Loureiro and Querol 1999). These are complex media, nutritionally rich, often supplemented with antibiotics against bacteria or compounds to inhibit the development of competitive molds (such as rose bengal or dichloran) and sometimes with an acidified pH and a pH indicator. These media give a global estimation of the total yeast contamination, but selective or differential media are used for the enumeration of particular yeast species. Thus, selective media have been developed to assess the presence of yeasts that are resistant to ethanol, preservatives, or reduced water activity, and differential media have been designed to take into account the capacity of yeasts to degrade certain groups of macromolecules, such as polysaccharides, proteins, pectins, or lipids (Loureiro and Querol 1999). However, although the detection and enumeration of yeasts by traditional plating techniques are discriminative and can detect low contamination levels, this requires 3–7 days of incubation and the results are not relevant enough for yeast identification.

Traditionally, the identification and characterization of yeast species have been based on morphological traits and physiological capabilities. Rapid kit identification methods, such as the API 20 C AUX, the API rapid ID32 C (both of bioMèrieux, France), or the RapID Yeast Plus System (Remel, U.S.), have been widely employed, but lack effectiveness because they were designed for clinical diagnosis purposes (Arias et al. 2002). Other methods described for yeast classification include the use of long-chain fatty acid profiling and electrophoretic isoenzyme profile analysis (Loureiro and Querol 1999).

In the last few decades, yeast identification has undergone a revolutionary change through the introduction of methods based on DNA analysis. Several techniques based on molecular polymorphisms have been used to improve yeast strain identification, such as those based on the analysis of nucleic acid sequences, karyotyping electrophoresis, microsatellites, mitochondrial DNA (mtDNA) restriction patterns, ribosomal DNA (rRNA) restriction patterns, and random amplified polymorphic DNA (Maqueda et al. 2010).

For species identification, methods based on the analysis of ribosomal regions are widely used. One of the most successful methods is restriction fragment length polymorphism (RFLP) analysis of the 5.8S rRNA gene and the two flanking internal transcribed sequences (ITS). This technique consists of direct polymerase chain reaction amplification using conserved oligonucleotide primers against the 26S and 18S rRNA genes, followed by an endonuclease restriction analysis of the amplified product. Because ribosomal regions evolve in a concerted manner, they have low intraspecific polymorphism and high interspecific variability. Consequently, RFLP analysis of the 5.8S-ITS region is an excellent tool for yeast identification (Arias et al. 2002). However, the list of methods based on molecular biology used in the characterization of yeast species or strains is quite long, and reviews of these methods, in foods and other substrates, are found in Loureiro and Malfeito-Ferreira (2003), Orberá (2004), Beh et al. (2006), Fernández-Espinar et al. (2006), and Pincus et al. (2007).

15.5.2 *ALICYCLOBACILLUS* SPP. ANALYSIS

During the past 10 years, many direct plating methods and agar media have been developed for the detection and quantification of *Alicyclobacillus* spp. Two frequently used enumerating media are the *Bacillus acidocaldarius* medium (BAM) and the *Bacillus acidoterrestris* medium (BAT), also called *B. acidoterrestris* thermophilic medium, which has the same composition as BAM with the exception of the amount of yeast extract, which is 2 g/L; twice the amount of that of BAM.

Other media frequently used are the *Alicyclobacillus acidocaldarius* medium (AAM), the *Alicyclobacillus* medium (ALI), the yeast starch glucose medium (YSG), the acidified potato dextrose agar medium (PDA at pH 3.5), the orange serum agar medium (OSA), the K agar medium, and the SK agar medium (Smit et al. 2011). It is suggested that spread plating is more effective than pour plating as surface colonies are larger and easier to enumerate.

Alicyclobacillus isolation procedures have mostly been performed using plating media, but have also been combined with membrane filtration (0.20 or 0.45 μm filters, depending on the method used) when product characteristics allow. *A priori* filtration is more sensitive and has a lower detection limit than conventional spread plating, as larger samples can be passed through the filter. However, membrane filtration is not suitable for all products, as many cannot be filtered. Because filters' capabilities vary, it is recommended to test the retention of *Alicyclobacillus* endospores on the filter membranes to be employed before using them in quality-control processes (Smit et al. 2011).

Since *Alicyclobacillus* spp. are endospore-forming microorganisms, isolation procedures are often combined with a heat-shock treatment in order to activate dormant endospores and promote germination and growth. *Alicyclobacillus* counts are often higher after a heat-shock treatment if the microbes are mostly present as endospores. Various heat-shock regimes have been investigated and the most commonly recommended are 80°C/10 min, 70°C/10 min, 70°C/20 min, and 60°C/30 min. While the differences between heat treatments are probably minimal, the application of some form of heat treatment is essential to ensure a true reflection of the contamination level in samples. Heat-shock treatments are usually followed by preenrichment procedures of incubation at 40°C–50°C for 48 h.

There are several standardized methods for the analysis of *Alicyclobacillus* spp. in foods and beverages. The American Public Health Association proposes the use of K agar and incubation at 43°C for 3 days, whereas the Japanese Fruit Juice Association (JFJA) recommends the use of acidified YSG agar with incubation at different temperatures according to the *Alicyclobacillus* species searched (Steyn et al. 2011).

In 2008, AIJN issued its "*Alicyclobacillus* Best Practice Guideline." The guideline recommends the use of the International Federation of Fruit Juice Producers (IFU) (2007) method no. 12 (Method on the detection of taint producing *Alicyclobacillus* in fruit juices) or alternative methods such as the JFJA method. IFU method no. 12 recommends the use of BAT (pH 4.0), YSG (pH 3.7), or K agar (pH 3.7), incubated at 45°C for 2–5 days. The method prescribes a heat-shock treatment at 80°C/10 min that is followed by direct plating or enrichment procedures. A filtration step is optional and requires 100 mL of a heat-shocked diluted sample and membranes of 0.45 μm pore size (Steyn et al. 2011). For the characterization and identification of the *Alicyclobacillus* isolates, the AIJN recommends several methods, such as growth in selective media, guaiacol detection, DNA sequence analysis, DNA ribotyping, genotyping, and gas chromatography–mass spectrometry (GC–MS) detection of guaiacol, 2,6-DBP, and 2,6-DCP (AIJN 2008).

The Australian Fruit Juice Association and South African fruit processors also support IFU method no. 12, with several extra recommendations.

As culture methods take up to 12 days to detect *Alicyclobacillus* species, a number of rapid methods have been developed: flow cytometry, real-time PCR, the foodproof *Alicyclobacillus* detection kit, gene probe technology, the Vermicon VIT-*Alicyclobacillus* detection test using VIT gene probe technology, and the use of an electronic nose (Gobbi et al. 2010; Mermelstein 2012).

REFERENCES

AIJN. (2008). *Alicyclobacillus* Best Practice Guideline. A guideline for the reduction and control of thermophylic, sporeforming bacteria (*Alicyclobacillus* species, ACB) in the production, packing and distribution of fruit juices, juice concentrates purees and nectars. http://www.unipektin.ch/docus/public/AIJN_Alicyclobacillus_Best_Practice_Guideline_July_2008.pdf (accessed February 25, 2013).

Alwazeer, D., C. Delbeau, C. Divies, R. Cachon. (2003). Use of redox potential modification by gas improves microbial quality, color retention, and ascorbic acid stability of pasteurized orange juice. *International Journal of Food Microbiology* 89: 21–29.

Arias, C.R., J.K. Burns, L.M. Friedrich, R.M. Goodrich, M.E. Parish. (2002). Yeast species associated with orange juice: Evaluation of different identification methods. *Applied and Environmental Microbiology* 68: 1955–1961.

Barnett, J., R.W. Payne, D. Yarrow. (1983). *Yeast: Characteristics and Identification*. Cambridge: Cambridge University Press.

Baysal, A.H., F. Icier. (2010). Inactivation kinetics of *Alicyclobacillus acidoterrestris* spores in orange juice by ohmic heating: Effects of voltage gradient and temperature on inactivation. *Journal of Food Protection* 73: 299–304.

Beh, A.L., G.H. Fleet, C. Prakitchaiwattana, G.M. Heard. (2006). Evaluation of molecular methods for the analysis of yeasts in foods and beverages. *Advances in Experimental Medicine and Biology* 571: 69–106.

Bevilacqua, A., M.R. Corbo, M. Sinigaglia. (2008a). Inhibition of *Alicyclobacillus acidoterrestris* spores by natural compounds. *International Journal of Food Science and Technology* 43: 1271–1275.

Bevilacqua, A., M. Sinigaglia, M.R. Corbo. (2008b). *Alicyclobacillus acidoterrestris*: New methods for inhibiting spore germination. *International Journal of Food Microbiology* 125: 103–110.

Bevilacqua, A., M.R. Corbo, M. Sinigaglia. (2012). High-pressure homogenisation and benzoate to control *Alicyclobacillus acidoterrestris*: A possible way? *International Journal of Food Science and Technology* 47: 879–883.

Coton, E., M. Coton. (2003). Microbiological origin of "Framboisé" in French ciders. *Journal of the Institute of Brewing* 109: 299–304.

Coton, M., J.M. Laplace, Y. Auffray, E. Coton. (2006). "Framboisé" spoilage in French ciders: *Zymomonas mobilis* implication and characterization. *LWT—Food Science and Technology* 39: 972–979.

Dicks, L.M.T., A. Endo. (2009). Taxonomic status of lactic acid bacteria in wine and key characteristics to differentiate species. *South African Journal of Enology and Viticulture* 30: 72–90.

Drilleau, J.F. (1977). Le framboisé dans les cidres. *BIOS* 12: 37–44.

Durak, M.Z., J.J. Churey, M.D. Danyluk, R.W. Worobo. (2010). Identification and haplotype distribution of *Alicyclobacillus* spp. from different juices and beverages. *International Journal of Food Microbiology* 142: 286–291.

Feng, G., J.J. Churey, R.W. Worobo. (2010). Thermoaciduric *Clostridium pasteurianum* spoilage of shelf-stable apple juice. *Journal of Food Protection* 73: 1886–1890.

Fergus, C.L. (1967). Resistance of spores of some thermophilic actinomycetes to high temperature. *Mycopathologia* 32: 205–208.

Fernández-Espinar, M.T., P. Martorell, R. De Llanos, A. Querol. (2006). Molecular methods to identify and characterize yeasts in foods and beverages. In: A. Querol and G.H. Fleet (eds), *Yeasts in Food and Beverages*, pp. 55–82. Berlin: Springer-Verlag.

Gobbi, E., M. Falasconi, I. Concina, G. Mantero, F. Bianchi, M. Mattarozzi, M. Musci, G. Sberveglieri. (2010). Electronic nose and *Alicyclobacillus* spp. spoilage of fruit juices: An emerging diagnostic tool. *Food Control* 21: 1374–1382.

Goto, K., H. Matsubara, K. Mochida, T. Matsumura, Y. Hara, M. Niwa, K. Yamasato. (2002). *Alicyclobacillus herbarius* sp. nov., a novel bacterium containing ω-cycloheptane fatty acids, isolated from herbal tea. *International Journal of Systematic and Evolutionary Microbiology* 52: 109–113.

Goto, K., K. Mochida, M. Asahara, M. Suzuki, H. Kasai, A. Yokota. (2003). *Alicyclobacillus pomorum* sp. nov., a novel thermo-acidophilic, endospore-forming bacterium that does not possess ω-alicyclic fatty acids, and emended description of the genus *Alicyclobacillus*. *International Journal of Systematic and Evolutionary Microbiology* 53: 1537–1544.

Hippchen, B., A. Röll, K. Poralla. (1981). Occurrence in soil of thermo-acidophilic bacilli possessing ω-cyclohexane fatty acids and hopanoids. *Archives of Microbiology* 129: 53–55.

Hosoya, K., M. Nakayama, T. Matsuzawa, Y. Imanishi, J. Hitomi, T. Yaguchi. (2012). Risk analysis and development of a rapid method for identifying four species of *Byssochlamys*. *Food Control* 26: 169–173.

Hutzler, M., R. Riedl, J. Koob, F. Jacob. (2012). Fermentation and spoilage yeasts and their relevance for the beverage industry—A review. *Brewing Science* 65: 33–52.

International Federation of Fruit Juice Producers (IFU). (2007). Method on the detection of taint producing *Alicyclobacillus* in fruit juices: IFU Method No. 12. Paris: IFU.

Jensen, N., F.B. Whitfield. (2003). Role of *Alicyclobacillus acidoterrestris* in the development of a disinfectant taint in shelf-stable fruit juice. *Letters in Applied Microbiology* 36: 9–14.

Justé, A., B. Lievens, I. Frans, M. Klingeberg, C.W. Michiels, C.A. Willems. (2008). Present knowledge of the bacterial microflora in the extreme environment of sugar thick juice. *Food Microbiology* 25: 831–836.

Juvonen, R., V. Virkajärvi, O. Priha, A. Laitila. (2011). Microbiological spoilage and safety risks in non-beer beverages. VTT Tiedotteita-Research notes 2599. http://www.vtt.fi/inf/pdf/tiedotteet/2011/T2599.pdf (accessed February 20, 2013).

Kalia, A., E.P. Gupta. (2006). Fruit microbiology. In: Y.H. Hui (ed.), *Handbook of Fruits and Fruit Processing*, pp. 3–28. Oxford: Blackwell Publishing.

Karavaiko, G.I., T.I. Bogdanova, T.P. Tourova, T.F. Kondrat'eva, I.A. Tsaplina, M.A. Egorova, E.N. Krasil'nikova, L.M. Zakharchuk (2005). Reclassification of 'Sulfobacillus thermosulfidooxidans subsp. thermotolerans' strain K1 as *Alicyclobacillus tolerans* sp. nov. and *Sulfobacillus disulfidooxidans* Dufresne et al. 1996 as *Alicyclobacillus disulfidooxidans* comb. nov., and emended description of the genus *Alicyclobacillus*. *International Journal of Systematic and Evolutionary Microbiology* 55: 941–947.

Khalesi, M., S.M. Deckers, K. Gebruers, L. Vissers, H. Verachtert, G. Derdelinckx. (2012). Hydrophobins: Exceptional proteins for many applications in brewery environment and other bio-industries. *Cerevisia* 37: 3–9.

Komitopoulou, E., I.S. Boziaris, E.A. Davies, J. Delves-Broughton, M.R. Adams. (1999). *Alicyclobacillus acidoterrestris* in fruit juices and its control by nisin. *Journal of Food Science and Technology* 34: 81–85.

Kusano, K., H. Yamada, M. Niwa, K. Yamasoto. (1997). *Propionibacterium cyclohexanicum* sp. nov., a new-tolerant ω-cyclohexyl fatty acid-containing propionibacterium isolated from spoiled orange juice. *International Journal of Systematic Bacteriology* 47: 825–831.

Loureiro, V., M. Malfeito-Ferreira. (2003). Spoilage yeasts in the wine industry. *International Journal of Food Microbiology* 86: 23–50.

Loureiro, V., A. Querol. (1999). The prevalence and control of spoilage yeasts in foods and beverages. *Trends in Food Science and Technology* 10: 356–365.

Lucas, R., M.J. Grande, H. Abriouel, M. Maqueda, N. Ben Omar, E. Valdivia, M. Martínez-Cañamero, A. Gálvez. (2006). Application of the broad-spectrum bacteriocin enterocin AS-48 to inhibit *Bacillus coagulans* in canned fruit and vegetable foods. *Food and Chemical Toxicology* 44: 1774–1781.

Maqueda, M., E. Zamora, N. Rodríguez-Cousiño, M. Ramírez. (2010). Wine yeast molecular typing using a simplified method for simultaneously extracting mtDNA, nuclear DNA and virus dsRNA. *Food Microbiology* 27: 205–209.

McKnight, I.C., M.N.U. Eiroa, A.S. Sant'Ana, P.R. Massaguer. (2010). *Alicyclobacillus acidoterrestris* in pasteurized exotic Brazilian fruit juices: Isolation, genotypic characterization and heat resistance. *Food Microbiology* 27: 1016–1022.

Merle, J., T.J. Montville. (2012). *Alicyclobacillus acidoterrestris*: The organism, the challenge, potential interventions. *Journal of Food Processing and Preservation*. Published electronically June 19, 2012. doi:10.1111/j.1745-4549.2012.00758.x (accessed February 26, 2013).

Mermelstein, N.H. (2012). Preventing juice spoilage. *Food Technology* 66(11): 62–67.

Orberá, T. (2004). Métodos moleculares de identificación de levaduras de interés biotecnológico. *Revista Iberoamericana de Micología* 21: 15–19.

Orr, R.V., L.R. Beuchat. (2000). Efficacy of disinfectants in killing spores of *Alicyclobacillus acidoterrestris* and performance of media for supporting colony development by survivors. *Journal of Food Protection* 63: 1117–1122.

Peña, W.E.L., P.R. De Massaguer, L.Q. Teixeira. (2009). Microbial modeling of thermal resistance of *Alicyclobacillus acidoterrestris* CRA7152 spores in concentrated orange juice with nisin addition. *Brazilian Journal of Microbiology* 40: 601–611.

Pettipher, G.L., M.E. Osmundson, J.M. Murphy. (1997). Methods for the detection and enumeration of *Alicyclobacillus acidoterrestris* and investigation of growth and production of taint in fruit juice and fruit juice-containing drinks. *Letters in Applied Microbiology* 24: 185–189.

Pincus, D.H., S. Orenga, S. Chatellier. (2007). Yeast identification—Past, present, and future methods. *Medical Mycology* 45: 97–121.

Pitt, J.I., A.D. Hocking. (1985). *Fungi and Food Spoilage*. London: Academic Press.

Siegmund, B., B. Pöllinger-Zierler. (2007). Growth behavior of off-flavor-forming microorganisms in apple juice. *Journal of Agricultural and Food Chemistry* 55: 6692–6699.

Silva, F.V.M., P. Gibbs. (2004). Target selection in designing pasteurization processes for shelf-stable high-acid fruit products. *Critical Reviews in Food Science and Nutrition* 44: 353–360.

Smelt, J.P.P.M., J.G.M. Raatjes, J.S. Crowther, C.T. Verrips. (1982). Growth and toxin formation by *Clostridium* at low pH values. *Journal of Applied Bacteriology* 52: 75–82.

Smit, Y., M. Cameron, P. Venter, R.C. Witthuhn. (2011). *Alicyclobacillus* spoilage and isolation—A review. *Food Microbiology* 28: 331–349.

Solberg, P., H.B. Castberg, J.I. Osmundsen. (1990). Packaging systems for fruit juices and non-carbonated beverages. In: D. Hicks (ed.), *Production and Packaging of Non-carbonated Fruit Juices and Fruit Beverages*, pp. 330–351. London: Blackie and Son.

Splittstoesser, D.F., J.J. Churey, C.Y. Lee. (1994). Growth characteristics of aciduric spore-forming *Bacilli* isolated from fruit juices. *Journal of Food Protection* 57: 1080–1083.

Steyn, C.E., M. Cameron, R.C. Witthuhn. (2011). Occurrence of *Alicyclobacillus* in the fruit processing environment—A review. *International Journal of Food Microbiology* 147: 1–11.

Stratford, M. (2006). Food and beverage spoilage yeasts. In: A. Querol and H.H. Fleet (eds), *Yeasts in Food and Beverages*, pp. 335–379. Berlin: Springer-Verlag.

Tournas, V. (1994). Heat-resistant fungi of importance to the food and beverage industry. *Critical Reviews in Microbiology* 20: 243–263.

Tribst, A.A.L., A. de S. Sant'Ana, P.R. de Massaguer. (2009). Review: Microbiological quality and safety of fruit juices—Past, present and future perspectives. *Critical Reviews in Microbiology* 35: 310–339.

Uemura, K., I. Kobayashi, T. Inoue. (2009). Inactivation of *Alicyclobacillus acidoterrestris* in orange juice by high electric field alternating current. *Food Science and Technology Research* 15: 211–216.

Vasavada, P.C. (2003). Microbiology of fruit juice and beverages. In: T. Foster and P.C. Vasavada (eds), *Beverage Quality and Safety*, pp. 95–123. Boca Raton, FL: CRC Press.

Vercammen, A., B. Vivijs, I. Lurquin, C.W. Michiels. (2012). Germination and inactivation of *Bacillus coagulans* and *Alicyclobacillus acidoterrestris* spores by high hydrostatic pressure treatment in buffer and tomato sauce. *International Journal of Food Microbiology* 152: 162–167.

Vieira, M.C., A.A. Teixeira, F.M. Silva, N. Gaspar, C.L.M. Silva. (2002). *Alicyclobacillus acidoterrestris* spores as a target for Cupuaçu (*Theobroma grandiflorum*) nectar thermal processing: Kinetic parameters and experimental methods. *International Journal of Food Microbiology* 77: 71–81.

Walker, M.E., C.A. Phillips. (2007). The growth of *Propionibacterium cyclohexanicum* in fruit juices and its survival following elevated temperature treatments. *Food Microbiology* 24: 313–318.

Walker, M.E., C.A. Phillips. (2008). The effect of preservatives on *Alicyclobacillus acidoterrestris* and *Propionibacterium cyclohexanicum* in fruit juice. *Food Control* 19: 974–981.

Wareing, P., R.R. Davenport. (2004). Microbiology of soft drinks and fruit juices. In: P.R. Ashurst (ed.), *Chemistry and Technology of Soft Drinks and Fruit Juices*, pp. 279–299. Oxford: Blackwell Publishing.

Wisotzkey, J.D., P. Jurtshuk, G.E. Fox, G. Deinhard, K. Poralla. (1992). Comparative sequence analyses on the 16S rRNA (rDNA) of *Bacillus acidocaldarius*, *Bacillus acidoterrestris* and *Bacillus cycloheptanicus* and proposal for creation of a new genus, *Alicyclobacillus* gen. nov. *International Journal of Systematic Bacteriology* 42: 263–269.

Yaguchi, T., Y. Imanishi, T. Matsuzawa, K. Hosoya, J. Hitomi, M. Nakayama. (2012). Method for identifying heat-resistant fungi of the genus *Neosartorya*. *Food Protection Trends* 75: 1806–1813.

Yamazaki, K., M. Murakami, Y. Kawi, N. Inoue, T. Matsuda. (2000). Use of nisin for inhibition of *Alicyclobacillus acidoterrestris* in acidic drinks. *Food Microbiology* 17: 315–320.

16 Safety in Fruit Juice Processing
Chemical and Microbiological Hazards

Sonia Marín and Antonio J. Ramos

CONTENTS

16.1 Introduction 330
16.2 Biological Hazards.. 331
    16.2.1 Viruses... 332
    16.2.2 Bacterial Pathogens 333
    16.2.3 Parasites.. 334
    16.2.4 Control Measures for Biological Hazards 335
        16.2.4.1 Preventing Biological Hazards in Raw Material 335
        16.2.4.2 Preventing Biological Hazards in Postharvest Handling... 335
        16.2.4.3 Fruit Sorting... 335
        16.2.4.4 Fruit Cleaning and Washing 335
        16.2.4.5 Juicing.. 335
        16.2.4.6 Microbial Inactivation Processes 336
        16.2.4.7 Cooling... 336
        16.2.4.8 Distribution 336
    16.2.5 European Legislation... 337
16.3 Chemical Hazards... 337
    16.3.1 Pesticides 337
    16.3.2 Environmental Contaminants.. 339
    16.3.3 Mycotoxins 340
    16.3.4 Food Additives.. 340
    16.3.5 Processing Contaminants 341
    16.3.6 Control Measures for Chemical Hazards 341
    16.3.7 European Legislation... 342
16.4 Food Safety Management 342
References.. 344

16.1   INTRODUCTION

Food safety is of paramount importance. Food safety management aims to minimize the risk associated with either biological, chemical, or physical hazards. In high-throughput manufacture, if a safety hazard is not detected and corrected somewhere in the production/supply chain, many consumers can be adversely affected. In the case of fruit juices, microbial or chemical contaminants affecting a small amount of raw material can be blended into a large batch and be distributed and consumed over a wide area (Bates et al. 2001).

The European Commission's (EC) Rapid Alert System for Food and Feed (RASFF) notifications usually report on risks identified in food, feed, or food-contact materials that are placed on the market in the notifying country, or detained at an EU point of entry at the border with an EU-neighboring country. Since 2001, there has been a consistent increase in the number of notifications (either alerts, information notifications, or border rejections) for the fruit and vegetables category. Although fruit juices are not included in this category, the evolution of certain contaminants, such as pesticides, may reflect the situation for the raw materials used for fruit juice production, too. In the nonalcoholic beverages category, in which fruit juices are located, a low number of notifications have been reported in the last few years (Figure 16.1).

Regarding the causes of such notifications, the use either of unauthorized pesticides or at levels above the authorized dose were the main causes for fruit and vegetables and the use either of unauthorized food additives or at levels above the authorized dose were the main causes for nonalcoholic beverages. Mycotoxins appeared as the cause of 11%–22% of the notifications, while the presence of potentially pathogenic microorganisms accounted for 6%–9% (Figure 16.2).

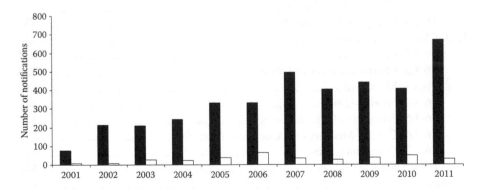

FIGURE 16.1   Evolution in the number of notifications reported by the RASFF for fruit and vegetables (■) and nonalcoholic beverages (□) categories. (From Rapid Alert System for Food and Feed [RASFF], Annual reports 2001–2011, Available at: http://ec.europa.eu/food/food/rapidalert/rasff_publications_en.htm.)

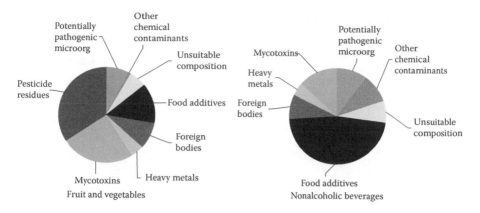

FIGURE 16.2 Notification causes in 2005–2011 (mean values) for fruit and vegetables and nonalcoholic beverages. (From Rapid Alert System for Food and Feed [RASFF], Annual reports 2005–2011, Available at: http://ec.europa.eu/food/food/rapidalert/rasff_publications_en.htm.)

16.2 BIOLOGICAL HAZARDS

A number of outbreaks caused by fruit juice-borne human pathogens were reported in the 1990s in the United States and other countries around the world. Orange juice, apple juice, and apple cider were usually involved, while the infectious agents were *Salmonella, Escherichia coli* O157:H7, and *Cryptosporidium* (Bates et al. 2001). In most cases the outbreaks were caused by the consumption of nonpasteurized juices (Vojdani et al. 2008).

Reports from organizations in charge of food-borne diseases surveillance indicate an increase in food borne outbreaks linked to the consumption of fruits and vegetables in general (including raw, fresh-cut, or processed), although few data refer specifically to fruit juices. At present, in the EU, the category "Fruit, berries and juices, and other products thereof" has a low contribution to food-borne diseases, and may be linked to between 1% and 3% of the total number of food-borne outbreaks in 2009–2010 (EFSA 2005, 2006, 2007, 2009a, 2010a, 2011a, 2012a; Figure 16.3), most of them being caused by viruses (50%–65%), followed by *Salmonella* (4.7%–8.6%), *Bacillus* toxins (2.9%–4.7%), and *Clostridium* toxins (0%–11.6%). This category accounted for 3%–51% of calicivirus outbreaks in 2008–2010, and 0.2% of *Salmonella* outbreaks were caused by consumption of these foodstuffs, while 0.6%–1.7% of *Salmonella* outbreaks were due to vegetables and juices and other products thereof.

Moreover, surveillance of microbial contamination of food products shows low levels or the absence of most pathogens in fruit and vegetables, with ready-to-eat fruits and vegetables being those most often contaminated (EFSA 2005, 2006, 2007, 2009a, 2010a, 2011a, 2012a).

Besides the problems associated with most common acidic fruit juices (pH < 4.5), the increasing consumption of higher pH fruit juices and the increase in exotic fruit

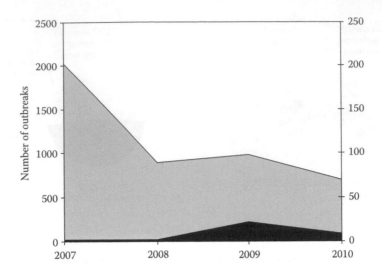

FIGURE 16.3 Total number of strong evidence outbreaks (gray) and those attributed to consumption of fruit, berries, and juices, and other products thereof (black). (From EFSA, *EFSA Journal*, 271, 1–128,2009a; EFSA, *EFSA Journal*, 8, 1496, 2010a; EFSA, *EFSA Journal*, 9, 2090, 2011a; EFSA, *EFSA Journal*, 10, 2597, 2012a)

juices may lead to new issues in food safety, as the risk related to these fruits is mostly unknown. The increasing consumption of fresh fruit juices as a result of changing dietary habits, and the emergence of pathogens associated with fruit juices, such as *Listeria monocytogenes*, plus their adaptation to survive and grow under acidic conditions and to resist to existing preservation techniques of previously reported pathogens, may explain the increased involvement of fruits/fruit juices as vehicles of disease outbreaks (Tribst et al. 2009).

16.2.1 VIRUSES

Caliciviruses (including noroviruses) cause approximately 90% of epidemic non-bacterial outbreaks of gastroenteritis around the world and are responsible for many food-borne outbreaks of gastroenteritis. These viruses are transmitted by food or water contaminated with human feces and by person-to-person contact. Many norovirus outbreaks have been traced to food that was handled by one infected person. Norwalk and Norwalk-like viruses are reported as being the most common acute gastroenteritis agents and their transmission via contaminated food is increasingly recognized. These viruses cause malaise, abdominal pain, pyrexia, diarrhea, and vomiting and can debilitate people in 2–3 weeks. Viruses cannot multiply in foods but some can cause illness via ingestion of a few viral particles. It been estimated that 10–100 particles of norovirus are sufficient for this, whereas infected persons can excrete several millions of infection particles in feces or vomit (EC 2002a).

Rotaviruses are the leading single cause of severe diarrhea among infants and young children. Rotaviruses are also transmitted by the fecal–oral route. Finally, the hepatitis A virus is distinguished from other viral agents by its prolonged (2–6 weeks) incubation period and its ability to spread beyond the stomach and intestines into the liver. The virus has often been associated with the consumption of contaminated fresh-cut vegetables and fruit.

As most viruses are host specific (calicivirus and hepatitis A virus), food-borne outbreaks caused by viruses are, in most cases, caused by fruits and vegetables that have direct or indirect contact with feces, and may also be present on fruit and vegetables following handling by an infected person (Seymour and Appleton 2001).

16.2.2 Bacterial Pathogens

Salmonellae are Gram-negative bacteria belonging to the family Enterobacteriaceae. The genus *Salmonella* contains two species (*Salmonella enterica* and *S. bongori*) based on phenotypic criteria. Human salmonellosis comprises several clinical syndromes including enteric (typhoid) fever, localized enterocolitis, and systemic infections by nontyphoid microorganisms. The infectious dose of salmonellae can vary, depending on the bacterial strain ingested as well as on the immunocompetence of individuals. The principal reservoir for salmonellae is the gastrointestinal tract of mammals, reptiles, and birds. In the case of poor agricultural practices, such as the collection of "windfalls," and particularly the use of contaminated irrigation water, fruit can be contaminated with salmonellae (EC 2003a). The incidence in juices has been associated with the poor hygiene of food handlers (Keller and Miller 2006) and with acid-tolerant serovars (Yuk and Schneider 2006).

Escherichia coli is a species within the Gram-negative family Enterobacteriaceae. The species is a normal constituent of the intestinal flora of humans and warm-blooded animals. Verotoxigenic *E. coli* (VTEC) is a group of *E. coli* that produces one or more verocytotoxins. Only a small fraction of all VTEC-types isolated from animals, food, and the environment are associated with human illness. However, VTEC O157 is an important cause of bloody diarrhea and kidney failure. Food-borne VTEC O157 infections originate from ingestion of foods contaminated by ruminant or human fecal material and where the conditions in the food chain thereafter enable survival. The infectious dose for VTEC O157 is very low and an infection may result from consumption of contaminated foods in which the bacteria have survived but have not necessarily grown. Fruits can become contaminated with VTEC O157 while growing in fields, or during harvest, handling, washing/cleaning, processing, distribution, retail, preparation, and final use. Due to its acid tolerance, *E. coli* O157:H7 has more potential to be associated with outbreaks caused from juice. Contamination in the field may be due to the use of improperly treated manure as fertilizer, exposure to fecally contaminated irrigation or washing water, or contact with animals, birds, or insects pre- and postharvest (EC 2003b).

These pathogenic bacteria are not normally present on fruit and vegetables or their environment, and tend to decline once introduced on fruits and vegetables during their primary production (Girardin et al. 2005). Moreover, those that survive are usually killed by the pasteurization process. As a consequence, most reported cases of contamination of juices by *Salmonella* and *E. coli* O157:H7 were due to fresh, unpasteurized juices. In this case, once contamination occurs, the pathogens may either just survive or even grow if the conditions in the juice are suitable. Acid fruit juices below pH 4.6 were once deemed a minor health threat due to their high acidity. Furthermore, refrigeration temperatures (below 5°C) represented an additional hurdle to pathogen growth, until the discovery that *L. monocytogenes* can grow at temperatures as low as 2°C (Tribst et al. 2009). To date, *L. monocytogenes* is not well established as a relevant fruit juice-borne pathogen; however, this pathogen can be considered to be of concern in fresh fruits and fruit juices, due to its ability to survive under a variety of adverse conditions (Caggia et al. 2009).

Spores from *Bacillus cereus* and *Clostridium* are common in soil. Bacterial spores are highly resistant and persist for long periods in the soil or on plant surfaces during primary production (Girardin et al. 2005). *B. cereus* may produce emetic and diarrheagenic toxins. Depending on the type of toxin, *B. cereus* may cause severe nausea, vomiting, and watery diarrhea. The emetic toxin of *B. cereus* has high heat tolerance and cannot be destroyed by normal heat treatment. *Clostridium botulinum* toxin is the cause of a rare but potentially deadly intoxication and occurs when the anaerobic bacterium grows in foods and produces botulinum toxin, a powerful paralytic toxin. *Clostridium perfringens* toxins cause abdominal cramps and diarrhea (EFSA 2009a). Spore-forming bacterial pathogens can be frequent on raw fruits and vegetables and their origin has been traced back to the soil where the fruits/vegetables were grown (Guinebretière and Nguyen-The 2003).

16.2.3 PARASITES

Cryptosporidium parvum is a highly infectious protozoan parasite that causes persistent diarrhea (Keller and Miller 2006). *Cryptosporidium* oocysts are persistent in the environment and are mainly water borne. They can be resistant to 3% sodium hypochlorite (Skovgaard 2007) and to acid. Heating (65°C/2 min or 74°C/1 min) and drying seem to be the most effective techniques to inactivate the oocysts (Laberge and Griffiths 1996). It is important to highlight that a mere 10 oocysts are enough to cause human infection (Tribst et al. 2009).

Trypanosoma cruzi is another important protozoan that can be especially found in Latin America (Steindel et al. 2008). *T. cruzi* is the etiologic agent of Chagas' disease, which develops irreversible lesions of the autonomous nervous system in the heart, esophagus, and colon (Steindel et al. 2008). In the Amazon region of Brazil, oral contamination is associated with the consumption of unpasteurized acai palm fruit juice; acai palm trees are the habitat of the triatomine vector, and the contamination of acai palm fruit juice by *T. cruzi* is related to the crushing of this insect during juice preparation (Valente et al. 1999). Freezing and pasteurization inactivate this parasite and other common protozoans, thus they may not pose a problem in industrialized juices (Tribst et al. 2009).

Finally, the presence of *Toxoplasma gondii* oocysts in raw fruits has been identified as a risk factor in epidemiological studies (Pereira et al. 2010); therefore, this hazard must not be disregarded in unpasteurized juices.

16.2.4   CONTROL MEASURES FOR BIOLOGICAL HAZARDS

16.2.4.1   Preventing Biological Hazards in Raw Material

Raw materials are the main source of biological hazards in the final juice product. Good agricultural practices (GAP) are the basis for the safety of fruits used as raw materials. The contamination of fruits with pathogens through fruit contact with feces highlights the failure to follow GAP (Bates et al. 2001). Particular attention must be paid to: (i) the use of manure as fertilizer; (ii) the use of fruit contaminated by insects, wildlife, or fruit that has fallen on the ground; (iii) fruit contamination by insects and wildlife; and (iv) contamination by field workers.

16.2.4.2   Preventing Biological Hazards in Postharvest Handling

Good manufacturing practices (GMP) are of the utmost importance at this point in order to prevent further pathogen contamination and later bacterial pathogen proliferation. Packing for transport should be gentle and sanitary, preventing juicing during transit and fermentation due to delayed delivery (Bates et al. 2001). Unfortunately, fruit intended for juice does not receive the care in packing, transport, or postharvest treatment reserved for fresh market and solid pack fruit (Fellows 1997).

16.2.4.3   Fruit Sorting

Inspection for exclusion of damaged, wormy, decayed, or rotten fruits is required before washing. This step will decrease the initial microbial load.

16.2.4.4   Fruit Cleaning and Washing

Cooling and cleaning can involve physical removal of surface debris by brushes or air-jet separation prior to washing with water. Temperature differentials between the fruits and the water (if the fruits have a higher temperature than the water) can be considered as the main cause of water being suctioned into the fruits (Eblen et al. 2004). Therefore, equipment and water sanitation via chlorination or the use of other sanitizers is critical, and recycling is usually necessary (Bates et al. 2001). Seymour and Appleton (2001) recommended chlorination to inactivate the Norwalk (10 mg/L) and hepatitis A viruses (5 mg/L), and also concluded that ozone was an efficient antiviral agent. However, other authors have reported that these viruses are resistant to the majority of disinfectants (Niu et al. 1992; Koopmans and Duizer 2004). Similarly, some parasite oocysts are not inactivated by chlorinated water. By contrast, chlorine and other sanitizers reduce populations of bacterial cells exposed on the surface of produce by up to 2 or 3 log10 units. In conclusion, these treatments still allow for the potential presence of low levels of pathogens in the juice, which poses a small risk if the juice is to be consumed without a further treatment, such as pasteurization.

16.2.4.5   Juicing

Generally, a whole fruit is more stable than the juice; therefore, fruit should not be committed to juice until the material can rapidly be stabilized or the process goes to completion. Attention to quality at the prejuicing step is extremely critical (Bates et al. 2001). Moreover, other sources of fruit juice contamination include equipment that is used to process the juice, such as presses, mills, extractors, pipelines, and filling machines (Jay and Anderson 2001).

16.2.4.6 Microbial Inactivation Processes

Unheated juice is subjected to rapid microbial, enzymatic, chemical, and physical deterioration. For long-life juice, UHT treatments are used. On the other hand, pasteurization inactivates viruses, parasites, and vegetative bacteria, although bacterial spores are not destroyed. Pasteurization processes should be designed in order to inactivate *C. parvum* oocysts, which may be more resistant to thermal processing than vegetative bacterial pathogens. Over the years, fruit juice preservation has relied mainly on pasteurization, low pH levels, refrigeration, and the addition of preservatives. Frequently, two or three of these methods were required to provide stability for ready-to-drink industrialized fruit juices (Tribst et al. 2009). In order to avoid or minimize pasteurization and prevent the use of preservatives, researchers have directed their studies to finding preservation techniques that are able to assure the safety of the juice without severely compromising the nutritional and sensory aspects. Several nonthermal methods such as high-pressure processing (HHP), ultraviolet light (UV), pulsed electric fields (PEF), electron beam irradiation, and high carbon dioxide processing have been assayed. Among these technologies, HHP is the best one developed for juice treatment (with 5-log reductions or greater of *E. coli* O157:H7 and *Salmonella* Enteritidis according to Bayindirli et al. [2006] at 350 MPa/5 min/30°C in apricot, orange, sour cherry, and apple juices.) Slifko et al. (2000) achieved the same level of inactivation for *C. parvum* using 550 MPa/1 min. PEF also displayed good results in the inactivation of pathogens, with a reduction of around 5 log cycles of *Salmonella* Enteritidis, *E. coli* O157:H7, *E. coli*, and *Listeria innocua* in orange and apple juices (Evrendilek et al. 2000; Lu et al. 2001; McDonald et al. 2000; Mosqueda-Melgar et al. 2008). These authors applied an electric field between 34 and 80 kV/cm combined with a temperature of 40°C–50°C, indicating that the PEF process is only efficient when combined with a mild heat treatment.

16.2.4.7 Cooling

Growth of surviving spore-forming bacteria is prevented through the refrigeration of juices after pasteurization processes. Moreover, improper sanitation procedures will result in recontamination of juice after pasteurization (Tribst et al. 2009).

16.2.4.8 Distribution

In acidic pH conditions in juice (pH < 4.5), pathogen growth should not be observed, while survival, although possible, would be improbable (Tribst et al. 2009). However, *E. coli* O157:H7 and some *Salmonella* serovars have caused illnesses with the ingestion of a few bacterial cells, without these having grown in the orange juice during shelf life (Vojdani et al. 2008), while spore-forming bacteria need to reach sufficiently high numbers in the food to cause illness to consumers. As a consequence, pasteurized juices (or juices treated with other technologies for an equivalent treatment) may be either distributed under refrigeration or not, while for unpasteurized, nontreated juices, refrigerated distribution is mandatory and a key step to guarantee juice safety.

Emerging high pH juices provide good conditions not only for the survival, but also for the growth of food-borne pathogens (Tribst et al. 2009). Even if a pasteurization process is undergone, they will require refrigerated distribution to prevent growth of heat-resistant spore-forming bacteria and toxin production during shelf life.

16.2.5 EUROPEAN LEGISLATION

Fruit juice production is subject to Regulation (EC) no. 852/2004 of April 29, 2004 on the hygiene of foodstuffs (EC 2004), in which procedures based on the hazard analysis and critical control points (HACCP) principles, together with the application of good hygiene practices (GHP) are imposed on food business operators. Pasteurized/treated juices produced according to the hygiene requirements in this regulation do not have any specific microbiological criteria to conform with, as they are considered to be microbiologically stable. In contrast, Regulation 2073/2005 sets the microbiological criteria in Table 16.1 for unpasteurized fruit and vegetable juices (EC2005a). A "food safety criterion" means one defining the acceptability of a product or a batch of foodstuff applicable to products placed on the market, while a "process hygiene criterion" is one indicating the acceptable functioning of the production process. Such a criterion is not applicable to products placed on the market. It sets an indicative contamination value above which corrective actions are required in order to maintain the hygiene of the process in compliance with food law.

16.3 CHEMICAL HAZARDS

Chemical substances play an important role in the production and distribution of food. Pesticides allow for improvement in crop yields, thus achieving lower costs of production. Food additives are intentionally added to food for a technological purpose, using materials such as plastics, paper, cardboard, and so on, to help to maintain hygienic conditions and allow food distribution, so as to improve its presentation. However, their use leads to the presence of chemicals in foods, constituting a potential risk that needs to be analyzed in an efficient manner to ensure consumer safety of such foods. The presence of chemicals in food can also have an unintended source, produced by environmental pollution (air, water, soil), or by fungi (natural toxins) in raw materials, whose risk should also be the subject of analysis.

16.3.1 PESTICIDES

Pesticides are widely applied in the field and postharvest to a variety of fruits and vegetables to control weeds, insects, and diseases. As a consequence, residues of these substances can be found in food, thus constituting a potential risk for human health, considering their toxicity and the exposure to these compounds. The pesticide residues tend to deposit on the fruit peels and transfer from peels into pulps and juices in long-term processes and pose some risk to human health (Bates et al. 2001). Unauthorized or excessive pesticide chemicals are the most common and avoidable contaminants readily preventable by GAP.

TABLE 16.1
Microbiological Criteria for Unpasteurized Fruit Juices

| Food Category | Microorganisms | Sampling Plan | | Limits | | Analytical Reference Method | Stage Where the Criterion Applies | Action in Case of Unsatisfactory Results |
		n	c	m	M			
Food Safety Criterion								
Unpasteurized fruit and vegetable juices (ready-to-eat)	Salmonella	5	0	Absence in 25 g		EN/ISO 6579	Products placed on the market during their shelf life	
Process Hygiene Criterion								
Unpasteurized fruit and vegetable juices (ready-to-eat)	E. coli	5	2	100 cfu/g	1000 cfu/g	ISO 16649-1 or 2	Manufacturing process	Improvements in production hygiene, selection of raw materials

Source: European Commission (EC), *Official Journal of the European Union* L 338, 1–26, 2005a.

Note: n, number of units comprising the sample.

c, number of sample units giving values between m and M.

m, samples over m are marginally acceptable; M, samples over M are unacceptable

In 2009, 21 different pesticides were found in 655 samples of orange juice from different countries in the EU. The most frequent pesticides were carbendazim and benomyl, followed by imazalil and thiabendazole. No maximum residue level (MRL) exceedances were reported (EFSA 2011b). Recently, the pesticides acephate, acetamiprid, imidaclorprid, ametryne, bromacil, carbofuran, diazinon, and difeconazole were also found in concentrations above the maximum allowed in orange juice samples sold in Brazil. It was observed that the occurrence of pesticides in industrialized juices is significantly higher than in fresh natural juices, possibly due to the preconcentration of the pulp during the production process, which is subsequently added to the juices (Bedendo et al. 2012). A total diet study on pesticide residues in France revealed that postharvest fungicides, such as chlorpyrifos, iprodione, carbendazim, and imazalil could be frequently detected in fruit and fruit juices. Diphenylamine was detected in 37.5% of compote samples and 36% of fruit samples. In soft drinks (including fruit juices), five fungicides were detected: 2-phenylphenol (OPP), imazalil, metalaxyl-M (mefenoxam), pyrimethanil, and thiabendazole, with mean estimated levels for the last four lower than in fruit. The foods contributing most to exposure (more than 5% of the total intake) were most frequently vegetables and beverages, including fruit juices (Nougadère et al. 2012).

Some pesticides such as fluazinam are partially removed in the washing water and also remain in the pomace, while a small proportion remains in the juices (EFSA 2012b).

16.3.2 Environmental Contaminants

Arsenic is a metalloid that occurs in different inorganic and organic forms that is found in the environment both from natural occurrence and from anthropogenic activity. The inorganic forms are more toxic as compared to the organic arsenic. The main adverse effects reported to be associated with long-term ingestion of inorganic arsenic in humans are skin lesions, cancer, developmental toxicity, neurotoxicity, cardiovascular diseases, abnormal glucose metabolism, and diabetes. There is emerging evidence of negative impacts on fetal and infant development, particularly reduced birth weight, and there is a need for further evidence regarding the dose–response relationships and critical exposure times for these outcomes. A total of 962 fruit juice samples were taken in the EU in 2003–2008 and analyzed; arsenic was detected in 20%, with mean levels of total arsenic of 0.002–0.010 mg/kg (EFSA 2009b).

Lead is a metal that occurs naturally, but whose presence in the environment has greatly increased as a result of anthropogenic activities. The inorganic forms predominate in the environment. Inorganic lead compounds were classified by the International Agency for Research on Cancer (IARC) as probably carcinogenic to humans (group 2A) in 2006. A total of 1011 fruit juice and nectar samples were taken in the EU in 2003–2009 and analyzed; lead was detected in 31%, with mean levels of 0.01–0.03 mg/kg (EFSA 2010b).

Cadmium is a heavy metal found as an environmental contaminant, both through natural occurrence and from industrial and agricultural sources. The IARC classified cadmium and cadmium compounds as carcinogenic to humans (group 1) in 2003. Foodstuffs are the main source of cadmium exposure for the nonsmoking general population. A total of 2357 fruit juice samples were taken in the EU in 2003–2007 and analyzed; cadmium was detected in 42%, with mean levels of 0.002–0.008 mg/kg (EFSA 2009c).

16.3.3 Mycotoxins

Mycotoxins are fungal metabolites that usually accumulate in raw materials such as fruits. Patulin and ochratoxin A are considered the most important fruit juice-associated mycotoxins (Tribst et al. 2009).

Patulin is a secondary metabolite produced by a number of fungal species in the genera *Penicillium*, *Aspergillus*, and *Byssochlamys*, of which *P. expansum* is probably the most commonly encountered species. There is no clear evidence that patulin is carcinogenic; however, it has been shown to cause immunotoxic effects and is neurotoxic in animals. Patulin has been found as a contaminant in many moldy fruits, vegetables, cereals, and other foods; however, the major sources of contamination are apples and apple products. From 7820 apple juice samples collected in the EU, 60% contained detectable amounts of patulin, with a mean level of 15.6 µg/kg, while in 551 samples of other fruit juices, 26% of samples were found to be positive, with a mean level of 11.3 µg/kg (EC 2002b).

Ochratoxin A is a mycotoxin produced by several fungal species of the genera *Penicillium* and *Aspergillus*. Exposure to ochratoxin A has been associated with distinct renal diseases endemic in the Balkans, referred to as Balkan endemic nephropathy (BEN) and urinary tract tumors (UTT). The IARC evaluated ochratoxin A in 1993, and classified it as possibly carcinogenic to humans (group 2B), based on sufficient evidence for carcinogenicity in animal studies and inadequate evidence in humans (IARC 1993). Contamination has been detected in many food commodities, including grape juice. Mean levels of 0.39 and 0.55 µg/kg have been reported in grape juice samples by Joint FAO/WHO Expert Committee on Food Additives (JEFCA) and Scientific Cooperation (SCOOP) reports, respectively (Bates et al. 2001).

Other natural toxins have been reported in fruit juices, such as *Alternaria* toxins. In general, less than 20% of samples were reported positive for apple, orange, grape, and grapefruit juices. Mean concentrations of alternariol and alternariol monomethyl ether in such fruit juices ranged from values of 0.01 to 3 µg/L. Tenuazonic acid was present in mean concentrations up to 20 µg/L, while alternariol methyl ether was not found in any of the samples analyzed (EFSA 2011c).

Finally, citrinin concentrations up to 0.2 µg/L in fruit and vegetable juices have been reported (EFSA 2012c).

16.3.4 Food Additives

Building on the hurdle principle, antimicrobials can effectively extend shelf life. Sulfur dioxide is quite effective in inhibiting both microbial growth and enzymatic and nonenzymatic browning, although it triggers sensitive reactions in some individuals. Other preservatives such as benzoates, sorbates and ascorbic and citric acid can be used individually or synergistically to extend the shelf life of minimally processed juice drinks. Moreover, a number of sweeteners are used in energy-reduced or no-added-sugar fruit nectars. Their use, however, should not surpass the legal maximum levels, and unauthorized additives must be avoided due to their toxicity.

Dimethylpolysiloxane is widely used as an antifoaming agent in fruit and vegetable juices and other foods. It has been related to ocular toxicity, and consequently maximum levels have been established (FAO/WHO 2009).

16.3.5 PROCESSING CONTAMINANTS

The use of non-food-grade equipment in the processing line, containing copper, bronze, aluminum, iron, and galvanized steel (except stainless), which are easily attacked by fruit acids and contribute toxic metal ions to the juice (lead, mercury, cadmium, and zinc), is a relatively minor safety concern (Bates et al. 2001). As regards inorganic tin, levels of 150 mg/kg in canned beverages and 250 mg/kg in other canned foods may cause gastric irritation in some individuals (EC 2001).

Furan, which can be formed in a variety of heat-treated commercial foods, has been shown to be carcinogenic in animal experiments. Mean values between 2.2 and 4.6 µg/kg for fruit juices (86% of samples over the limit of detection (LOD)) have been reported. Fruit juices are major contributors to furan exposure in toddlers and other children (EFSA 2011d).

16.3.6 CONTROL MEASURES FOR CHEMICAL HAZARDS

As regards pesticide residues, GAP are crucial for their prevention. Primary producers must adhere to (i) permitted pesticides, (ii) convenient dose applications, and (iii) no treatment close to the harvest date. For contaminants, including mycotoxins, GAP may play a role in prevention of ochratoxin A accumulation in vineyards, including prevention of lesions on the berries and skin damage caused by diseases, insects, phytotoxicity, and sunburn, and pesticide treatments.

Regarding postharvest steps, for the particular case of patulin contamination, GMP/GHP should ensure that cold storage does not lead to fungal growth. Moreover, storage of fruits at room temperature prior to processing must be limited to prevent further mycotoxin accumulation. Selection of fruits intended for juice production, in order to remove moldy and faulty fruits, is a critical control measure. In addition, seriously contaminated lots must be avoided before further processing.

Moreover, washing, peeling, and juicing can largely reduce the level of pesticide residues (Li et al. 2012), mycotoxins, and other environmental contaminants.

Patulin is relatively temperature stable, particularly at acid pH levels. High-temperature (150°C), short-term treatments have been reported to result in an approximately 20% reduction in patulin concentrations, and ochratoxin A is also highly thermostable. Thus, thermal processing alone is not sufficient to ensure a product free of mycotoxins.

Finally, GMP should ensure safe levels of food additives and processing contaminants in the final products.

16.3.7 EUROPEAN LEGISLATION

Increasing public concern about health risks from pesticide residues in the diet has led to strict regulation of the MRL and total dietary intake of pesticide residues in foodstuffs. Annexes II and III of Regulation (EC) no. 396/2005 of February 23, 2005, on maximum residue levels of pesticides in or on food and feed of plant and animal origin (EC 2005b) harmonize all MRLs of pesticide/commodity combinations within the EU member states. The MRLs can be easily accessed in the EU pesticides database (EC 2013). The MRLs in this regulation apply to raw materials and not finished products, thus processing factors are required to apply such MRLs to final products (Article 20.1). Such factors will be issued in Annex VI of Regulation 396/2005 in the near future.

As regards contaminants and food additives, Table 16.2 summarizes the maximum levels set for fruit juice categories, in particular Commission Regulation 1881/2006 of December 19, 2006, which sets maximum levels for certain contaminants in foodstuffs (EC 2006), and Commission Regulation 1129/2011 of November 11, 2011 (EC 2011a), which amends Annex II to Regulation 1333/2008 by establishing a union list of food additives (EC 2008a). Moreover, a specific list has recently been issued on food flavorings (Commission Implementing Regulation 872/2012 of October 1, 2012 (EC 2012), adopting the list of flavoring substances provided for by Regulation 2232/96 of the European Parliament and of the Council, introducing it in Annex I to Regulation 1334/2008) to be applied in accordance with GMP, with some exceptions. On the other hand, a Community list of approved food enzymes, with conditions of use in foods under Regulation 1332/2008 (EC 2008b), is still pending.

According to Recommendation 2011/516/EC (EC 2011b), member states should perform random monitoring of the presence of dioxins, dioxin-like polychlorinated biphenyls (PCBs), and non-dioxin-like PCBs in feed and food proportionate to their production, use, and consumption thereof. In cases where levels of dioxins and furans and/or dioxin-like PCBs in fruit are in excess of 0.3 and 0.1 pg/g, respectively, member states should, in cooperation with operators, (a) initiate investigations to identify the source of contamination and (b) take measures to reduce or eliminate the source of contamination.

16.4 FOOD SAFETY MANAGEMENT

As stated in previous sections, GAP, GHP, and GMP are the basis for safe fruit juice production. Farmers should control production so that contamination of the crop through water or organic manure, proliferation of pests, and diseases of animals and plants does not compromise food safety. GAP, including GHP where appropriate, to ensure suitable picking (avoiding rotten fruits and soil-picking), handling (to prevent bruises), and hygienic transport, should be adopted to make sure that the harvested fruit commodity will not present a food hazard to the consumer in terms of either biological or chemical risks. While management of chemical hazards in the juice industries relies mainly on GAP and raw material selection on reception, plus an adequate washing step, management of biological risks involves further implementation of HACCP systems, including the control measures mentioned above as part of the hygiene requisites or the management of critical control points (CCPs) (Figure 16.4). Hygiene prerequisites of

TABLE 16.2
Maximum Permitted Levels of Contaminants and Food Additives in Fruit Juices and Nectars

	Foodstuffs	Maximum Levels
Food Additives		
Calcium carbonate	Grape juice	*Quantum satis*
Sulfur dioxide/sulfites	Orange, grapefruit, apple, and pineapple juice	50 mg/L
	for bulk dispensing in catering establishments	350 mg/L
	Lime and lemon juice	
Lactic acid	Fruit nectars	5000 mg/L
Malic acid	Pineapple juice	3000 mg/L
Ascorbic acid	Fruit juices and nectars	*Quantum satis*
Citric acid	Fruit juices	3000 mg/L
	Fruit nectars	5000 mg/L
Potassium tartrates	Grape juice	*Quantum satis*
Pectins	Pineapple and passion fruit juice and nectar	3000 mg/L
Dimethylpolysiloxane	Pineapple juice	10 mg/L
Acesulfame K	Energy-reduced or no-added-sugar fruit nectars	350 mg/L
Aspartame	Energy-reduced or no-added-sugar fruit nectars	600 mg/L
Cyclamates	Energy-reduced or no-added-sugar fruit nectars	250 mg/L
Saccharins	Energy-reduced or no-added-sugar fruit nectars	80 mg/L
Sucralose	Energy-reduced or no-added-sugar fruit nectars	300 mg/L
Neohesperidin DC	Energy-reduced or no-added-sugar fruit nectars	30 mg/L
Neotame	Energy-reduced or no-added-sugar fruit nectars	20 mg/L
Salt of aspartame-acesulfame	Energy-reduced or no-added-sugar fruit nectars	350 mg/L
Steviol glycosides	Energy-reduced or no-added-sugar fruit nectars	100 mg/L
Mycotoxins		
Ochratoxin A	Grape juice	$2 \mu g/kg$
Patulin	Fruit juices	$50 \mu g/kg$
	Apple juice for infants and young children	$10 \mu g/kg$
Metals		
Lead	Fruit	0.10 mg/kg
	Fruit juices	0.05 mg/kg
Cadmium	Fruit	0.05 mg/kg
Tin (inorganic)	Fruit juices	100 mg/kg

Source: European Commission (EC), *Official Journal of the European Union* L 364, 5–24, 2006; European Commission (EC), *Official Journal of the European Union* L 295, 1–177, 2011a.

relevance in the fruit juice industries include raw material control, sanitation, maintenance, water control, and personnel training programs, as well as traceability systems. The raw material control program must enable the rejection of damaged lots, which are more prone to contain both biological hazards and mycotoxins, after inspection. Sanitary design of the equipment is required, while the sanitation program must allow

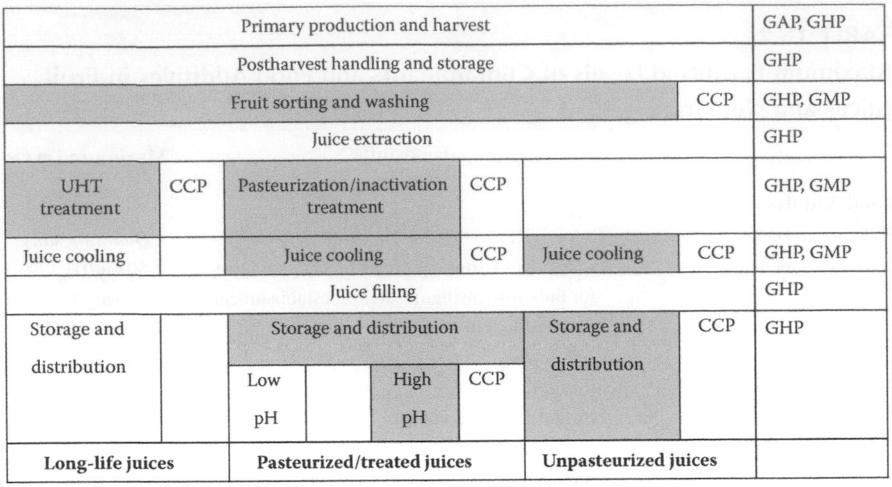

Primary production and harvest						GAP, GHP
Postharvest handling and storage						GHP
Fruit sorting and washing					CCP	GHP, GMP
Juice extraction						GHP
UHT treatment	CCP	Pasteurization/inactivation treatment	CCP			GHP, GMP
Juice cooling		Juice cooling	CCP	Juice cooling	CCP	GHP, GMP
Juice filling						GHP
Storage and distribution		Storage and distribution		Storage and distribution	CCP	GHP
		Low pH		High pH	CCP	
Long-life juices		**Pasteurized/treated juices**		**Unpasteurized juices**		

FIGURE 16.4   Scheme of food safety management in fruit juice production.

for clean and sanitized equipment, free of residues. The water control program must guarantee good-quality water for the washing step, and GMP must ensure an adequate level of antimicrobial agents. Personnel training programs will engage employees in practicing good hygiene with respect to washing of hands, clothing, and hair restraints, and eating and smoking behavior. Moreover, GMP will prevent an excess of food additives or processing contaminants. On top of these GHP and GMP, a number of CCP are required to finally achieve safe fruit juice production; these differ depending on the processing technologies implemented (Figure 16.4).

In conclusion, a certain number of both chemical and biological hazards may threaten the safety of fruit juices, and put consumers' health at risk. However, if both farmers and producers are aware of these risks and understand the importance of maintaining GAP, GHP, and GMP, such risks can be minimized. Finally, particular attention must be paid to monitoring the performance of those processing steps (CCPs) that guarantee the safety of the final product.

REFERENCES

Bates, R.P., J.R. Morris, P.G. Crandall. (2001). *Principles and Practices of Small- and Medium-Scale Fruit Juice Processing.* FAO Agricultural Services Bulletin 146. Rome: FAO.

Bayindirli, A., H. Alpas, F. Bozoğlu, M. Hizal. (2006). Efficiency of high pressure treatment on inactivation of pathogenic microorganisms and enzymes in apple, orange, apricot and sour cherry juices. *Food Control* 17: 52–58.

Bedendo, G.C., I.C. Jardim, E. Carasek. (2012). Multiresidue determination of pesticides in industrial and fresh orange juice by hollow fiber microporous membrane liquid–liquid extraction and detection by liquid chromatography-electrospray-tandem mass spectrometry. *Talanta* 88: 573–580.

Caggia, C., G.O. Scifò, C. Restuccia, C.L. Randazzo. (2009). Growth of acid-adapted *Listeria monocytogenes* in orange juice and in minimally processed orange slices. *Food Control* 20: 59–66.

Eblen, B.S., M.O. Walderhaug, S. Edelson-Mammel, S.J. Chirtel, A. De Jesus, R.I. Merker, R.L. Buchanan, A.J. Miller. (2004). Potential for internalization, growth, and survival of *Salmonella* and *Escherichia coli* O157:H7 in oranges. *Journal of Food Protection* 67: 1578–1584.

EC (European Commission). (2001). Opinion of the Scientific Committee on Food on acute risks posed by tin in canned foods. Available at: http://ec.europa.eu/food/fs/sc/scf/out110_en.pdf (accessed March 2013).

EC (European Commission). (2002a). Opinion of the Scientific Committee on Veterinary Measures relating to Public Health on Norwalk-like viruses. Available at: http://ec.europa.eu/food/fs/sc/scv/out49_en.pdf (accessed March 2013).

EC (European Commission). (2002b). Assessment of dietary intake of patulin by the population of EU member states. Directorate-General Health and Consumer Protection, European Commission. Available at: http://ec.europa.eu/food/fs/scoop/3.2.8_en.pdf (accessed March 2013).

EC (European Commission). (2002c). Assessment of dietary intake of ochratoxin A by the population of EU member states. Directorate-General Health and Consumer Protection, European Commission. Available at: http://ec.europa.eu/food/fs/scoop/3.2.7_en.pdf (accessed March 2013).

EC (European Commission). (2003a). Opinion of the Scientific Committee on Veterinary Measures relating to Public Health on salmonellae in foodstuffs. Available at: http://ec.europa.eu/food/fs/sc/scv/out66_en.pdf (accessed March 2013).

EC (European Commission). (2003b). Opinion of the Scientific Committee on Veterinary Measures relating to Public Health on verotoxigenic *E. coli* (VTEC) in foodstuffs. Available at: http://ec.europa.eu/food/fs/sc/scv/out58_en.pdf (accessed March 2013).

EC (European Commission). (2004). Regulation (EC) No 852/2004 of the European Parliament and of the Council of 29 April 2004 on the hygiene of foodstuffs. *Official Journal of the European Union* L 139: 1–54.

EC (European Commission). (2005a). Commission Regulation (EC) No 2073/2005 of 15 November 2005 on microbiological criteria for foodstuffs. *Official Journal of the European Union* L 338: 1–26.

EC (European Commission). (2005b). Regulation (EC) No 396/2005 of the European Parliament and of the Council of 23 February 2005 on maximum residue levels of pesticides in or on food and feed of plant and animal origin and amending Council Directive 91/414/EEC. *Official Journal of the European Union* L 70: 1–16.

EC (European Commission). (2006). Commission Regulation (EC) No 1881/2006 of 19 December 2006 setting maximum levels for certain contaminants in foodstuffs. *Official Journal of the European Union* L 364: 5–24.

EC (European Commission). (2008a). Regulation (EC) No 1333/2008 of the European Parliament and of the Council of 16 December 2008 on food additives. *Official Journal of the European Union* L 354: 16–33.

EC (European Commission). (2008b). Regulation (EC) No 1332/2008 of the European Parliament and of the Council of 16 December 2008 on food enzymes and amending Council Directive 83/417/EEC, Council Regulation (EC) No 1493/1999, Directive 2000/13/EC, Council Directive 2001/112/EC and Regulation (EC) No 258/97. *Official Journal of the European Union* L 354: 7–15.

EC (European Commission). (2011a). Commission Regulation (EU) No 1129/2011 of 11 November 2011 amending Annex II to Regulation (EC) No 1333/2008 of the European Parliament and of the Council by establishing a union list of food additives. *Official Journal of the European Union* L 295: 1–177.

EC (European Commission). (2011b). Commission Recommendation of 23 August 2011 on the reduction of the presence of dioxins, furans and PCBs in feed and food. *Official Journal of the European Union* L 218: 23–25.

EC (European Commission). (2012). Commission Implementing Regulation (EU) No 872/2012 of 1 October 2012 adopting the list of flavouring substances provided for by Regulation (EC) No 2232/96 of the European Parliament and of the Council, introducing it in Annex I to Regulation (EC) No 1334/2008 of the European Parliament and of the Council and repealing Commission Regulation (EC) No 1565/2000 and Commission Decision 1999/217/EC. *Official Journal of the European Union* L 267: 1–161.

EC (European Commission). (2013). EU pesticides database. http://ec.europa.eu/sanco_pesticides/public/index.cfm.

EFSA (European Food Safety Authority). (2005). Trends and sources of zoonoses, zoonotic agents and antimicrobial resistance in the European Union in 2004. *EFSA Journal* 310.

EFSA (European Food Safety Authority). (2006). The community summary report on trends and sources of zoonoses, zoonotic agents, antimicrobial resistance and foodborne outbreaks in the European Union in 2005. *EFSA Journal* 94: 1–288.

EFSA (European Food Safety Authority). (2007). The community summary report on trends and sources of zoonoses, zoonotic agents, antimicrobial resistance and foodborne outbreaks in the European Union in 2006. *EFSA Journal* 130: 1–352.

EFSA (European Food Safety Authority). (2009a). Food-borne outbreaks in the European Union in 2007. *EFSA Journal* 271: 1–128.

EFSA (European Food Safety Authority). (2009b). Scientific opinion on arsenic in food. *EFSA Journal* 7(10): 1351.

EFSA (European Food Safety Authority). (2009c). Scientific opinion on cadmium in food. *EFSA Journal* 980: 1–139.

EFSA (European Food Safety Authority). (2010a). Trends and sources of zoonoses and zoonotic agents and food-borne outbreaks in the European Union in 2008. *EFSA Journal* 8(1): 1496.

EFSA (European Food Safety Authority). (2010b). Scientific opinion on lead in food. *EFSA Journal* 8(4): 1570.

EFSA (European Food Safety Authority). (2011a). Scientific report of EFSA and ECDC. The European Union summary report on trends and sources of zoonoses, zoonotic agents and food-borne outbreaks in 2009. *EFSA Journal* 9(3): 2090.

EFSA (European Food Safety Authority). (2011b). The 2009 European Union report on pesticide residues in food. *EFSA Journal* 9(11): 2430.

EFSA (European Food Safety Authority). (2011c). Scientific opinion on the risks for animal and public health related to the presence of *Alternaria* toxins in feed and food. *EFSA Journal* 9(10): 2407.

EFSA (European Food Safety Authority). (2011d). Update on furan levels in food from monitoring years 2004–2010 and exposure assessment. *EFSA Journal* 9(9): 2347.

EFSA (European Food Safety Authority). (2012a). Scientific report of EFSA and ECDC. The European Union summary report on trends and sources of zoonoses, zoonotic agents and food-borne outbreaks in 2010. *EFSA Journal* 10(3): 2597.

EFSA (European Food Safety Authority). (2012b). Reasoned opinion on the modification of the existing MRL for fluazinam in apples. *EFSA Journal* 10(5): 2710.

EFSA (European Food Safety Authority). (2012c). Scientific opinion on the risks for public and animal health related to the presence of citrinin in food and feed. *EFSA Journal* 10(3): 2605.

Evrendilek, G.A., K.T. Ruhlman, X. Qiu, Q.H. Zhang, and E.R. Richter. (2000). Microbial safety and shelf-life of apple juice and cider processed by bench and pilot PEF systems. *Innovative Food Science and Emerging Technologies* 1: 77–86.

FAO/WHO (Food and Agriculture Organization/World Health Organization). (2001). Ochratoxin A. In *Safety Evaluation of Certain Mycotoxins in Food*, Prepared by the 56th Meeting of the Joint FAO/WHO Expert Committee on Food Additives (JECFA). WHO Food Additives Series 47, pp. 281–387. Geneva: World Health Organization.

FAO/WHO (Food and Agriculture Organization/World Health Organization). (2009). Polydimethylsiloxane. In *Safety Evaluation of Certain Food Additives*, Prepared by the 69th Meeting of the Joint FAO/WHO Expert Committee on Food Additives (JECFA). WHO Food Additives Series 60, pp. 165–181. Geneva: World Health Organization.

Fellows, P.J. (1997). *Traditional Foods: Processing for Profit.* London: Intermediate Technology Publications.

Girardin, H., C.E. Morris, C. Albagnac, N. Dreux, C. Glaux, C. Nguyen-The. (2005). Behaviour of the pathogen surrogates *Listeria innocua* and *Clostridium sporogenes* during production of parsley in fields fertilized with contaminated amendments. *FEMS Microbiology Ecology* 54: 287–295.

Guinebretière, M.H. C. Nguyen-The. (2003). Sources of *Bacillus cereus* contamination in a pasteurised zucchini puree processing plant, differentiated by two PCR-based methods. *FEMS Microbiology Ecology* 43: 207–215.

IARC (International Agency for Research on Cancer). (1993). *IARC Monographs on the Evaluation of Carcinogenic Risks to Humans, Some Naturally Occurring Substances. Food Items and Constituents, Heterocyclic Aromatic Amines and Mycotoxins*, vol. 56. Lyon, France: International Agency for Research on Cancer.

Jay, S. J. Anderson. (2001). Fruit juice and related products. In: C.J. Moir, C. Andrew-Kabilafkas, G. Arnold, B.M. Cox, A.D. Hocking, and I. Jenson (eds), *Spoilage of Processed Foods: Causes and Diagnosis*, pp. 187–197. Waterloo, NSW, Australia: Australian Institute of Food Science and Technology.

Keller, S.E. A.J. Miller. (2006). Microbial safety of fresh citrus and apple juices. In G.M. Sapers, J.R. Gorny, and A.E. Yousef (eds), *Microbiology of Fruits and Vegetables*. Boca Raton, FL: Taylor & Francis.

Koopmans, M. E. Duizer. (2004). Foodborne viruses: An emerging problem. *International Journal of Food Microbiology* 1: 23–41.

Laberge, I. M.W. Griffiths. (1996). Prevalence detection and control of *Cryptosporidium parvum* in food. *International Journal of Food Microbiology* 32: 1–26.

Li, Y., B. Jiao, Q. Zhao, C. Wang, Y. Gong, Y. Zhang, W. Chen. (2012). Effect of commercial processing on pesticide residues in orange products. *European Food Research and Technology* 234: 449–456.

Lu, J., G.S. Mittal, M.W. Griffiths. (2001). Reductions in levels of *Escherichia coli* O157:H7 in apple cider by pulsed electric fields. *Journal of Food Protection* 64: 964–969.

McDonald, C.J., S.W. Lloyd, M.A. Vitale, K. Petersson, F. Innings. (2000). Effect of pulsed electric fields on microorganisms in orange juice using electric field strengths of 30 and 50 kV/cm. *Journal of Food Science* 65: 984–989.

Mosqueda-Melgar, J., R.M. Raybaudi-Massilia, O. Martín-Belloso. (2008). Non-thermal pasteurization of fruit juices by combining high-intensity pulsed electric fields with natural antimicrobials. *Innovative Food Science and Emerging Technologies* 9: 328–340.

Niu, M.T., L.B. Polish, B.H. Robertson, B.K. Khanna, B.A. Woodruff, C.N. Shapiro, M.A. Miller, et al. (1992). Multistate outbreak of hepatitis A associated with frozen strawberries. *Journal of Infectious Diseases* 166: 518–524.

Nougadère, A., V. Sirot, A. Kadar, A. Fastier, E. Truchot, C. Vergnet, F. Hommet, J. Baylé, P. Gros, J.C. Leblanc. (2012). Total diet study on pesticide residues in France: Levels in food as consumed and chronic dietary risk to consumers. *Environment International* 45: 135–150.

Pereira, K.S., R.M.B. Franco, D.A.G. Leal. (2010). Transmission of toxoplasmosis (*Toxoplasma gondii*) by foods. *Advances in Food and Nutrition Research* 60: 1–19.

Rapid Alert System for Food and Feed (RASFF). (2001). Annual report 2001. Available at: http://ec.europa.eu/food/food/rapidalert/rasff_publications_en.htm.

Rapid Alert System for Food and Feed (RASFF). (2002). Annual report 2002. Available at: http://ec.europa.eu/food/food/rapidalert/rasff_publications_en.htm.

Rapid Alert System for Food and Feed (RASFF). (2003). Annual report 2003. Available at: http://ec.europa.eu/food/food/rapidalert/rasff_publications_en.htm.

Rapid Alert System for Food and Feed (RASFF). (2004). Annual report 2004. Available at: http://ec.europa.eu/food/food/rapidalert/rasff_publications_en.htm.

Rapid Alert System for Food and Feed (RASFF). (2005). Annual report 2005. Available at: http://ec.europa.eu/food/food/rapidalert/rasff_publications_en.htm.

Rapid Alert System for Food and Feed (RASFF). (2006). Annual report 2006. Available at: http://ec.europa.eu/food/food/rapidalert/rasff_publications_en.htm.

Rapid Alert System for Food and Feed (RASFF). (2007). Annual report 2007. Available at: http://ec.europa.eu/food/food/rapidalert/rasff_publications_en.htm.

Rapid Alert System for Food and Feed (RASFF). (2008). Annual report 2008. Available at: http://ec.europa.eu/food/food/rapidalert/rasff_publications_en.htm.

Rapid Alert System for Food and Feed (RASFF). (2009). Annual report 2009. Available at: http://ec.europa.eu/food/food/rapidalert/rasff_publications_en.htm.

Rapid Alert System for Food and Feed (RASFF). (2010). Annual report 2010. Available at: http://ec.europa.eu/food/food/rapidalert/rasff_publications_en.htm.

Rapid Alert System for Food and Feed (RASFF). (2011). Annual report 2011. Available at: http://ec.europa.eu/food/food/rapidalert/rasff_publications_en.htm.

Seymour, I.J. H. Appleton. (2001). Foodborne viruses and fresh produce. *Journal of Applied Microbiology* 91: 759–773.

Skovgaard, N. (2007). New trends in emerging pathogens. *International Journal of Food Microbiology* 120: 217–224.

Slifko, T.R., E. Raghubeer, J.B. Rose. (2000). Effect of high hydrostatic pressure on *Cryptosporidium parvum* infectivity. *Journal of Food Protection* 63: 1262–1267.

Steindel, M., L.K. Pacheco, D. Scholl, M. Soares, M.H. de Moraes, I. Eger, C. Kosmann, et al. (2008). Characterization of *Trypanossoma cruzi* isolated from human vectors and animal reservoirs following an outbreak of acute human Chagas disease in Santa Catarina State, Brazil. *Diagnostic Microbiology and Infectious Disease* 60: 25–32.

Tribst, A.A.L., A. De Souza Sanfana, P.R. De Massaguer. (2009). Review: Microbiological quality and safety of fruit juices past, present and future perspectives microbiology of fruit juices. *Critical Reviews in Microbiology* 35: 310–339.

Valente, S.A.S., V.C. Valente, H. Fraiha Neto. (1999). Consideration of the epidemiology and transmission of Chagas disease in the Brazilian Amazon. *Memórias do Instituto Oswaldo Cruz* 94: 395–398.

Vojdani, J.D., L.R. Beuchat, R.V. Tauxe. (2008). Juice-associated outbreaks of human illness in the United States, 1995 through 2005. *Journal of Food Protection* 71: 356–364.

Yuk, H.G. K.R. Schneider. (2006). Adaptation of *Salmonella* spp. in juice stored under refrigerated and room temperature enhances acid resistance to simulated gastric fluid. *Food Microbiology* 23: 694–700.

17 Public and Private Standards and Regulations Concerning Fruit Juices

Antonio Martínez, Dolores Rodrigo,
Josep Arbós, and Yvonne Colomer

CONTENTS

17.1 Food Safety Regulations 350
    17.1.1 General Principles of Food Safety (Regulation 178/2002)...............350
    17.1.2 Traceability 353
    17.1.3 Risk Assessment (HACCP) 354
    17.1.4 Codex Alimentarius 357
    17.1.5 Legislation 358
        17.1.5.1 General Interest 358
        17.1.5.2 Sectorial 358
17.2 Product Authenticity Regulations (Fruit Juice) 360
    17.2.1 AIJN Standards 360
    17.2.2 Royal Decree 1518/2007 362
    17.2.3 Specialized Laboratory Standards 362
17.3 Management Standards for Food Quality 362
    17.3.1 ISO 9000 362
    17.3.2 ISO 22000 363
    17.3.3 BRC 364
    17.3.4 Standard IFS 364
17.4 Norms of Quality Assessment of a Juice or Puree 365
    17.4.1 Physical–Chemical Quality 365
    17.4.2 Organoleptic Quality 365
    17.4.3 Microbiological Quality 366
17.5 Biological Hazards 366
    17.5.1 Bacterial Contamination 366
    17.5.2 Mold Contamination 369
    17.5.3 Yeast Contamination 369
17.6 HACCP and Industrial Assessment to Control Microbial Hazards 370
References 371

17.1   FOOD SAFETY REGULATIONS

Food Security is, according to:

- The United Nations Food and Agriculture Organization (FAO):
  - Access (whether physical, social, and economic) for all people at all times, to sufficient, safe, and nutritious food to meet their nutritional needs and cultural preferences for an active and healthy life.
- The U.S. Department of Agriculture (USDA):
  - Access at all times for all members of a household to enough food for an active and healthy life. This access includes at least:
    - The immediate availability of nutritionally adequate and safe foods
    - Assured ability to dispose of such food in a sustainable and socially acceptable way (i.e., without having to rely on emergency food supplies, scavenging, stealing, or using other coping strategies)
- The European Economic Community:
  - The guarantee of a high level of:
    - Food quality
    - Health, welfare, and animal feed
    - Plant health

In the European Union, the implementation and monitoring of coherent "farm to table" measures ensure the effective functioning of the internal market.

For this, the European Economic Community has developed legislative action and other measures to:

- Ensure effective control systems (traceability of food from the farm to the table) and assess compliance with the Community rules on food quality, health, welfare, and plant health and animal feed.
- Manage international relations with third countries and international organizations with regard to food safety, health, animal welfare, animal nutrition, and plant health.
- Ensure scientific risk management.

The food chain is a cycle that begins in primary production and ends with consumption. The way to ensure food safety, in other words, is to avoid hazards arising in food and consider the food chain holistically.

17.1.1   GENERAL PRINCIPLES OF FOOD SAFETY (REGULATION 178/2002)

The objectives of the Food Safety Legislation under Regulation EEC 178/2002 are:

- To pursue one or more of the general objectives of achieving a high level of protection of people's life and health, and to protect consumer interests, including fair practices in food trade, taking into account, where appropriate, the protection of health and animal welfare, plant health and the environment

- To achieve the free movement of food and feed manufactured or marketed according to the principles and requirements of Food Safety
- To consider existing international standards, or those soon to be applied, to the development or adaptation of food law, unless such standards or relevant parts thereof are ineffective or inappropriate to comply with the legitimate objectives of the food law or there is a scientific justification, or the level of protection offered is different from that determined to be appropriate by the community

These are based on the following principles:

1. Risk analysis
   Risk analysis is a process made up of three interconnected components:

   ### Risk assessment
   A science-based process consisting of four steps:
   - Identification of the risk factor
   - Characterization of the risk factor
   - Measurement of exposure
   - Characterization of the risk

   Risk assessment is based on the available scientific evidence and undertaken independently, objectively, and transparently.

   ### Risk management
   Risk management is a different process from the above for weighing policy alternatives in consultation with interested parties, considering risk assessment and other legitimate factors, and, if needed, selecting appropriate options for prevention and control.

   ### Risk communication
   Risk communication is the process that involves the interactive exchange of information and opinions regarding the possible hazards and risks, risk-related factors and risk perceptions throughout the risk analysis process, which is established between risk assessors and those responsible for risk management, including consumers, food companies, the scientific community, and other interested parties. This exchange includes the explanation of the results of the risk assessment and the reasons for decisions related to risk management.

2. Caution
   In special circumstances, when the possibility of adverse health effects appears following an assessment of available information, but scientific uncertainty persists, provisional risk-management measures may be taken to ensure a high level of health protection pending further scientific information to allow a more comprehensive risk assessment.

   These interim measures must be proportionate and no more restrictive of trade than is required to achieve the high level of health protection chosen, taking into account the technical and economic feasibility and together with other factors regarded as legitimate in the question in hand. These measures should be reviewed within a reasonable time, depending on the nature of the risk to life or health, and the type of scientific information needed to clarify the uncertainty and lead to a more comprehensive risk assessment.

3. Protection of consumer interests

The protection of consumer interests is based on avoiding:
  • Fraudulent or deceptive practices
  • Adulteration of food
  • Practices that may mislead the consumer

This Food Safety Legislation:

• Contributes to
  • The development of international technical standards for food and development of health and plant health standards
  • Reaching agreements on recognition of the equivalence of certain food-related measures
• Promotes
  • Coordination of standardization work related to food undertaken by international governmental and nongovernmental organizations
  • Consistency between international technical standards while also ensuring that the high level of protection for a given country or state is not reduced
• Pays particular attention to the special needs of developing countries in development, finance, and trade, in order to avoid international standards creating unnecessary obstacles to exports from developing countries

It also establishes the following qualifications:

1. Do not sell unsafe food.
2. A food is considered not to be safe when it is
   a. Harmful to health.
   b. Unsuitable for human consumption.
3. To determine whether a food is safe, the following will be taken into account:
   a. Normal conditions for the use of the food by the consumer and at each stage of production, processing, and distribution processes.
   b. The information provided to consumers, including that contained on the label, or other data that is generally available to the consumer for the prevention of certain adverse health effects that result derived from a specific foodstuff or food category.
4. In determining whether any food is injurious to health, the following is taken into account.
   a. The probable immediate, short- and long-term effects of that food not only for the health of the person consuming it, but also for their descendants.
   b. The possible cumulative toxic effects.

    c. The particular health sensitivity of a specific category of consumers, when the food is intended for them.

5. When determining whether a food is unfit for human consumption, it is taken into account if the food is unacceptable for human consumption according to the use for which it is intended, by being contaminated by undesired material or otherwise, or through putrefaction, deterioration, or decay.

6. When a food that is unsafe belongs to a batch or consignment of food of the same class or description, it is assumed that all the food in that batch, lot, or consignment is also unsafe, unless a detailed assessment demonstrates that there no evidence that the rest of the lot or consignment is unsafe.

7. Food that complies with specific Community provisions governing food safety is considered safe with respect to the matters covered by those provisions.

8. The conformity of a food with specific provisions applicable to it does not prevent the competent authorities from taking appropriate measures to impose restrictions on the market or to require its withdrawal from the market when there is reason to think that, despite such conformity, the food is unsafe.

9. In the absence of specific provisions, it is considered that a food is safe when it conforms to the specific provisions of national food law of the country or state where the food is sold.

17.1.2 TRACEABILITY

Traceability is the set of established and self-sufficient procedures that provide insight into the history, location, and trajectory of a product or batch of products through the supply chain at any given time, with certain tools.

Food traceability is the ability to find and follow the trail through all stages of production, processing, and distribution of a food or a substance incorporated into a food.

As a result, it is clear that to ensure the traceability of a product, the trace that the product leaves as it moves through the chain must be identified and recorded, either in the normal direction or in the reverse direction (as reverse logistics), specifying and determining clearly for any product:

- The origin of its components
- The history of the processes applied to the product
- The distribution and location after delivery

This allows at any time to know "everything" related to the product, in this case food, at any time during the production process, thus greatly facilitating any decision-making before a food safety problem.

The concept of traceability is divided into two types:

- Internal traceability, which consists of obtaining the trace that a product leaves in the internal processes of a company, with manipulation, composition, the machinery used, the shift, temperature, batch, and so on; in other words, all the evidence that can vary or may vary the product for the final consumer

- External traceability, consisting of externalizing internal tracing data and, if necessary, adding more, such as rupture of the package, a change in temperature chain, and so on

There are many ways of registering the data, such as temperature and humidity sensors, but there are few methods to transmit this evidence in a standardized, secure, and reliable way between different actors in the chain, notable among which are the different coding systems.

17.1.3   RISK ASSESSMENT (HACCP)

The Hazard Analysis and Critical Control Points (HACCP) is a systematic prevention process to ensure food safety, logically and objectively.

It is based on the following principles:

1. Hazard identification
   Identify all potential hazards (physical, chemical, and biological) that can appear at each stage in the process and the prevention measures to avoid these. However, it only studies those hazards that are potentially dangerous for the consumer, or takes into account those dangers that jeopardize the quality of the product.
2. Identify the *critical control points* (CCP)
   Identify critical control points, that is, those stages of the production process in which "control is essential to safeguard the safety of the product for the consumer," using the decision tree showed in Figure 17.1.
3. Definition of critical limits
   The critical limits of the control measures that will make the difference between what is safe and what is not are defined in detail for each CCP.
   When a value is outside the limits, it indicates a deviation, and therefore the process is out of control, so that the product can be dangerous for the consumer.
4. Establish a system of monitoring CCPs
   This identifies the actions to be implemented to establish if the process is being conducted under the conditions laid down, and is thus under control.
      These actions are performed for each CCP, also establishing monitoring frequency, that is, how often these should be tested, and who should carry out the monitoring or surveillance.
5. Definition of corrective actions
   It details the corrective actions to be taken when the monitoring system detects that a CCP is not under control. In addition to these actions, it must specify who is responsible for carrying them out. These actions will be those that lead the process back to normal and thus work under safe conditions.
6. Implementation of a verification system
   The verification system allows it to be confirmed that the HACCP system is working correctly, that is, that the HACCP system identifies and reduces all significant hazards for food to acceptable levels.

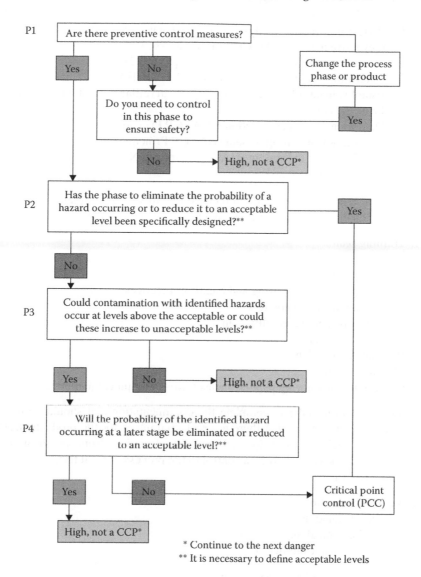

P1 Are there preventive control measures?

Yes   No   Change the process phase or product

Do you need to control in this phase to ensure safety?   Yes

No   High, not a CCP*

P2 Has the phase to eliminate the probability of a hazard occurring or to reduce it to an acceptable level been specifically designed?**   Yes

No

P3 Could contamination with identified hazards occur at levels above the acceptable or could these increase to unacceptable levels?**

Yes   No   High, not a CCP*

P4 Will the probability of the identified hazard occurring at a later stage be eliminated or reduced to an acceptable level?**

Yes   No   Critical point control (PCC)

High, not a CCP*

* Continue to the next danger
** It is necessary to define acceptable levels

FIGURE 17.1 Identifying the critical control points (CCPs).

7. Creating a documentation system

This documentation system can record everything related to the HACCP system. There are 12 elements in the implementation of a HACCP system:

1. Training of the team
2. Description of the products
3. Identification of the expected use of the product by the consumer
4. Development of a flowchart and the description of the process

5. Performing hazard analysis associated with production and identify preventive measures (HACCP Principle No. 1)
6. Identification of CCPs (HACCP Principle No. 2)
7. Determination of critical limits for each CCP (HACCP Principle No. 3)
8. Establishment of a monitoring and surveillance system (HACCP Principle No. 4)
9. Definition of corrective actions (HACCP Principle No. 5)
10. Registration and filing of data (HACCP Principle No. 6)
11. Verification of the system (HACCP Principle No. 7)
12. Review of the system

Every good HACCP system is reinforced by so-called "support plans" that should be defined to ensure the proper hygienic habits. They are as follows:

1. Training plan
2. Sanitation plan
3. Pest control plan
4. Plan for good manufacturing and handling practices
5. Plan for approval of suppliers
6. Identification and traceability plan
7. Water control plan
8. Residue control plan
9. Maintenance plan
10. Control and monitoring plan for measurement equipment (calibration)

In addition and in order to complete the documentation that should be part of the system and thus ensure that there are real guarantees for the products, testing procedures are established to help detect possible deviations from specifications to enable corrective measures to regain control to the process without the need to reject the product, and they are as follows:

1. Visual observation
2. Sensory evaluation
3. Physical/chemical measurement
4. Microbiological examination

Legal obligations of food business operators are:

1. Food liability
   The food business operator is legally responsible for food security and may not sell food that is unsafe according to established rules, and failing these, on the basis of scientific knowledge.
2. Self-control
   Operators of food businesses must
   • Create, implement, and maintain the necessary permanent set of procedures that make up self-control to ensure food security in their food products, in the terms prescribed by the applicable regulations.

- Prove that, at all stages of production, processing, and distribution that take place within the premises under their control, the food meets the requirements of the food safety legislation.
- Ensure proper removal, destruction, or channeling of food that is spoiled, past the sell-by date, seizures or products unfit for human or animal consumption or circuits to companies established and authorized under applicable legal frameworks, so that it cannot be reintroduced as part of food, or cause pollution of the environment.

3. Traceability

Operators of food businesses must ensure traceability of food from any other substance intended to be, or likely to be, incorporated into a food, at all stages of production, processing, and distribution.

4. Transparency

The food business operator must maintain updated information at all times on their activity that can have an impact, from the perspective of health protection related to the stages of production, processing, and distribution in which it operates, and transmit the corresponding information, where appropriate, to the various operators in the food chain. This information should always be available to the authority responsible for carrying out official controls, which have access to it at all times. For reasons of health protection, the health authorities will have access, directly and immediately, to such information, including computer-based information, regardless of the stage where the food business operates.

5. Emergency, prevention, and cooperation

When the food business operator considers or has reason to believe that there is or may be a risk to the health and safety of citizens in relation to any of the foods that have been imported, produced, processed, or distributed, they should immediately withdraw this food from the market and must inform the health authorities of the reasons for adopting the measure to which the provision refers. This obligation must also be assumed for the consumers if the food or products have been distributed. In the latter case, the food business operator must inform the health authorities of the measures adopted to protect consumers.

17.1.4 Codex Alimentarius

The Codex Alimentarius is a collection of internationally recognized standards, codes of practice, guidelines, and other recommendations relating to food, food production, and security with the objective of consumer protection. Officially, this code is maintained by the Codex Alimentarius Commission, a body set with the Food and Agriculture Organization (FAO), an agency within the United Nations and the World Health Organization (WHO).

The General Standard or base standard is the Codex General Standard for Fruit Juices and Nectars (CODEX STAN 247-2005), supplemented and modified according to the decisions taken in the various committees of the Codex Alimentarius that meet regularly, and distributed into the following sections:

1. Scope
2. Description
   a. Product definition
   b. Species
3. Essential composition and quality factors
   a. Composition
   b. Quality criteria
   c. Authenticity
   d. Verification of the composition, quality, and authenticity
4. Food additives
5. Processing aids
6. Contaminants
7. Hygiene
8. Labeling
9. Methods of analysis and sampling
10. Annex (minimum Brix level for juice and minimum reconstituted juice and/or puree in nectars [%v/v] 15°C–20°C)

17.1.5   LEGISLATION

17.1.5.1   General Interest

General interest legislation is specific to each country and based on

- Consumer protection
- General product safety

17.1.5.2   Sectorial

17.1.5.2.1   General

Classified as:

1. Rules related to additives (colorants, sweeteners, etc.), aromas, and food enzymes
2. Rules for storage and transport
   a. Frozen food
   b. Cold storage
   c. Nonrefrigerated storage
   d. Irradiation of foods
   e. Transport
3. Trade regulations
   a. Retail
   b. Restaurants
   c. Sale outside a permanent commercial establishment
4. Regulations on radioactive contamination

5. Regulations on contaminants in food (general legislation applicable)
   a.   Acrylamide
   b.   Dioxins and PCBs
   c.   Polycyclic aromatic hydrocarbons (PAHs)
   d.   Spanish legislation on specific pollutants
   e.   Heavy metals and other environmental and industrial pollutants
   f.   Mycotoxins
   g.   Nitrates
   h.   Contaminants
6. Official control regulations
   a.   General character of control
   b.   Control of products of animal origin
7. Labeling and advertising regulations
   a.   Labeling foodstuffs
   b.   Labeling nutritional properties
   c.   Nutrition and health
8. General regulations on food hygiene
   a.   Public water consumption
   b.   Microbiological criteria
   c.   Cleaning products, disinfection, and insect and pest removal
9. Regulations on materials in contact with food
   a.   Rubber: N-nitrosamines
   b.   Regenerated cellulose
   c.   Ceramics
   d.   Epoxy derivatives: BADGE, BFDGE, NOGE
   e.   Polymeric material
   f.   Plastics
10. Regulations concerning novel foods and novel ingredients
   a.   Foods that can be put on the EU market under Article 4.2, first draft of
        Regulation (EC) No 258/97
   b.   Authorization to market novel foods and novel food ingredients
   c.   Denial of permission to market novel foods and novel food ingredients
11. Regulations on genetically modified organisms (GMOs)
12. Regulations on organisms and procedures
   a.   Food Safety Agency
   b.   General health registry of food and food companies
   c.   External health
   d.   Request for reports from the scientific committee
13. Animal Protection Regulations
14. Waste Regulations
   a.   Veterinary drug residues and certain substances prohibited in animal
        production
   b.   Pesticide residues
15. Food safety legislation
16. By-product regulations

17.1.5.2. By-Sectors

There are specific rules for each sector, so there are many rules; the aim of this article is to focus on specific food safety standards in the sector of fruit and vegetable juices (national, EU, U.S.).

Royal Decree 1050/2003

This approves the Technical Health Regulation of fruit juices and certain similar products intended for human consumption. It is a result of the transposition of Directive 2001/112/EC and Directive 2009/106/EC.

Royal Decree 667/1983

This approves the Technical Health Regulation for the development and sale of juices from fruit and other plants and their derivatives.

Directive 2001/112/EC as amended by Directive 2012/12/CE
Directive 2009/106/EC

...

17.2   PRODUCT AUTHENTICITY REGULATIONS (FRUIT JUICE)

17.2.1   AIJN STANDARDS

The International Association of Juices and Nectars (AIJN) is the representative of the fruit juice industry in the European Union.

Its aim is to work toward the best possible policy, regulatory, and economic framework in the EU to add value and promote the growth of the fruit juice industry. More specifically, the AIJN is designed to:

1. Represent the interests and promote the image of the European fruit juice industry in all contacts with EU officials, EU institutions, and other relevant organizations.
2. Support and lobby EU institutions in all aspects of policy and legislation on the production, marketing, sales and trade in fruit juices and nectars in the EU.
3. Promote and maintain fair competition and commercial viability of the juices and nectars in the EU.
4. In collaboration with the Quality Control System European (EQCS), provide mechanisms and tools to ensure safety and authentic products in order to maintain and boost consumer confidence in a good healthy image of fruit vegetable juices and nectars.
5. Inform and advice the fruit juice industry in all aspects of European legislation that may affect their business.

Because the law does not cover all aspects of the chain of fruit juice processing and bottling in detail and the laws sometimes leave room for different interpretations, the AIJN has developed guidelines and standards. These include the AIJN

Code of Practice for evaluating the quality and authenticity of fruit and vegetable juices, traceability guidelines, aroma guidelines, and so on, which currently contains benchmarks for 21 different fruit and vegetable juices, and is based on:

- Criteria for quality
- Criteria of identity and authenticity

1. Quality criteria
    a. Industrial requirements
        i. Gravity
        ii. Brix
    b. Hygiene requirements
        i. Ethanol
        ii. Acid D/L lactic
        iii. Mycotoxins (patulin)
    c. Environmental requirements
        i. Arsenic and heavy metals
    d. Compositional requirements
        i. Hydroxymethylfurfural
2. Criteria for identity and authenticity
    a. Total acidity
    b. Citric acid
    c. Isocitric acid
    d. Citric acid/isocitric acid
    e. L-Malic acid
    f. D-Malic acid
    g. Fumaric
    h. Ash
    i. Sodium
    j. Potassium
    k. Calcium
    l. Magnesium
    m. Phosphorus
    n. Nitrates
    o. Sulfates
    p. Number of formaldehyde
    q. Glucose/fructose
    r. Sucrose
    s. Sugar-free extract
    t. Sorbitol
    u. Amino acids
        i. Aspartic acid
        ii. Threonine
        iii. Serine
        iv. Asparagine
        v. Glutamic acid

    vi. Glutamine
    vii. Proline
   viii. Glycine
    ix. Alanine
    x. Valine
    xi. Methionine
    xii. Iso-leucine
   xiii. Leucine
   xiv. Tyrosine
    xv. Phenylalanine
   xvi. Gamma-aminobutyric acid
  xvii. Ornithine
 xviii. Lysine
   xix. Histidine
   xx. Arginine
   xxi. Aspartic acid+asparagines
  xxii. …
 xxiii. Isotopic values
 xxiv. Water or Delta O18
  xxv. (D/H) I Etanol2H-NMR
 xxvi. Delta 13C or sugar
xxvii. Delta 13C or ethanol

17.2.2 ROYAL DECREE 1518/2007

This legislation establishes minimum quality parameters for fruit juices and analysis methods.

17.2.3 SPECIALIZED LABORATORY STANDARDS

Specialized laboratories have been set up in various countries to carry out extensive studies of fruit juices, going beyond the rules themselves, and databases have been created with their own methods, based on the DNA of their own fruit, anthocyanins, carotenoids, disaccharides, glycosides, and so on, which, while not yet official, or legally recognized, are of high value given the prestige of these laboratories in firms in the fruit juice sector (manufacturers, bottlers, importers, etc.).

17.3 MANAGEMENT STANDARDS FOR FOOD QUALITY

17.3.1 ISO 9000

These are standards and quality management protocols, developed by the International Organization for Standardization (ISO), which specify the requirements for a Management System (QMS) and can be used for internal application by organizations, whether the product or service is provided by a public or private company, whatever its size, for certification or contractual purposes.

Chief among these is the ISO 9001:2008 standards containing the specification of the management model. It contains the "requirements" of the model, and is divided into the following chapters:

- Chapters 1 through 3: Guidelines and general descriptions.
- Chapter 4. Management system: the general requirements and requirements for managing records.
- Chapter 5. Management responsibilities: requirements to be met by organizational leadership, such as defining the policy, ensuring that responsibilities and authorities are defined, approving objectives, management commitment to quality, etc.
- Chapter 6. Resources management: the Standard distinguishes three types of resources to act on: HR, infrastructure, and work environment. This contains the requirements for managing these.
- Chapter 7. Making product/service: the requirements purely for what is produced or provided as a service (the standard includes service when it is called "Product"), from customer service to delivery of the product or service.
- Chapter 8. Measurement, analysis, and improvement: the requirements for the processes that collect, analyze, and act accordingly. The goal is continuously to improve the organization's ability to deliver products and/or services that meet the requirements. The objective stated in the Standard is that the organization relentlessly seeks customer satisfaction through the fulfillment of the requirements.

17.3.2   ISO 22000

However, it is of particular importance to ISO 22000, which is an ISO standard series focused on food. This standard defines and specifies the requirements for developing and implementing a Safety Management System for food, to achieve international harmonization leading to better food security throughout the supply chain. Its objectives are to

- Ensure *consumer protection* and strengthen their confidence
- Strengthen food security
- Promote cooperation between industries and governments
- Improve performance costs throughout the food supply chain

And pick the "key elements" completely covering industrial safety requirements, forming the basis of any approved food safety standard, these requirements, in no way meant to replace legal and regulatory requirements, are:

- Requirements for developing a HACCP system according to the principles of the Codex Alimentarius
- Requirements for GMP or prerequisite program
- Requirements for a management system

17.3.3 BRC

The BRC is a food safety standard established by the British Retail Association or British Retail Consortium (BRC).

Its main interests and objectives are to

- Strengthen food security
- Ensure compliance with legal liabilities
- Provide consumer protection to offer a safe, high-quality product
- Provide a common basis for evaluation and audits of suppliers
- Reduce production costs
- Limit the inflation of food prices

This standard is based on the following sections:

1. Management responsibility
2. System quality management
3. Assessment of the environment and production process facilities
4. Control product
5. Process control
6. Staff

The IFS system provides a certification that can offer a number of benefits to companies striving for excellence in food safety, quality, and customer satisfaction and the pursuit of a competitive advantage on the market:

- Facilitates compliance with applicable law
- Reduces the cost of the possible errors of any production
- Provides an organized and effective communication with all stakeholders
- Provides consumer confidence
- Improved documentation
- Allows more efficient and dynamic control of food safety hazards
- Prerequisite programs incorporate the management system of the organization

17.3.4 STANDARD IFS

The IFS is a food quality and safety standard developed by the German federation of retail companies (Einzelhandels Hauptverband des deutschen, HDE) and its French counterpart (Fédération des Entreprises du Commerce et de la Distribution, FCD) of retail branded food products, named IFS Food, which is designed to assess food safety and supplier quality systems according to standardized criteria. This standard applies to all stages from the farm to postprocessing of foods.

Its main interests and objectives are to establish a common standard with a uniform evaluation system, to work with accredited certification bodies and qualified auditors to ensure comparability and transparency throughout the supply chain to reduce costs and time, for both suppliers and retailers.

This standard is based on the following sections:

1. Responsibility of senior management
2. Quality and food management systems
3. Resource management
4. Production process
5. Measurement, analysis and improvements.
6. Food defense

The IFS system provides a certification that can offer a number of benefits to companies striving for excellence in food safety, quality, and customer satisfaction and the pursuit of a competitive advantage in their market:

- Better understanding between management and staff based on good practices, standards, and procedures
- Monitoring of compliance with food regulations
- More efficient use of resources
- Reduced need for customer audits
- Independent third-party audits
- Ability to reduce total audit time by combining multiple audits
- Increasing flexibility by individual application due to a risk-based approach improving the company's reputation as a manufacturer of high-quality and safe products

17.4 NORMS OF QUALITY ASSESSMENT OF A JUICE OR PUREE

17.4.1 PHYSICAL–CHEMICAL QUALITY

1. °Brix
2. Acidity
3. Ratio (Brix/acidity)
4. pH
5. Pulp content
6. Viscosity (Bostwick)
7. Color (L, a, b)
8. Color (transmittance, absorbance)
9. Turbidity.
10. …

17.4.2 ORGANOLEPTIC QUALITY

1. Color
2. Taste
3. Flavor
4. Aroma
5. General appearance

17.4.3   Microbiological Quality

1. Total number of bacteria
2. Total number of yeasts and fungi
3. Total acid-tolerant microorganisms
4. Total thermophilic acid bacteria
5. ...

17.5   BIOLOGICAL HAZARDS

One of the major growth segments in the food retail industry is fresh and minimally processed fruits and vegetables. This was stimulated largely by consumer demand for fresh, healthy, convenient, and additive-free foods that are safe and nutritious.

With the growing demand for fresh fruits and vegetables, the Centers for Disease Control and Prevention (CDC) reported an increase in the frequency of fruit and vegetables associated to food-borne disease outbreaks (Bean et al., 1997; Mead et al., 1999). The potential for contamination increases as the fruits and vegetables moves from farm to table that is, irrigation water, improperly composted manure, wash water systems, soiled equipment, unsanitary practices, and so on can contribute to contamination of the product. Fruits and vegetables carry a natural nonpathogenic epiphytic microflora and at the same time contain the nutrients necessary to support the rapid growth of food-borne pathogens, yet outbreaks of illness caused by consumption of fruits and vegetables are less frequent than outbreaks involving other foods. This higher level of protection is due in part to proper pasteurization and to the presence of external barriers such as the peels and rind of fruits, which prevent microorganisms from entering and subsequently growing in the interior of the fruit or vegetables (Burnet and Beuchat, 2001; Trifirò et al., 1997; Abdul-Raouf et al., 1993).

17.5.1   Bacterial Contamination

Fruits and vegetables have an important pathogenic and nonpathogenic microbiological load coming from soil, water, insects, and handling by man. Mesophilic bacteria from plate count studies typically will vary depending on seasonal and climatic variation and range from 10^3 to 10^8 CFU/g (Beuchat, 1996), while total counts on products after processing range from 10^3 to 10^6 CFU/g (Nguyen-the and Carlin, 1994). In general, the common microbial flora is composed by Gram-negative bacteria and belongs either to the *Pseudomonas* genus or to the Enterobacteriaceae. Many of these organisms are normally nonpathogenic for humans. The inner tissues of fruits and vegetables are usually regarded as sterile (Lund, 1992). However, bacteria can be present in low numbers as a result of the uptake of water through certain irrigation or washing procedures. If these waters are contaminated with human pathogens, these may also be introduced. However, in recent decades, juices have become a frequent vehicle for transmitting pathogens, such as enterohaemorrhagic *Escherichia coli* O157:H7 (American Public Health Association, 2001), *Salmonella* (CDC, 1997a),

Shigella, Listeria monocytogenes, and *Campylobacter*. A study focused on the microbiological quality of the fruit juices sold in Greece showed that *E. coli* O157:H7 was detected in four of the analyzed samples (3.34%), and *Staphylococcus aureus* in four different samples (3.34%), while all of them were negative for *Lactobacillus, Clostridium perfrigens, Salmonella* spp., *Bacillus cereus*, total coliforms, *E. coli*, and *Listeria monocytogenes* (Vantarakis et al., 2011). Ghenghesh et al. (2005) analyzed 146 fruit juice samples sold in Tripoli. Total bacterial counts (TBC) of samples examined ranged between <1 and 3×10^5 CFU/ml (mean = 5×10^4). Almond juice showed the highest TBC, ranging between 1.8×10^3 and 3×10^5 (mean = 1.7×10^5). *S. aureus* was detected in 8 (5.5%) samples, *Streptococcus* spp. in 4 (2.7%), coliforms in 33 (22.6%), *E. coli* (none were of serogroup O157) in 3 (2.1%), *Klebsiella pneumonia* in 17 (11.6%), *Aeromonas* spp. in 3 (2.1%), and *Pseudomonas aeruginosa* in 6 (4.1%). Thus, the belief that high-acid foods are of minimal concern with regard to pathogenic bacteria has been challenged (Cheringuene et al., 2007). However, the prevalence of food-borne pathogens on fruits and vegetables and their involvement in outbreaks are not well documented from a European perspective. In the United States, between 1990 and 2002, 56 outbreaks with 6762 cases were linked to fruits. Four percent of the cases were caused by berries, 2% by melon, and 94% by other fruits. In fruits, *Salmonella* and *E. coli* represented the most significant hazards (Smith DeWaal and Barlow, 2002). Salmonellosis outbreaks have been associated with contaminated fresh fruits (CDC, 1991) such as strawberries (Niu et al., 1992; CDC, 1997b) and raspberries (Ramsay and Upton, 1989).

Temperature is the environmental factor that affects the activity and microbial growth the most. The minimum and maximum temperatures for growth of a microorganism depend on factors such as pH and water activity (Aw). If these factors concerning the environment (pH and Aw) are outside the optimum values, the minimum temperature increases and the maximum decreases, thus narrowing the range of growth (Garbutt, 1997), as shown in Table 17.1.

Processes, include pasteurization, are intended to reduce the microbial load, but even after some processing, ready-to-eat vegetables retain much of their original microbiota. This is a serious health issue, because pathogens may be part of that microbiota.

Soil is the major source of microorganisms. Pathogens within soil may contaminate crops directly when heavy rain or water gun irrigation cause leaf splash. The ability of the pathogen to survive in the environment will impact on the likelihood of crop contamination and pathogen viability at harvest and through to consumption.

It has long been known that the improper use of manure can transfer pathogens onto crops, resulting in human disease. Raw manure should not be applied to crops. In addition to the hazard of pathogen transmission, it is well recognized that salt injury to sensitive vegetable crops and transfer of viable weed seed may result unless the manure is subjected, at least, to a period of unmanaged (no thorough mixing or pile inversion) composting. In places where noncomposted animal manure as fertilizer and untreated water are used to wash fresh products or to irrigate vegetable crops, *Salmonella, Shigella, B. cereus*, and *Clostridium botulinum* are easily observed. Health problems due to the consumption of Swiss chard, lettuce, cabbage, and watercress contaminated with *Salmonella* and *Shigella* are being reported.

TABLE 17.1

Major Environmental Conditions for Microbial Growth

Pathogens	Parameters					
	T_{min} (°C)	T_{max} (°C)	pH_{min}	pH_{max}	$a_{w\ min}$	$NaCl_{max}$
C. jejuni	32	45	4.9	9.0	0.98	2
C. botulinum type A or B proteolytic	10	50	4.6	8.5	0.93	10
C. botulinum type E nonproteolytic	3	45	4.6	8.5	0.97	5
E. coli	7	46	4.4	9.0	0.95	6.5
L. monocytogenes	0	45	4.39	9.4	0.92	10
Salmonella spp.	5	47	4.2	9.5	0.94	8
Shigella spp.	7	47	4.9	9.3	0.97	5.2
Y. enterocolitica	−1	42	4.2	9.6	0.97	7

Source: FDA, Survey of imported fresh produce, URL: http://www.cfsan.fda.
gov/~dms/prodsur6.html, 2001; ICMSF, *Microorganisms in Foods: Their
Significance and Methods of Enumeration*, 2nd edn., University of Toronto
Press, Toronto, 1986.

According to Frank and Takeushi (1999), fresh produce, especially lettuce, was identified as a carrier of pathogenic bacteria relevant to human health, such as *Salmonella*, *Shigella*, *L. monocytogenes*, *Yersinia enterocolitica*, enteropathogenic *E. coli*, enterotoxigenic *E. coli* and enterohaemorrhagic *E. coli* (O157:H7), as well as protozoa, parasites, and hepatitis A virus (Nascimento et al., 2003).

The National Advisory Committee on Microbiological Criteria for Foods (NACMCF) lists 11 agents associated with produce-borne outbreaks. Foremost among them are *E. coli* O157:H7 and various *Salmonella* serotypes (Tauxe, 1997). Health officials at a recent national food safety meeting disclosed preliminary data, which demonstrate that food-borne illness associated with fresh produce in the United States is related predominantly to pathogens of animal origin. Illness attributed to imported produce predominantly aligns with human sources of contamination. The prevalence of *E. coli* O157:H7 and *Salmonella* spp. in manure also varies with the source animal. *E. coli* O157:H7 colonizes cattle and other ruminants but generally not poultry. The prevalence of cattle pathogen shedding varies among different studies. Cassin et al. (1998) projected that the number of *E. coli* O157:H7 shedding animals varies from 0.3% to 0.8%, but may be considerably higher in a population consisting exclusively of young or stressed animals. In addition, survey results may be strongly influenced by regional and seasonal variation.

Bacteria such as *C. botulinum*, *B. cereus*, and *L. monocytogenes*, all capable of causing illness, are normal inhabitants of many soils, whereas *Salmonella*, *Shigella*, *E. coli*, and *Campylobacter* reside in the intestinal tracts of animals, including humans, and are more likely to contaminate raw fruits and vegetables through contact with feces, sewage, untreated irrigation water, and surface water. The contamination of fruits and vegetables can occur also at some stage of food processing. For example, the slicing step may increase the risk of contamination because the cutting of surfaces exude nutrients, which become available to the microorganisms naturally present in the produce, that is, growth of pathogens. So, all this processing contributes to microorganism multiplication and eventually increases bacterial counts (Berbari et al., 2001). Therefore, the prevention of risks of contamination by pathogens may occur from the realization of good agricultural practices ranging from planting to harvesting and other important aspects, even in the process of farming, such as water quality used for irrigation, employment practices adequate sanitation by producers in handling, and care of plants in the farmer's field as well observing the Good Manufacture Practices in the industry avoiding cross-contamination and maintaining a good control of processes.

17.5.2 Mold Contamination

Some fruits, including oranges, are susceptible to attack by pathogenic fungi for example, *Aspergillus* because of their low pH, higher moisture content, and nutrient composition (Little and Mitchell, 2004). Molds and yeasts tolerate conditions of high osmotic pressure and low pH and can grow at refrigerator temperatures (two factors that generally prohibit the growth of competitive bacteria) and can therefore cause spoilage in the processed product. About two-thirds of the spoilage of fruits is caused by molds (ICMSF, 1986). Members of the genera *Penicillium*, *Aspergillus*, *Sclerotinia*, *Botrytis*, and *Rhizopus* are commonly involved in this process. The spoilage is usually associated with cellulolytic or pectinolytic activity, which causes softening, and weakening of plant structures. These structures are important barriers to prevent growth in the products by contaminating microbes. Tournas et al. (2006) analyzed 38 fruit salad samples and 65 pasteurized fruit juice samples from local supermarkets in Washington, DC. Low numbers of *Penicillium* spp. were found in pineapple salads, whereas *Cladosporium* spp. were present in mixed fruit and cut strawberry salads. At the same time low counts of *Penicillium* and *Fusarium* spp. (1.70 and 1.60 $\log_{10}$ cfu/mL, respectively) were present in grapefruit juice.

17.5.3 Yeast Contamination

Frequently isolated yeast species found in citrus juices are *Candida parapsilosis*, *Candida stellata*, *Saccharomyces cerevisiae*, *Torulaspora delbrueckii*, and *Zygosaccharomyces rouxii*, although species from the genera *Rhodotorula*, *Pichia*, *Hanseniaspora*, and *Metschnikowia* are also common. Ghenghesh et al. (2005) analyzed 146 fruit juice samples sold in Tripoli. They found *Candida albicans* in 18 (12.3%), *Candida* spp. in 109 (74.7%), and other yeasts in 85 (58.2%). Tournas et al. (2006) analyzed 38 fruit salad samples including cantaloupe, citrus fruits, honeydew, pineapple, cut strawberries, and mixed fruit salads, and 65 pasteurized fruit juice samples (apple, carrot, grapefruit, grape and orange juices, apple cider, and soy milk) from local supermarkets in the Washington, DC area and tested for yeast contamination. The majority of fruit salad samples (97%) were contaminated with yeasts at levels ranging from <2.0 to 9.72 $\log_{10}$ of colony-forming units per gram (cfu/g). Frequently encountered yeasts were *Pichia* spp., *Candida pulcherrima*, *C. lambica*, *C. sake*, *Rhodotorula* spp., and *Debaryomyces polymorphus*.

17.6 HACCP AND INDUSTRIAL ASSESSMENT TO CONTROL MICROBIAL HAZARDS

The proactive use of HACCP requires a long way to recognize the microbiological risks and the requirements for dealing with them. However, in recent years, scientists and managers of food safety in both government and industry have been seeking additional scientific tools more robust that can be used to support the HACCP. Therefore, knowing the number of microorganisms in the final stages of the production process is important for the food industry because it is an objective way to determine a critical control point to be checked.

The "Codex Microbiological Risk Assessment" (MRA), as one of the three components of the Codex Hazard Analysis (the others are risk management and risk communication), is an approach that has been used at both the national and international levels to improve objective assessment of microbiological risks. Risk assessment is defined by the Codex as "a process that has a scientific basis," which consists of the following steps: (i) hazard identification, (ii) hazard characterization, (iii) exposure assessment, and (iv) risk characterization.

Exposure assessment and predictive microbiology are areas that have developed rapidly; they use mathematical models that, in combination with Monte Carlo simulation techniques, can be useful tools for predicting the number of pathogens that survive an inactivation treatment, their growth or their presence in food. This is important for industry because it can be an objective way to detect CCPs and which of them should be controlled.

Although this methodology has been used almost exclusively in risk assessment by managers, these tools can also be of interest to the food industry in those cases where it is necessary to predict the effect of preservation treatment on microorganisms that cause spoilage on foods or pathogenic microorganism.

The Monte Carlo simulation can also be performed to determine which factors are most influential in the final number of microorganisms after a preservation process. This tool may be of interest to the food industry in the design of appropriate treatments for inactivation of target microorganisms and selected technologies. With this method it is possible to work with stochastic models based on data to predict the lifetime, as a result of changes in environmental factors and to address the variability and uncertainty.

The food industry can benefit from the concepts of Risk Assessment to manage the safety of food produced. It is clear that the industry does not need to carry the various stages of risk assessment with the same intensity as would be necessary in the event that such an assessment was required by a public authority.

For example, hazard identification, microbial toxin, or microorganism of interest tend to be "default" data that can be derived from, for example, a risk analysis, an HACCP study, expert opinion, or an outbreak. Most risk assessments at industry level are essentially exposure assessments. A food manufacturer may change the level of microorganisms or microbial toxins in foods at the time of consumption, changing ingredients or processing or storage parameters. An evaluation of the dose-response cannot be performed as part of an industrial risk assessment, as the resources needed are too large. Instead you should consult the scientific literature and experts to find the current opinion regarding a particular hazard.

The result of an industrial risk assessment is not "an estimate of the probability of adverse health effects occurring in a given community." Instead, it tends to be an estimate of how safe the food is that is currently processed. This evaluation can be absolute or comparative with the product of an existing production process. The estimate will tend to be qualitative or quantitative as necessary to obtain a useful result.

REFERENCES

Abdul-Raouf, U.M., Beuchat, L.R., Ammar, M.S. (1993). Survival and growth of *Escherichia coli* O157:H7 on salad and vegetables. *Appl Environ Microbiol.* 59: 1999–2006.

American Public Health Association. (2001). *Compendium of Methods for the Microbiological Examination of Foods,* 4th edn. Washington DC: APHA.

Bean, N.H., Goulding, J.S., Daniels, M.T., Angulo, F.J. (1997). Surveillance for foodborne disease outbreaks—United States, 1998–1992. *J Food Prot.* 60: 1265–1286.

Berbari, S.A.G., Paschoalino, J.E., Silveira, N.F.A. (2001). Efeito do cloro na água de lavagem para desinfecção de alface minimamente processada. *Cien Tecnol Aliment.* 21: 197–201.

Beuchat, L.R. (1996). Pathogenic microorganisms associated with fresh produce. *J Food Prot.* 59: 204–216.

Burnett, S.L. Beuchat, L.R. (2001). Human pathogens associated with raw produce and unpasteurized juices, and difficulties in decontamination. *J Ind Microb Biotechnol.* 27: 104–110.

Cassin, M.H., Lammerding, A.M., Todd, E.C.D., Ross, W., McColl, R.S. (1998). Quantitative risk assessment for *Escherichia coli* O157:H7 in ground beef hamburgers. *Int J Food Microbiol.* 41: 21–44.

CDC (Center for Disease Control) (1991). Multistate outbreak of *Salmonella poona* infections—United States and Canada, 1991. *Morb Mortal Wkly Rep.* 40: 549 552.

CDC (Center for Disease Control) (1997a). Outbreak of *Escherichia coli* O157:H7 infections associated with eating alfalfa sprouts—Michigan and Virginia, June–July 1997. *Morb Mortal Wkly Rep.* 46(32): 741–744.

CDC (Center for Disease Control) (1997b). Outbreaks of *Escherichia coli* O157:H7 infection and cryptosporidiosis associated with drinking unpasteurized apple cider: Connecticut and New York, October 1996. *Morb Mortal Wkly Rep.* 46(01): 4–8.

Cheringuene, A., Chougrani, F., Bekada, A.M.A., El Soda, M., Bensoltane, A. (2007). Enumeration and identification of lactic microflora in Algerian goats' milk. *Afr J Biotechnol.* 6(15): 1854–1861.

FDA (Food and Drug Administration, USA) (2001). FDA Survey of imported fresh produce. URL: http://www.cfsan.fda.gov/~dms/prodsur6.html.

Frank, J.F. Takeushi, K. (1999) Direct observation of *Escherichia coli* O157:H7 inactivation on lettuce leaf using confocal scanning laser microscopy. In: Tuitjelaars et al. (eds), *Food Microbiology and Food Safety into the Next Millennium.* Proceedings of 17th International Conference of International Committee on Food Microbiology and Hygiene (ICFMH), pp. 795–797. Vendhoven, The Netherlands, 13–17, September, 1999.

Garbutt, J. (1997). *Essentials of Food Microbiology.* Londres, Reino Unido: Arnold.

Ghenghesh, K.S., Belhaj, K., El-Amin, W.B., El-Nefathi, S.E., Zalmum, A. (2005). Microbiological quality of fruit juices sold in Tripoli-Libya. *Food Control.* 16: 855–858.

ICMSF (International Commission on Microbiological Specifications for Foods) (1986). *Microorganisms in Foods: Their Significance and Methods of Enumeration*, 2nd edn., vol. 1. Toronto: University of Toronto Press.

Little, C.L. Mitchell, R.T. (2004). Food standards agency; local authorities coordinators of regulatory services; health protection agency. Microbiological quality of precut fruit, sprouted seeds, and unpasteurised fruit and vegetable juices from retail and production premises in the UK, and the application of HAACP. *Commun Dis Public Health.* 7(3): 184–190.

Lund, B.M. (1992). Ecosystems in vegetable foods. *J Appl Bact.* 73(Suplement 21): 115S–135S.

Mead, P.S., Slutsker, L., Dietz, V., McCaig, L.F., Bresee, J.S., Shapiro, C., Griffin, P.M., Tauxe, R.V. (1999). Food-related illness and death in the United States. *Emerg Infect Dis.* 5(5): 607–625.

Nascimento, M.S., Silva, N., Okazaki, M.M. (2003) Avaliação comparativa da eficácia de cloro, vinagre, ácido acético e ácido peracético na redução da população de microrganismos aeróbios mesófilos em verduras e frutas. REV NET- DTA Online. v. 3, n. 6, 3 de novembro de 2003.

Nguyen-the, C. Carlin, F. (1994) The microbiology of minimally processed fresh fruits and vegetables. *Crit Rev Food Sci Nutr.* 34(4): 371–401.

Niu, M.T., Polish, L.B., Robertson, B.H., Khanna, B.K., Woodruff, B.A., Shapiro, C.N., Miller, M.A., et al. (1992). Multistate outbreak of hepatitis A associated with frozen strawberries. *J Infect Dis.* 166: 518–524.

Ramsay, C.N. Upton, P.A. (1989). Hepatitis A and frozen raspberries. *Lancet.* 1: 43–44.

Smith DeWaal, C. Barlow, K. (2002). *Outbreak Alert! Closing the Gaps in Our Federal Food Safety Net*, 5th edn. Washington DC: Center for Science in the Public Interest.

Tauxe, R.V. (1997). Emerging foodborne diseases: An evolving public health challenge. *Dairy Food Environ Sanit.* 17(12): 788–795.

Tournas, V.H., Heeres, J., Burgess, L. (2006). Moulds and yeasts in fruit salads and fruit juices. *Food Microbiol.* 23: 684–688.

Trifirò, A., Saccani, G., Gherardi, S., Vicini, E., Spotti, E., Previdi, M.P., Ndagijimana, M., Cavalli, S., Reschiotto, C. (1997). Use of ion chromatography for monitoring microbial spoilage in the fruit juice industry. *J Chromatogr.* 770: 243–252.

Vantarakis, A., Affifi, M., Kokkinos, P., Tsibouxi, M., Papapetropoulou, M. (2011). Occurrence of microorganism of public health and spoilage significance in fruit juices sold in retail markets in Greece. *Anaerobe.* 17: 288–291.

Index

A

AAB, *see* Acetic acid bacteria (AAB)
Açaí, 29
Acerola, 18, 29, 36
Acetic acid bacteria (AAB), 315
Active packaging, 308
Adulteration
  analytical methods, 80
  berry juice, 79–80
  chemical markers, 78
  contaminants, 76–77
  isotopic analysis, 77–78
  labeling legislation, 76
  lemon and apple juices, 79
  orange juice, 78–79
  pomegranate juice, 79
  sugar, 77
  water, 76
Affective methods, 141
AIJN, *see* International Association of Juices
    and Nectars (AIJN)
Alicyclobacillus spp., 317–321
  detection and quantification, 323–325
Amino acids, 78
Amylases, 161–162
Anion-exchange membranes, 277
Antimicrobial food packaging, 308
Antioxidant capacity (AOC), 28, 36
APIB treatment, 65, 67
Apple juices
  adulteration, 79
  composition effects, fruit juice
    rheology, 122
  enzymatic mash treatment, 166
  enzyme immobilization, 165
  global consumption, 6, 7
  unit operations, fruit juice rheology, 129
Arbutin, 78, 79
Aroma recovery
  experimental studies, 290–291
  pervaporation, 289
  polymeric materials, 289, 292
Arsenic, 339
Ascorbic acid degradation pathways, 182
Aseptic processing, 4, 306
Asymmetric membranes, 273
Avocado, 29

B

Bacillus cereus, 334
Bacteria, 333–334
Berry juice, adulteration, 79–80
Bingham plastic fluids, 89
Bioactive compounds
  HHP, storage stability, 250
  HPH, 248–249
    in vitro bioaccessibility, 251–252
  HPP, 248
    storage stability, 249
    in vitro bioaccessibility, 251
Bioethanol, 62–63
Biological hazards
  bacteria, 333–334, 366–369
  control measures
    cooling, 336
    fruit sorting and cleaning, 335
    juicing, 335–336
    microbial inactivation, 336
    raw materials and postharvest handling, 335
    refrigerated distribution, 336–337
  European legislation, 337
  molds, 369
  parasites, 334
  viruses, 332–333
  yeasts, 369–370
Bipolar membrane electrodialysis, 277–278
Blackberry, 29
Blackcurrant, 29–30
Blueberry juice, 30
  HPH, 254
British Retail Consortium (BRC) standard,
    24, 364
Burger model, 104
By-products
  animal feed, 22–23
  citrus fruits
    bioethanol, 62–63
    dietary fiber, 47–52
    essential oil recovery, 57–60
    limonene, 60–62
    pectin, 43–47
    pulp, 52–57
  grape juice
    lees, 66
    seeds, 65–66

skins, 63–65
stalks, 66–67
phenolic fractions, 22–23, 23
Byssochlamys, 322

C

Cadmium, 339–340
Caliciviruses, 332
Canning, 305
Cation-exchange membranes, 277
Cellulases, 161
Cellulose, 153–154
Cell wall structure
 cell turgor, 152
 components, distribution of, 151–152
 polysaccharides
  cellulose, 153–154
  hemicelluloses, 154
  pectin, 152–153
  starch, 154
Centers for Disease Control and Prevention
 (CDC), 366
Chemical hazards
 control measures, 341
 environmental contaminants, 339–340
 European legislation, 342
 food additives, 340–341
 mycotoxins, 340
 pesticides, 337, 339
 processing contaminants, 341
Cherry juices, 30, 162
Chilled ready-to-serve (RTS) juice, 4
Citrus essential oil recovery
 one centrifuge
  flow diagram, 61
  process description, 59–60
 two centrifuges
  flow diagram, 60
  process description, 57–59
Citrus juices
 by-products
  bioethanol, 62–63
  dietary fiber, 47–52
  essential oil recovery, 57–60
  limonene, 60–62
  pectin, 43–47
  pulp, 52–57
  temperature effects, fruit juice rheology,
   105, 107
Citrus pulp recovery process, 52–57
Clarification, 267
 membrane technology, 281–287
Clarified juices
 processing steps, 7
  clarification, 9, 11
  evaporation and cooling, 11–12

preconcentration stage, 9
selection, grinding and pressing steps, 9
washing, 8–9
standard process flow diagram, 8
Clean label product, 18
Clostridium botulinum toxin, 334
Clostridium butyricum, 316
Clostridium pasteurianum, 315–316
Clostridium perfringens toxins, 334
Cloudy juices, processing steps, 7
Codex Alimentarius, 2, 357–358
Codex Microbiological Risk Assessment
 (MRA), 370
Cold atmospheric plasma, 230
Concentration, 267
 membrane technology, 287–288
Concentration polarization, 270–272
Consumer expectations, 143–144
Continuous radio-frequency electric field
 process, 211
Control measures
 biological hazards
  cooling, 336
  fruit sorting and cleaning, 335
  juicing, 335–336
  microbial inactivation, 336
  raw materials and postharvest
   handling, 335
  refrigerated distribution, 336–337
 chemical hazards, 341
Cox–Merz rule, 101
Cranberries, 30
Creep and recovery procedure, 102–104
Cross-flow membrane filtration, 275
Cross-linked enzyme aggregates (CLEAs), 164
Cryptosporidium parvum, 334

D

Dates, 30
Deacidification, 288–289
Dead-end membrane filtration, 275
Deaerator, 181–184
 schema and installation, 183
 structure, 181
Decimal reduction time, 176
Descriptive analysis, 140–141
Dielectric heating
 loss factor spectrum, dissipation effects of,
  204–206
 penetration depth, 206
Dietary fiber
 definition, 47
 industrial production, 48–52
Dilatant fluids, 88
Dimethylpolysiloxane, 341
Dimple tube design, 190

front view, 191
    lateral view, 192
Dipolar rotation, 204
Direct osmosis concentration (DOC), 279–280
Direct steam infusion, 179
Direct steam injection, 177–179
Discrimination methods, 140
DOC, *see* Direct osmosis concentration (DOC)
Dynamic oscillatory shear procedure, 97–102
Dynamic pressure treatments, *see* High-pressure
    homogenization (HPH)

E

ED, *see* Electrodialysis (ED)
EFSA, *see* European Food Safety Agency
    (EFSA)
Electric field technology
    engineering and industrial aspects, 223–225
    fruit juice components, effects on, 221–222
Electrodialysis (ED), 276–278
Electromagnetic phenomena, 203–204
Endopolygalacturonases, 160
E numbers, 17
Environmental contaminants, 339–340
Enzymatic browning, 181, 267
Enzymatic mash treatment, 166
Enzyme immobilization, 164–165
Enzyme inactivation
    HHP, 246
    HPH, 242, 245
    HPP, 245–246
Enzymes
    amylases, 161–162
    cellulases and hemicellulases, 161
    glucose oxidase, 162
    immobilization, 164–165
    mash treatment, 166
    pectinases, 158, 160–161
Eriocitrin, 78
Escherichia coli, 333
Euromonitor International, 36
European Economic Community, 350
European Food Safety Agency (EFSA), 23
European legislation
    biological hazards, 337
    chemical hazards, 342
Exopolygalacturonases, 160
External traceability, 354

F

Falguera–Ibarz model, 90
Fast Blue BB method, 35
Fig fruits, 31
Fin deflectors, 189–190
Flavor Profile method, 140

Florida Citrus Commission, 3
Flow behavior index, 107–108
Folin–Ciocalteu method, 35
Food additives, 340–341
Food and Drug Administration (FDA), 79
Food colorings, 18
Food safety management, 342–344
Food Safety (Regulation 178/2002), 350–353
Food safety regulations
    Codex Alimentarius, 357–358
    Regulation 178/2002
        objectives, 350–351
        principles, 351–352
        qualifications, 352–353
    risk assessment, 354–357
    traceability, 353–354
Four-wing tube in-tube pasteurizer, 190
Fran Rica (JBT) flash cooler, 178
FreshNote system, 293
Frozen concentrated orange juice (FCOJ), 3–4
Fruit purees, processing steps, 7, 12
Fungal acid protease, 162
Furan, 341

G

Gamma radiation technique, 212
GAP, *see* Good agricultural practices
Generally recognized as safe (GRAS), 17
GHP, *see* Good hygiene practices
Glass packaging, 303
Global fruit juice and nectar sales, 4–7
Glucose oxidase, 162
GMP, *see* Good manufacturing practices
Guji, 31
Good agricultural practices (GAP), 335, 341
Good hygiene practices (GHP), 337
Good manufacturing practices (GMP), 335, 341
Grape juice, 31
    composition effects, fruit juice
        rheology, 120
    by-products
        lees, 66
        seeds, 65–66
        skins, 63–65
        stalks, 66–67
    HPP, 249
GRAS, *see* Generally recognized as safe
    (GRAS)
Guarana fruit, 31–32
Guava fruit, 31

H

Hazard Analysis and Critical Control Points
    (HACCP), 370–371
    implementation, 355–356

legal obligations, 356–357
   principles, 354–355
   support plans, 356
   testing procedures, 356
Heat injector, 178
Heat transfer coefficient *K* factor, 180
Hemicellulases, 161
Hemicelluloses, 154
Hepatitis A virus, 333
Hermetic containers, 302–303
Herschel–Bulkley (HB) model, 89
HHP, *see* High hydrostatic pressure technology
High-energy irradiation, *see* Irradiation
High hydrostatic pressure (HHP) technology
   application, 229
   bioactive compounds, storage stability, 250
   chemical reactions, 228
   drawbacks, 229
   enzyme inactivation, 246
   microorganism inactivation, 243
   microorganisms, 227–228
   principle, 227
   product processing devices, 228–229
High-pressure homogenization (HPH)
   bioactive compounds, 248–249
      in vitro bioaccessibility, 251–252
   blueberry juice, 254
   enzyme inactivation, 242, 245
   equipment, 241
   juice rheology, 124–126
      alginate and carrageenan, 129
      cashew apple juice, 129
      tomato juice, 127, 128
   microorganism inactivation, 242, 243–244
High-pressure processing (HPP), 239–241
   bioactive compounds, 248
      storage stability, 249
      in vitro bioaccessibility, 251
   enzyme inactivation, 245–246
   mode of action, 240
   principles, 240
   probiotics and digestibility, 241
Hollow-fiber membranes, 274
Hollow-fiber ultrafiltration (HFUF), 165
Homogalacturonan (HG), 152
Hot fill, 305–306
HPH, *see* High-pressure homogenization
   (HPH)
HPP, *see* High-pressure processing (HPP)

I

IFS, *see* International Food Safety (IFS)
   standard
Immunoglobulin A (IgA), 252
Indulleida, 20
Industrial enzyme preparations, 155–158

Infrared (IR) heating, 212
Innocent Drinks, 15–17
Integrated membrane process, 293–296
Intelligent packaging, 308
Internal traceability, 353
International Agency for Research on Cancer
   (IARC), 339
International Association of Juices and Nectars
   (AIJN), 360–362
International Food Safety (IFS) standard,
   24, 364–365
International Organization for Standardization
   (ISO) 9001:2008, 24
Ionic conductivity, 204
Irradiation, 230
   fruit juice rheology, 130
   preservation, 307
ISO 9000, 362–363
ISO-22000, 363
ISO 22000:2005, 24
Isostatic pressure, 240

K

Kiwifruit, 32
Krieger–Dougherty equation, 116

L

LAB, *see* Lactic acid bacteria (LAB)
Lactic acid bacteria (LAB), 315
Laminates, 304
Lead, 339
Lees, 66
Lemon juice
   adulteration, 79
   industrial fiber, 48–52
Limonene, 60–62
Limoninase, 162

M

Magnetic field technology
   engineering and industrial aspects, 225
   fruit juice components, effects on, 223
Mandarin juice, low homogenization pressure,
   252–253
Mangoes, 32
Mangosteen, 32
Mannans, 154
Man–Rogosa–Sharpe medium, 322
Maxwell–Wagner effect, 205
Mayonnaise, 89
Membrane concentration factor, 271
Membrane distillation, 280
Membrane fouling, 272–273
Membrane technology

application
 aroma recovery, 289–292
 clarification, 281–287
 concentration, 287–288
 deacidification, 288–289
 vs. conventional separation technologies, 266
 disadvantage, 266
 driving forces, 269
 electrodialysis, 276–278
 integrated membrane process, 293–296
 novel techniques
  direct osmosis concentration, 279–280
  membrane distillation, 280
  osmotic distillation, 280–281
 pervaporation, 278–279
 pressure-driven processes, 275–276
Metal packaging, 303–304
Microorganism inactivation
 HHP, 243
 HPH, 242, 243–244
Microwave heating
 applications, 206–208
 dipolar rotation and ionic conductivity, 204
 equipment, 208–209
 pomegranate, 208
 vitamin C degradation, 200
Molds, 321–322
Multitubular heat exchanger with flange, 193
Mycotoxins, 340

N

Nanofiltration (NF), 276
Naringin, 78
Naringinase, 162
National Advisory Committee on
  Microbiological Criteria for Foods
  (NACMCF), 368
Nectars, 7–8
New product development, 143
Nine-point hedonic scale, 141
Nonenzymatic browning, 267
Noni, 33
Non-Newtonian fluids, 86
Nonporous membranes, 273
Nonthermal technologies
 cold atmospheric plasma, 230
 electric and magnetic fields, 221–225
 high-energy irradiation, 230
 high hydrostatic pressure, 227–229
 pulsed light, 220–221
 sonication, 225–227
  cavitation, 227
 supercritical/dense phase processing,
  230–231
 ultraviolet radiation, 218–220
Norwalk viruses, 332

Not-from-concentrate (NFC) juices, 4
Nutraceuticals, 42
Nutrient bioaccessibility, 250

O

Ochratoxin A, 340, 341
Ohmic heating
 applications, 200–202
 flow sheet, 202
 PME inactivation, 201
 PPO, 201
 schematic diagram, 199
 system design, 202–203
 theoretical basis, 198–199
Oil-holding capacity (OHC), 50
One centrifuge essential oil extraction systems
  flow diagram, 61
 process description, 59–60
Orange juices, 33
 adulteration, 78–79
 concentration effects, fruit juice rheology,
  113–114
 global consumption, 6
 industrial fiber production, 48–52
 integrated membrane process, 295
 ohmic heating, 200–201
 viscosity *vs.* temperature diagram, 184
Osmotic dehydration coupled reverse-osmosis
  concentration process, 294–295
Osmotic distillation, 280–281
Ostwald–de Waele model, 87
Oxygen
 deaerator, 183–184
 negative influence of, 181
 pasteurization, 174

P

Packaging
 active packaging, 308
 intelligent packaging, 308
 materials
  glass, 303
  laminates, 304
  metal, 303–304
  PET, 304
 nutrients, preservation of, 307–308
 preservation
  high pressures, 306
  ionizing radiation, 307
  pulsed electric fields, 306–307
 primary containers
  hermetic containers, 302–303
  materials, 303–304
  requirements, 302
 secondary containers, 302

techniques, 302
    aseptic processing, 306
    canning, 305
    hot fill, 305–306
    sterile filtration, 305
Paired preference, 141
Papain, 35
Papaya, 33
Parasites, 334
Pasteurization
    affecting factors
        juice, rheology of, 175
        oxygen, 174
        pH and water activity, 174
        raw material, 175
    direct heating/cooling
        steam infusion, 179
        steam injection, 177–179
    indirect heating/cooling
        deaeration process, 180–184
        energy regeneration, 185
        flow types, heat exchanger, 184
        heat transfer coefficient, 180
        holding time, 180
        materials, 179–180
        PHE, 185–188
        THE, 185–195
    microorganisms, 173–174
    process steps, 180
    reference microorganisms, 176
Patulin, 340, 341
PDMS, see Polydimethylsiloxane (PDMS)
Peach juice
    concentration effects, fruit juice rheology,
        111–112, 115
    temperature effects, fruit juice rheology, 106
Peclet number, 88–89
Pectin, 152–153
    characteristics, 43–44
    industrial production, 44–47
Pectinases, 158, 160–161
Pectinesterase activity (PE), 163
Pectinesterases, 160
Pectin methylesterase (PME), 245–246
    inactivation, 201
PEF, see Pulsed electric fields (PEF)
        technology
Penetration depth, 206
Permeation flux, 269
Pervaporation, 278–279
    feed temperature and permeate
        pressure, 292
Pesticides, 337, 339
PET, see Polyethylene terephthalate (PET)
pH value, 312
    vs. apparent viscosity, 117
    ethanol-producing bacteria, 316

pasteurization, 174
pectin, 43–44
PHE, see Plate heat exchanger (PHE)
Pineapple juice
    composition effects, fruit juice
        rheology, 118
    unit operations, fruit juice rheology, 125
Pineapple juices, global consumption, 7
Plate and frame membranes, 274
Plate count agar (PCA) medium, 322
Plate heat exchanger (PHE)
    application, 186
    plate shape and thickness, 188
    process description, 185–186
    schema, 187
PME, see Pectin methylesterase (PME)
Polyamide membranes, 287
Polydimethylsiloxane (PDMS), 292
Polyethylene terephthalate (PET), 304
Polygalacturonases, 160
Polygalacturonic acid (PGA), 152–153
Polymethylgalacturonases, 160
Polyphenolics, 35
Polyphenol oxidase (PPO), 201
Polysaccharides
    activity determination, 162–164
    cellulose, 153–154
    fruit juice problems caused by, 155
    hemicelluloses, 154
    pectin, 152–153
    starch, 154
Pomegranate juice, 33–34
    adulteration, 79
    microwave heating, 208
Porous membranes, 273
Potato puree, 123, 124
PPO, see Polyphenol oxidase (PPO)
Preservation techniques
    high pressures, 306
    ionizing radiation, 307
    pulsed electric fields, 306–307
Pressure-driven membrane processes, 275–276
Pressure treatments
    applications, 238
    bioactive compounds, 247–252
    blueberry juice, 254
    dynamic pressures, 241–242
    enzyme inactivation, 244–246
    mandarin juice, 252–253
    microbial inactivation, 242–244
    static pressures, 239–241
    types, 238
Primary containers
    hermetic containers, 302–303
    materials, 303–304
    requirements, 302
Processing contaminants, 341

Product authenticity regulations
  AIJN Standards, 360–362
  Royal Decree 1518/2007, 362
  specialized laboratory standards, 362
Product innovation
  food colorings, 18
  food safety issues, 24
  novel technologies, 21
  smoothies, 15–17
Propionibacterium cyclohexanicum, 317
Protopectinases, 160–161
Pseudoplastic fluids, 87
Pulsed electric fields (PEF) technology, 19–20,
    222–224
  fruit juice rheology, 126
  preservation, 306–307
  vs. pressure treatments, 249
Pulsed light (PL)
  engineering and industrial aspects, 221
  fruit juice components, effects on, 220–221

Q

Quality assessment, norms of
  microbiological quality, 366
  organoleptic quality, 365
  physical–chemical quality, 365
Quality management standards
  BRC, 364
  IFS, 364–365
  ISO 9000, 362–363
  ISO-22000, 363

R

Radio-frequency heating
  applications, 209
  beta dispersion, 205
  equipment, 209–211
  schematic arrangement, 210
Rapid Alert System for Food and Feed
    (RASFF), 330
Raspberry, 34
Raw material
  GAP, 335
  pasteurization, 175
Reconstituted from concentrate (RFC) juices, 147
Redox potential (Eh), 312
Refined juice sacs, 20
Reflexive consumption, 2
Restriction fragment length polymorphism
    (RFLP), 323
Retention coefficient, 270
Reverse osmosis (RO) membranes, 276, 287–288,
    293–295
  disadvantage, 279
Rhamnogalacturonan-II (RGII), 152

Rhamnogalacturonan-I (RGI), 152, 153
Rheological consistency index, 107
Rheological properties
  assessment
    steady-state shear procedures, 95–97
    time dependence, 97
    viscoelastic properties, 97–104
  composition effects
    apple juice, 122
    grape juice, 120
    hydrocolloids, 119–122
    particle mean size, jabuticaba pulp, 118
    pH, 117
    pineapple ripening, 118
    salt addition, 119
  concentration effects
    flow behavior index, 112
    frozen concentrated orange juice, 113–114
    particle size, 116
    peach juice, 111–112, 115
    tomato juice, 116
    viscosity, 111
  importance, 84
  pasteurization, 175
  steady-state shear properties
    Bingham plastic fluids, 89
    dilatant fluids, 88
    Newtonian fluids, 85
    non-Newtonian fluids, 86
    pseudoplastic fluids, 87
  temperature effects
    Arrhenius equation, 105–106
    citrus juices, 105, 107
    goldenberry yield stress, 108
    peach juice, 106
    rheological consistency index, 107
    siriguela pulp, 106
    sweet potato baby food consistency
      coefficient, 107, 110
  time dependence, 90–92
  unit operations
    cashew apple juice, 129
    freezing process and temperature, 123, 124
    HPH process, 124–129
    irradiation processing, 130
    lemon fiber dispersion, 123, 125
    pineapple juice, 125
    potato puree, 123, 124
    pulsed electric field (PEF) processing, 126
    rotational speed and sieve dimensions,
      121–122
    strawberry juice, 126
    thermal processing, 125
    tomato juice, 121–122, 126–128
    ultrasound processing, 130
    ultraviolet processing, 125
  viscoelastic material, 92–94

Rheometers, *see* Rotational viscometers
Rheopectic behavior, 90
Rotational viscometers, 94–95
Rotaviruses, 332
Royal Decree 1518/2007, 362

S

Salmonellae, 333
Scraped surface heat exchanger, 193–195
Seabuckthorn, 34
Secondary containers, 302
Selectivity, 270
Sensory evaluation
    advantages and disadvantages, 141–142
    affective methods, 141
    applications
        consumer expectations, 143–144
        new product development, 143
    consumer response, 141
    descriptive analysis, 140
    discriminative techniques, 140
    flavor, 138–139
    vs. instrumental measurements, 144–145
    product appearance, 138
    product properties, 146
    temperature, 145–146
    texture, 139
    unit operations, 146–147
Separation factor, 270
Siriguela pulp
    flow behavior index, 108
    frequency sweep, 100
    temperature effects, fruit juice rheology,
        106, 109
Smoothies, 15–17, 35–36
Solution-diffusion model, 276
Sonication
    cavitation, 227
    engineering and industrial aspects, 226–227
    fruit juice components, effects on, 225–226
Specialized Laboratory Standards, 362
Spiral wound membranes, 274
Spoilage microorganisms
    bacteria
        AAB, 315
        Alicyclobacillus spp., 317–321, 323–325
        ethanol-producing bacteria, 316–317
        LAB, 315
        Propionibacterium cyclohexanicum,
            323–325
        spore-forming bacteria, 315–316
    molds, 321–322
    yeasts, 313–314
        identification, 322–323
Sporolactobacillus inulinus, 316
Stalks, 66–67

Standard homogenization, *see* High-pressure
    homogenization (HPH)
Starch, 154
Static pressure treatments, *see* High-pressure
    processing (HPP)
Sterile filtration, 305
Storage modulus, 98
Strawberry juice, 34
    unit operations, fruit juice rheology, 126
Streptomyces griseus, 316
Sulfur dioxide, 340
Supercritical/dense phase processing, 230–231
Superfruits, 24
    antioxidant health benefits, 28
    market for, 36–37
    success elements, 28
Symmetric membranes, 273

T

Tangerine, industrial fiber, 52
THE, *see* Tubular heat exchangers (THE)
Thermal death time (TDT), 176
Thermally accelerated short time evaporator
    (TASTE), 10, 294
Thermal techniques
    dielectric heating
        loss factor spectrum, dissipation effects
            of, 204–206
        penetration depth, 206
    gamma radiation technique, 212
    IR heating, 212
    microwave heating, 206–208
        equipment, 208–209
    ohmic heating
        applications, 200–202
        schematic diagram, 199
        system design, 202–203
        theoretical basis, 198–199
    radio-frequency heating
        applications, 209
        equipment, 209–211
        schematic arrangement, 210
    UV treatment, 211–212
Thermal treatment technology, *see* Pasteurization
Thixotropic behavior, 90, 92, 93
Tomato juice
    concentration effects, fruit juice rheology, 116
    unit operations, fruit juice rheology, 121–122,
        126–128
Total antioxidant activity (TAA), 287
Total dietary fiber (TDF), 47
Toxoplasma gondii, 334
Traceability, 353–354
Trypanosoma cruzi, 334
Tubes in shell heat exchangers, 191–192
Tubular and capillary membranes, 274

Tubular heat exchangers (THE)
   characteristics, 188–189
   process description, 188
   tube in shell design, 191–192
   tube-in-tube design, 189–191
Two centrifuges essential oil extraction systems
   flow diagram, 60
   process description, 57–59

U

Ultrafiltration (UF), 165
Ultrasound processing; *see also* Sonication
   fruit juice rheology, 130
Ultraviolet (UV) radiation processing, 211–212
   drawback, 220
   engineering and industrial aspects, 219–220
   fruit juice components, effects on, 218–219
   fruit juice rheology, 125
Unit operations
   rheological properties, fruit juice
      cashew apple juice, 129
      freezing process and temperature,
         123, 124
      HPH process, 124–129
      irradiation processing, 130
      lemon fiber dispersion, 123, 125
      pineapple juice, 125
      potato puree, 123, 124
      pulsed electric field (PEF) processing, 126
      rotational speed and sieve dimensions,
         121–122
      strawberry juice, 126
      thermal processing, 125

tomato juice, 121–122, 126–128
   ultrasound processing, 130
   ultraviolet processing, 125
   sensory evaluation, 146–147
United Nations Food and Agriculture
      Organization (FAO), 350
U.S. Department of Agriculture (USDA), 3, 350
U.S. Food and Drug Administration (FDA), 17

V

Vacuum pervaporation, 279
Verotoxigenic *E. coli* (VTEC), 333
Viruses, 332–333
Viscoelastic behaviors, 92–94

W

Water activity, pasteurization, 174
Water-holding capacity (WHC), 49
Wine industry, *see* Grape juice

Y

Yeasts, 313–314
   identification, 322–323

X

Xyloglucan, 154

Z

Zymomonas mobilis, 316–317

Printed and bound by CPI Group (UK) Ltd, Croydon, CR0 4YY

18/10/2024

01776257-0013